titles in the Emergencies

nergencies

nesia
, Andrew McIndoe, and Iain H. Wilson

diology
yerson, Robin P. Choudhury, and Andrew Mitchell

bstetrics and Gynaecology
kumaran

gencies in Dentistry
d Jason Leitch

s in Palliative and Supportive Care
David Currow and Katherine Clark

cies in Psychiatry
Puri

gencies in Paediatrics and Neonatology
d by Stuart Crisp and Jo Rainbow

ergencies in Critical Care
dited by Martin Beed, Richard Sherman, and Ravi Mahajan

Emergencies in Respiratory Medicine
Edited by Robert Parker, Catherine Thomas, and Lesley Bennett

Emergencies in Primary Care
Chantal Simon, Karen O'Reilly, John Buckmaster, and Robin Proctor

Emergencies in Oncology
Edited by Martin Scott-Brown, Roy A.J. Spence, and Patrick G. Johnston

NIKKI

D1175503

Unsettled/crying child
headache
asthma
PR bleeding
lymphadenopathy
PT
abdo pain
constipation.

Published and forthcoming
in ... series:

Head, Neck and Dental Em
Edited by Mike Perry

Emergencies in Anaesth
Edited by Keith Allman

Emergencies in Card
Edited by Saul G. M

Emergencies in O
Edited by S. Arul

Medical Emerg
Nigel Robb a

Emergencie
Edited by D

Emergen
Basant P

Emer
Edite

Em
E

Nec

Emergencies in Paediatrics and Neonatology

Edited by

Stuart Crisp FRCPCH, FRACP (Paeds)

Consultant Paediatrician,
Wangaratta Paediatric Clinic,
Victoria, Australia

and

Jo Rainbow MRCPCH, FRACP (Paeds)

Staff Specialist,
Orange Base Hospital, Orange,
New South Wales, Australia

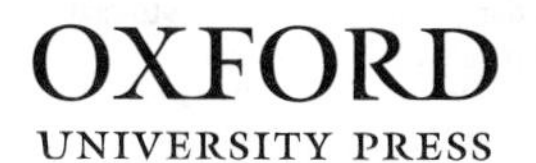

OXFORD
UNIVERSITY PRESS

Great Clarendon Street, Oxford OX2 6DP

Oxford University Press is a department of the University of Oxford.
It furthers the University's objective of excellence in research, scholarship,
and education by publishing worldwide in

Oxford New York

Auckland Cape Town Dar es Salaam Hong Kong Karachi
Kuala Lumpur Madrid Melbourne Mexico City Nairobi
New Delhi Shanghai Taipei Toronto

With offices in

Argentina Austria Brazil Chile Czech Republic France Greece
Guatemala Hungary Italy Japan Poland Portugal Singapore
South Korea Switzerland Thailand Turkey Ukraine Vietnam

Oxford is a registered trade mark of Oxford University Press
in the UK and in certain other countries

Published in the United States
by Oxford University Press Inc., New York

© Oxford University Press, 2007

The moral rights of the authors have been asserted
Database right Oxford University Press (maker)

First published 2007
Reprinted 2010
Reprinted 2011

All rights reserved. No part of this publication may be reproduced,
stored in a retrieval system, or transmitted, in any form or by any means,
without the prior permission in writing of Oxford University Press,
or as expressly permitted by law, or under terms agreed with the appropriate
reprographics rights organization. Enquiries concerning reproduction
outside the scope of the above should be sent to the Rights Department,
Oxford University Press, at the address above.

You must not circulate this book in any other binding or cover
and you must impose the same condition on any acquirer.

A catalogue record for this title is available from the British Library

Library of Congress Cataloging in Publication Data

Data available

Typeset by Newgen Imaging Systems (P) Ltd., Chennai, India
Printed in China
on acid-free paper through
Asia Pacific Offset

ISBN 978–019–856866–7 (flexicover: alk. paper)

10 9 8 7 6 5 4 3

Oxford University Press makes no representation, express or implied, that the drug dosages in this book are correct. Readers must therefore always check the product information and clinical procedures with the most up-to-date published product information and data sheets provided by the manufacturers and the most recent codes of conduct and safety regulations. The authors and the publishers do not accept responsibility or legal liability for any errors in the text or for the misuse or misapplication of material in this work. Except where otherwise stated, drug dosages and recommendations are for the non-pregnant adult who is not breast-feeding.

Preface

This book has been written for anyone who assesses and manages acutely unwell children. It has been written by doctors who do just that, day in, day out. It provides clear, simple, but definitive early management for paediatric conditions seen in the Emergency Department. Some children presenting will be seriously ill, but many will not. There is, therefore, a coding system of icons, indicating the likely severity and consequent urgency of treatment.

The book is symptom-based, as that is how children present. It covers resuscitation and immediate management in detail, to get you through those first nerve-racking minutes. Longer-term treatment is then discussed. For each condition, the key features of the history are described, along with the cardinal signs to be elicited on examination. The judicious use of investigations is also covered (as well as what the results mean!). Frequent re-assessment is emphasized to detect any clinical deterioration. Potential complications are listed, along with what to do next and when to seek further specialist advice.

Drug doses are included within the text. The doses have been taken from *BNF for Children* (2005, ISBN 978–0853696261, Royal Pharmaceutical Company of Great Britain).

Being an at-a-glance reference, the book is in the form of short notes and bullet points, with critical information highlighted. Flow diagrams guide you through the more complex areas. All are based on the best available evidence or on accepted best practice.

Topics are grouped by body system, with a detailed index to provide easy access to information. Cross references have been kept to a minimum to facilitate use at the bedside. Where a complex subject is mentioned, consultation of the forthcoming, more detailed *Oxford Handbook of Paediatrics* is recommended.

This book is ideal for any health professional or student who has to treat unwell children. Most of these will present to the Emergency Department, but some will be first seen by their local doctor (GP or LMO) or other specialists in related fields. The book is therefore aimed at:

- Paediatricians and doctors in the Emergency Department.
- Nurse practitioners, both paediatric and Emergency Department.
- Anaesthetists, surgeons.
- GP and GP trainees.
- Medical students.
- Allied health professionals.

We hope you find it useful, but please let us know if you have suggestions for improvement.

Dr Stuart Crisp
Dr Jo Rainbow
March 2007

Dedication

With love to Cari, Titch, Mopsy, Catie, Jack, Sophie, and Beeboo.

Contents

Contributors

Dr Steve Allen
Reader in Paediatrics
School of Medicine
Swansea University
Swansea, UK
Chapter 12

Dr Gordon D L Bates
Consultant Child and Adolescent Psychiatrist
Woodbourne Priory Hospital Birmingham, and Honorary Senior Clinical Lecturer
Department of Psychiatry
University of Birmingham, UK
Chapter 25

Dr Charlotte C Bennett
Consultant Neonatologist and Honorary Senior Clinical Lecturer
University Department of Paediatrics
John Radcliffe Hospital Oxford, UK
Chapter 3

Dr Stuart Crisp
Consultant Paediatrician
Wangaratta Paediatric Clinic
Victoria, Australia
Chapters 1, 2, 5, 8, 11, 13, 28, and appendices

Dr Patrick Davies
Specialist Registrar
Emergency Department
Bristol Children's Hospital
Bristol, UK
Chapter 27

Dr Julie Edge
Consultant Paediatrician
John Radcliffe Hospital
Headington, Oxford, UK
Chapter 24

Mr Paul Johnson
Reader in Paediatric Surgery and Honorary Consultant Paediatric Surgeon
John Radcliffe Hospital
Oxford, UK
Chapters 14 and 15

Ita Kelly
Paediatric Resuscitation Officer
Oxford Radcliffe Hospitals NHS Trust, Oxford, UK
Chapter 4

Miss Penny Lennox
Consultant Adult and Paediatric Otolaryngologist
John Radcliffe Hospital
Oxford, UK
Chapter 17

Dr Tom Millard
Consultant Dermatologist
Department of Dermatology
Gloucester Royal Hospital
Gloucester, UK
Chapter 23

Ms Sarah Passey
Commercial Business Manager
PO Box 1179, Wangaratta
Victoria 3676, Australia
Chapter 2

Dr Huw Pullen
Specialist Registrar
The Royal Gwent
Newport, UK
Chapters 6 and 18

Dr Jo Rainbow
Staff Specialist
Orange Base Hospital, Orange
New South Wales, Australia
Chapters 1, 2, 7, 9, 10, 16, 20, 26, and appendices

Dr Ingo Scholler
Consultant Paediatrician
Morriston Hospital
Swansea, UK
Chapter 12

Dr Tamsin Sleep
Consultant Ophthalmologist
Department of Ophthalmology
Torbay General Hospital
Torquay, Devon, UK
Chapter 19

Dr Denise Tritton
Associate Specialist in Paediatric Oncology and Haematology
John Radcliffe Hospital
Oxford, UK
Chapters 21 and 22

Mr Paul Williams
Consultant Trauma and Orthopaedic Surgeon
Morriston Hospital
Swansea, UK
Chapters 6 and 18

Symbols and abbreviations

📖	cross reference
1°	primary
2°	secondary
AAFB	acid alcohol-fast bacilli
ABC	airway, breathing, circulation
ABCD	airway, breathing, circulation, disability
ABCDE	airway, breathing, circulation, disability, exposure
ABG	arterial blood gas
ACL	anterior cruciate ligament
ACTH	adrenocorticotrophic hormone
ADD	attention deficit disorder
ADEM	acute disseminated encephalomyelitis
ADH	antidiuretic hormone
ADHD	attention deficit hyperactivity disorder
AED	automated external defibrillator
AGEP	acute generalized exanthemic pustulosis
AIDS	acquired immune deficiency syndrome
ALL	acute lymphocytic leukaemia
ALP	alkaline phosphatase
ALS	advanced life support
ALT	alanine transaminase
AML	acute myeloblastic leukaemia
ANA	antinuclear antibody
ANCA	antinuclear cytoplasmic antibody
AP	anterior–posterior
APP	acute phase protein
APTT	activated partial thromboplastin time
AR	aortic regurgitation
AS	aortic stenosis
ASD	atrial septal defect
ASOT	antistreptolysin O titre
AST	aspartate transaminase
AV	arteriovenous
AVM	arteriovenous malformation
AVPU	alert, (responsive to) voice, (responsive to) pain, unresponsive
AVSD	atrioventricular septal defect

AXR	abdominal X-ray
BCG	bacille Calmette–Guérin
bd	twice a day
β-HCG	beta human chorionic gonadotrophin
BLS	basic life support
BM stick	finger prick glucose
BMA	bone marrow aspirate
BMI	body mass index
BP	blood pressure
BSA	body surface area
BT	Blalock–Taussig shunt
BXO	balanitis xerotica obliterans
CAH	congenital adrenal hyperplasia
CAMHS	child and adolescent mental health service
CCF	congestive cardiac failure
CHARGE	coloboma, heart anomalies, choanal atresia, retardation of growth and development, genital, and ear anomalies
CF	cystic fibrosis
CK	creatinine kinase
cm	centimetre
CMV	cytomegalovirus
CNS	central nervous system
COA	coarctation of the aorta
CPAP	continuous positive airway pressure
CPR	cardiopulmonary resuscitation
CRP	C-reactive protein
CSF	cerebrospinal fluid
CT	computerized tomography
CTG	cardiotocography
CVA	cardiovascular accident
CVL	central venous line
CVS	cardiovascular system
CXR	chest X-ray
d	day
D & C	dilatation and curettage
DDAVP	1-deamino-8-D-arginine vasopressin
DDH	developmental dysplasia of the hip
DEFG	don't ever forget glucose
DIC	disseminated intravascular coagulation
DKA	diabetic ketoacidosis
DMSA	dimercaptosuccinic acid
DNH	disseminated neonatal haemangiomatosis

DOPES	displacement of endotracheal tube, obstruction of endotracheal tube or upper airway, pneumothorax, equipment failure, splinting of diaphragm by air in stomach
DSH	deliberate self-harm
DVT	deep vein thrombosis
EB	epidermolysis bullosa
EBV	Epstein–Barr virus
ECG	electrocardiogram
ECHO	echocardiogram
ED	emergency department
EDTA	ethylene diamine tetra-acetic acid
EEG	electroencephalogram
EMG	electromyogram
ENT	ear, nose, and throat
ESR	erythrocyte sedimentation rate
EUA	examination under anaesthesia
$etCO_2$	end-tidal carbon dioxide
ETT	endotracheal tube
Fab	antigen-binding fragment
FBC	full blood count
FDP	fibrin/fibrinogen degradation product
FEV_1	forced expiratory volume in 1 second
FFP	fresh frozen plasma
FII	fabricated and induced illness
FiO_2	fraction of inspired oxygen
Fr	French
FTT	failure to thrive
FVC	forced vital capacity
g	gram
GA	general anaesthetic
GAD	glutamic acid decarboxylase
Gal-1P-UT	galactose-1-phosphate-uridyltransferase
GBS	group B streptococcus
GCS	Glasgow coma scale
GFR	glomerular filtration rate
GGT	gamma glutamyl transferase
GI	gastrointestinal
GIT	gastrointestinal tract
GOR	gastro-oesophageal reflux
GP	general practitioner
G6PD	glucose-6-phosphate dehydrogenase

GU	genitourinary
h	hour
Hb	haemoglobin
HbS	sickle haemoglobin
HbSS	sickle cell anaemia
HCV	hepatitis C virus
HDU	high dependency unit
HEV	hepatitis E virus
HHV6	human herpes virus 6
HIE	hypoxic–ischaemic encephalopathy
HIV	human immunodeficiency virus
HLA	human leucocyte antigen
HMD	hyaline membrane disease
HMPV	human metapneumovirus
HOCM	hypertrophic obstructive cardiomyopathy
HSP	Henoch–Schönlein purpura
HSV	herpes simplex virus
HUS	haemolytic uraemic syndrome
IBD	inflammatory bowel disease
ICP	intracranial pressure
IDDM	insulin-dependent diabetes mellitus
IgA	immunoglobulin A
IM	intramuscular
IO	intraosseous
IRT	immunoreactive trypsinogen
ITP	idiopathic thrombocytopenic purpura
IV	intravenous
IVC	inferior vena cava
IVH	intraventricular haemorrhage
IVIg	intravenous immunoglobulin
IVP	intravenous pyelography
IVU	intravenous urogram
J	joule
JIA	juvenile idiopathic arthritis
kg	kilogram
KUB	plain abdominal X-ray (showing kidneys, ureters, and bladder)
l	litre
LAH	left atrial hypertrophy
LDH	lactate dehydrogenase

LFT	liver function tests
LKM	liver kidney microsomal (antibody)
LLSE	lower left sternal edge
LMP	last menstrual period
LP	lumbar puncture
LRTI	lower respiratory tract infection
LSCS	lower segment Caesarean section
LVF	left ventricular failure
mcg	microgram
MCH	mean corpuscular haemoglobin
M, C & S	microscopy, culture, and sensitivity
MCUG	micturating cystourethrography
MCV	mean cell volume
mg	milligram
MHA	mental health act
ml	millilitre
mmol	millimole
μmol	micromole
MPS	mucopolysaccharidoses
MR	mitral regurgitation
MRI	magnetic resonance imaging
MS	mitral stenosis *or* multiple sclerosis
MSE	mental state examination
MSUD	maple syrup urine disease
MVP	mitral valve prolapse
NAI	non-accidental injury
NBM	nil by mouth
NBT	nitroblue tetrazolium
NCA	nurse-controlled analgesia
NEC	necrotizing enterocolitis
NF1	neurofibromatosis type 1
NG	nasogastric
NGT	nasogastric tube
NICU	neonatal intensive care unit
NPA	nasopharyngeal aspirate
NPH	neutral protein Hagedorn (insulin)
NSAID	nonsteroidal anti-inflammatory drug
OCP	oral contraceptive pill
OFC	occipito-frontal head circumference
ORF	oral rehydration formula
OTC	ornithine transcarbamylase

$PaCO_2$	carbon dioxide tension measured by arterial gas
PaO_2	oxygen tension measured by arterial gas
PCA	patient-controlled analgesia
pCO_2	carbon dioxide tension measured by arterial or venous blood gas
PCR	polymerase chain reaction
PDA	patent ductus arteriosus
PE	pulmonary embolism
PEA	pulseless electrical activity
PEEP	positive end-expiratory pressure
PEF	peak expiratory flow
PEFR	peak expiratory flow rate
PICU	paediatric intensive care unit
PID	pelvic inflammatory disease
PKU	phenylketonuria
PNET	primitive neuroectodermal tumor
PNS	peripheral nervous system
PO	orally, by mouth
PPHN	persistent pulmonary hypertension of the newborn
PR	per rectum *or* pulmonary regurgitation
prn	as required
PS	pulmonary valve stenosis
PT	prothrombin time
PTH	parathyroid hormone
PTSD	post-traumatic stress disorder
PUJ	pelviureteric junction
PUO	pyrexia of unknown origin
qds	four times a day
RAH	right atrial hypertrophy
RAPD	relative afferent pupillary defect
RBBB	right bundle branch block
RBC	red blood cells
RhD	rhesus D (antigen)
RR	respiratory rate
RSI	rapid sequence induction
RSV	respiratory syncytial virus
RT	rapid tranquillization
RTA	renal tubular acidosis
RVH	right ventricular hypertrophy
SAFE	shout for help, approach with caution, free from danger, evaluate ABC

SaO_2	oxygen saturation measured by arterial gas
SBE	subacute bacterial endocarditis
SC	subcutaneous
SCIWORA	spinal cord injury without radiological abnormality
SIADH	syndrome of inappropriate anti-diuretic hormone secretion
SIDS	sudden infant death syndrome
SJS	Stevens–Johnson syndrome
SL	sublingual
SMA	smooth muscle antibody (against actin)
SPA	suprapubic aspirate
SpO_2	oxygen saturation measured by pulse oximetry
SSRI	selective serotonin re-uptake inhibitor
SSSS	staphylococcal scalded skin syndrome
STD	sexually transmitted disease
SUDI	sudden unexpected death of an infant
SVC	superior vena cava
SVR	systemic vascular resistance
SVT	supraventricular tachycardia
T_3	triiodothyronine
T_4	thyroxine
TAPVD	total anomalous pulmonary venous drainage
TB	tuberculosis
tds	three times a day
TEN	toxic epidermal necrolysis
TFT	thyroid function tests
TGA	transposition of great arteries
Ti	inspiratory time
TIBC	total iron binding capacity
TOF	tracheo-oesophageal fistula
TORCH	toxoplasma, other (HIV, syphilis, gonorrhoea) rubella, cytomegalovirus, herpes simplex virus
TPHA	*Treponema pallidum* haemagglutination assay
TPN	total parenteral nutrition
TR	tricuspid regurgitation
TSH	thyroid-stimulating hormone
TT	thrombin time
TTG	tissue transglutaminase
UAC	umbilical artery catheter
UEC	urea, electrolytes, creatinine
ULSE	upper left sternal edge
UMN	upper motor neuron

URSE	upper right sternal edge
URTI	upper respiratory tract infection
USS	ultrasound scan
UTI	urinary tract infection
UVC	umbilical venous catheter
VACTERL	vertebral defect, anal atresia, cardiac anomaly, tracheoesophageal fistula, (o)esophageal atresia, renal defects, and radial limb dysplasia
VBG	venous blood gas
VDRL	Venereal Disease Research Laboratory (test)
VF	ventricular fibrillation
VMA	vanillylmandelic acid
VSD	ventricular septal defect
VT	ventricular tachycardia
VUJ	vesicoureteric junction
vWF	von Willebrand factor
VZV	varicella zoster virus
WCC	white cell count
WPW	Wolff–Parkinson–White (syndrome)
ZN	Ziehl–Neelson

Detailed contents

Chapter 1

Introduction

When faced with an ill child and anxious parents, a feeling of panic is understandable. This book aims to help you gain confidence and competence in dealing with all paediatric life-threatening conditions, as well as more commonly seen presentations to the emergency department.

The assessment of an ill child who may be anxious, in pain, grumpy, tired or all of the above is a difficult skill. In addition, the fears and concerns of the parents must be addressed. Tips are provided on how to obtain useful information from children, as well as suggestions for eliciting clinical signs from the un-cooperative ones! How to communicate well with parents is discussed in Chapter 2.

Advanced Life Support advocates the systematic **ABCD** approach to the severely unwell patient, namely:

Airway.
Breathing.
Circulation.
Disability.

In children, **DEFG**—**D**on't **E**ver **F**orget **G**lucose—also applies. This approach is used throughout the book and is described in detail in Chapter 4. In addition, for each condition, the key facts of the history along with the cardinal clinical signs are covered. Relevant investigations and potential complications are also featured.

Management plans are based on the best available evidence or else on accepted best practice. Inevitably, there are grey areas where different regimens may be equally efficacious. In such cases, if local protocols or guidelines are not available, the medications suggested should be discussed with a consultant in the relevant subspecialty.

Drug doses are included within the text, where they are needed. The doses have been taken from *BNF for children* (ISBN 0 85369 626 8 Royal Pharmaceutical Company of Great Britain). Doses should be checked with whichever formulary is used in your hospital.

The composition of intravenous fluids varies between countries—this book cites fluids used in the UK. If the fluid is not available to you, a fluid with an equivalent amount of saline should be used (📖 p.506). This appendix also covers how to supplement fluids with glucose or potassium if required.

Finally, never forget to ask for help. Another pair of hands or clinical opinion can provide much needed reassurance and may expedite your patient's recovery.

Age groups have been quoted where possible in the handbook. The following age groups apply to the terms below.

- **Premmie**—under 36 weeks of gestation
- **Neonate**—under 8 weeks of age
- **Baby**—2 months to 1 year
- **Toddler**—1 to 3 years
- **Child**—1 to 12 years
- **Adolescent**—over 12 years

Chapter 2

Coping with patients and parents

Introduction

The consultation in paediatric emergency differs from that of adult emergency. There are the additional facts to incorporate into the history such as perinatal events and developmental milestones. But the style of the interview, and how we treat and even investigate the patients is also quite different.

Those of us who spend our working lives in a hospital have to remember how frightening it is to outsiders. Especially for the small child who is feeling unwell, and dreads the 'doctor with a needle'. So this chapter covers 'the art' of paediatric emergency, namely:

- the ability to conduct a consultation with the child and the parents that leaves all parties satisfied;
- the skill of dealing with a child in pain.

Consultation

> The good physician treats the disease; the great physician treats the patient who has the disease.
>
> Sir William Osler (1849–1919)

The 'great paediatrician', however, must treat the whole family. The worries of the carers and siblings must be addressed, as part of our holistic response to their presentation to hospital. Parental fears for their child may greatly exceed (or, less often, underestimate) the dangers associated with the disease or symptoms their child presents with. Moreover, parental anxiety may exacerbate the concerns of a fearful child, as they lie in a strange room with frightening noises, smells, and people all around.

We must, therefore endeavour to put ourselves in two sets of shoes—those of the patient and carer.

- How is the child feeling? Not their headache, but their fears and worries? Their pain will be worse if they have a fear (rational or not) that we fail to address. They may be concerned about their parents' feelings or who will feed the cat. They may think we will do something painful to them, or 'put them to sleep'.
- How are their parents coping? Outwardly brave, whilst screaming in fear within? Many will worry their child is dying. Can we make their child better? How quickly and will it hurt? What will it cost (time/money)? Why didn't their GP pick it up sooner? Why did they as parents not notice earlier?

How we address these issues and communicate the information to the child and family is an important part of the treatment we give—it is part of the healing process. Make the child better, but leave a poor impression and the family will leave the hospital dissatisfied. Help a family cope with a devastating diagnosis and they will be eternally grateful.

So what are the important factors in our interaction with patients and their family?

First impressions

- Dress.
  - Clothes and hair should be professional, smart, and appropriate. Nothing too extreme; save the trendy outfit for outside work, it will only get blood, wee, or poo on it!
- Welcome. Introduce yourself to parent and child (however young).
  - Spend a moment playing with teddy; get down to the child's eye level, even if that means kneeling or sitting on the floor.
- Smile—however trivial or annoying the presentation is. Be professional.
- Tone of voice. Always friendly, with no hint of blame (parent or GP).
- Be prompt. If there will be a delay, put your head around door and explain that you are busy and will be there as soon as possible.
- Interaction with nursing staff—parents will notice if you are rude or discourteous to other staff.

The critically ill child

Here, the priority is resuscitation, but that does not mean ignoring the parents, who have every right to be there with their child. If possible, assign a nurse to stay with the parents. He or she can assist with explanations.

- Introduce yourself.
  - If the child has arrested, resuscitate as you talk to the parents.
- Explain that their child is very ill and you need to get on and do a few things and that you will update them as soon as you can.
- Ask them to quickly recount the last hours/days, whilst asking nursing staff to put monitors on.
  - What symptoms have been noticed?
  - Is the child usually fit and thriving?
  - Is the child on any medications, or allergic to any?
  - Are there any illnesses that run in the family?
- When you get a chance to talk to the parents again:
  - go over the history in more detail;
  - explain the clinical situation. If you think their child might die, tell them so. If you don't know, admit it.
- Speak to the parents little and often, as most of what you say will not be fully absorbed.

History

- Don't be afraid to use a template as an *aide-mémoire*, nor to go back and ask the things you forgot.
- Direct your questions to the child—their answers are often more informative than their tender years might suggest. Allow the child and parents to answer without interruption.
- Observe the family as you talk—much of your examination is from these observations.
- Be gentle but persistent in your history-taking. If you do not understand the course of events, start again and take it day by day from when the child was last 100% well.
- Try to get the child/parents' views—not what they were told by the GP.
- When you are happy with your history, briefly recount it to the family—only then can they be sure that you understand what they thought they meant to tell you.

Examination

It cannot be overemphasized how important ***observation*** is. Most of what you need to know can be gleaned by careful observation of a child in the mother's arms.

- Go through each system in your head and look at the child, noting any abnormalities, before approaching the child.
- Get down to the child's level and talk to them. Examine their teddy, if they will let you (or mum's arm). Don't forget to smile, however ill they are and however scared/bored/tired/hungry you are. A minute spent playing with the child will save you time when they allow you to listen to their chest without a squawk!

- Do the important things first while maintaining the child's dignity and warmth.
  - In a baby, auscultate through their clothes, as undressing often produces crying. Feel the femoral pulses, before removing clothes/nappy.
  - Listen again once fully undressed.
- Save ENT until last, but do not forget.
- Persist or repeat later until happy that you have adequately covered all systems.
  - May need to return later, especially if child gets upset—do not persist when the child is distraught.

Investigations

- It is crucial that the child and family know what tests you are hoping to do and why. If it is going to hurt, say so—if you promised a pain-free cannulation and the magic cream does not work, the child will not forgive you.
- Explain the need to keep the child still—this is rarely possible on the parental lap. Lying the child on a bed gives you better control and therefore a higher chance of success.
- Experienced assistance is always a prerequisite to any procedure.
- Know when to get further help.
  - No more than 3 attempts should be made without discussing with a more senior doctor. If they wish you to persist, give everyone (especially yourself) a few minutes break, before trying again.
- Ask the parent if they wish to leave.
  - Fathers rarely want to stay! Tell them that their baby will scream just from being held still, so they should not stand outside the door listening—go right away and get a cup of tea.
  - If they do remain in the room, tell them what you are going to do and how they can help—by keeping calm and still and distracting the child.
- Don't forget to thank the staff after helping you with a procedure.

Note-taking

All notes must be legible, signed, and dated. If there is any concern of abuse, then ensure you have a witness and record who is present during consultation. Never move on to the next patient until your notes are complete—you will forget things. Always write a brief summary and your differential diagnosis. This enables you to collect your thoughts and, 10 years down the line, may convince the judge that you had considered all the relevant possibilities!

What if the consultation goes wrong

Even 'great paediatricians' occasionally have disputes with the families they are treating. Always discuss with a senior colleague before proceeding—a time out and a second opinion may ensure you don't dig an even bigger hole! If you have made a mistake, apologize and try to rectify matters. If the conflict cannot be resolved, ask the family if they would prefer to see one of your colleagues and arrange handover of their care as swiftly as possible. Document all actions concisely and non-emotively in the notes. Compose yourself before seeing your next patient.

If the experience was distressing for you, discuss it with a senior colleague and learn from it.

Dealing with the child in pain

Everyone is distressed when a child is in pain. How you respond to the child can greatly lessen the child's perception of pain. Dismissing the child as a wailing 'drama queen' may be part of the problem!

Contributory factors to the severity of pain include the following.

- Behavioural—sex; developmental stage; cultural norms of expression of emotion.
- Psychological—anxiety/fears of child (N.B. parents' role); fatigue; unfamiliar environment.
- Cognitive—understanding of circumstances; previous experience; co-existing medical conditions.

For children, the treatment of pain not only requires analgesia but also alleviation of anxiety. Reassurance can be provided by staff appearing empathic and calm and the surroundings being comfortable and, ideally, quiet. Distractions such as books and blowing bubbles are invaluable when dealing with a young child.

Pain assessment

Pain is subjective and requires frequent re-assessment by the child and by the observer. There are various validated pain scales for use in children, e.g. a selection of faces—smiling to grimacing. Be familiar with whichever is used in your hospital. Children over 7 years can reliably rank their pain on a scale of 1 to 10, where 1 is no pain and 10 is the worst pain ever.

Further assessment is by independent observation of physiological variables and behaviour.

- Physiological variables:
  - heart rate;
  - blood pressure;
  - sweating;
  - respiratory rate.
- Behavioural variables:
  - crying, irritability;
  - grimacing;
  - reluctance to move or eat;
  - withdrawal; minimal interaction.

Do not overlook the pale, motionless child who does not complain!

Treatment of pain

A combination of reassurance techniques and medication is used. Non-pharmacological therapy is particularly important for children.

- *Non-pharmacological*
  - Parental presence—if parents are calm and sensible.
  - Quiet environment—procedure room away from the hubbub of the ward.
  - Distraction—video, play therapist, story.
  - Soothing—breathing exercises, gentle massage, cold or warm compress.
  - Repositioning fractures—pillow, sling, plaster of Paris.

- *Pharmacological*. Medications are used for analgesia and sedation. Most emergency departments will have a policy for conscious sedation—do not upset anaesthetists by exceeding your expertise!

Analgesia

When deciding which analgesic is to be used, consider the speed of onset of action and which routes of administration are available to you. Intramuscular medications are seldom used in paediatrics.

Local

- **EMLA®** (2.5% prilocaine and lignocaine). Takes 60 minutes for full effect and analgesia persists for an hour. Can cause vasoconstriction, which will resolve 15 minutes after removal of dressing.
- **Ametop®** (amethocaine). Effective in 30–45 minutes and lasts 4–6 hours. ***Never*** on inflamed skin or mucous membranes.
- **Xylocaine®**. 1 or 2% lignocaine for subcutaneous infiltration. Neonate: <0.3mg/kg 1%; 1 month–12 years: <0.4ml/kg, 1%; >12 years, 20ml 1% or 10ml 2%. Rarely, CNS side-effects.
- **Bupivicaine**. For regional blocks (p.480); takes an hour for effect, but lasts up to 7 hours; usually with local anaesthetic.
- **Lignocaine gel**. For mouth ulcers, sore throat.
- **Ethyl chloride**. If old enough to differentiate cold from painful.

Oral

Oral preparations usually take 60 minutes to act. The exception is codeine phosphate, which works within 20 minutes.

- **Paracetamol**.
  - Neonate: 20mg/kg once, then 10–15mg/kg 8–12 hourly. Maximum 30mg/kg/day—halve if jaundiced or baby under 28 weeks' gestation.
  - Over 1 month: 20mg/kg once, then 15–20mg/kg 6 hourly. Maximum 90mg/kg/day and 1g/dose (maximum 60mg/kg/day in 1–3-month olds).
- **NSAIDs**.
  - **Ibuprofen**: 10mg/kg 8 hourly. Maximum 400mg/dose or 2.4g/day.
  - **Diclofenac**: 1mg/kg 8 hourly. Maximum 3mg/kg/day or 150mg/day.
  - **Naproxen**: 5–7.5mg/kg 12 hourly. Maximum dose 500mg.
  - NSAIDs are excellent for musculoskeletal or colicky pain. But use cautiously if:
    - — under 3 years;
    - — poorly controlled asthma;
    - — known sensitivity;
    - — impaired renal function;
    - — thrombocytopenia;
    - — coagulopathy;
    - — liver failure;
    - — IBD.
- **Codeine phosphate**: 1mg/kg 4 hourly; maximum <1 year 3mg/kg/day or 240mg/day; maximum >1 year, 6mg/kg/day.

Rectal

Absorption can be unreliable and takes up to 60 minutes before onset of action. This route is not to be used if the child is neutropenic.

- **Paracetamol**: Neonate: 30mg/kg then 20mg/kg 8 hourly. Maximum, 60mg/kg/day, Halve if jaundiced. Over 1 month: 40mg/kg loading dose (maximum 1g), then 15–20mg/kg 6 hourly. Maximum 90mg/kg/day or 4g/day.
- **Diclofenac**: loading dose up to 2mg/kg, 1mg/kg 8 hourly. Maximum, 3mg/kg/day or 150mg/day.

Intravenous

- **Morphine**
  - Commonly administered in a bolus, but use of infusions and patient/nurse controlled analgesia (PCA/NCA) becoming widespread.
  - Close observation, especially of neonates, is necessary because of side-effects:
    - — respiratory depression;
    - — sedation;
    - — nausea;
    - — hypotension—with bolus;
    - — pruritis;
    - — constipation—if prolonged use.
  - Bolus. Neonate: 25mcg/kg; 1–3 months: 50mcg/kg; >3 months: 100mcg/kg; then 20mcg/kg bolus until effective
  - IV infusion. N.B. Give a bolus dose before starting infusion. Infusion: 1mg/kg morphine made up to 50ml with 0.9% saline; 1ml/h is = 20mcg/kg/h.
  - Ventilated patient: infusion 20–40mcg/kg/h.
  - Non-ventilated: neonate, 5–10mcg/kg/h; >1 month, 10–20mcg/kg/h.
  - **Nurse-controlled analgesia**. Background infusion as above until adequate analgesia.
  - Neonate: bolus 10mcg/kg. Lockout 45 minutes.
  - >1 month: bolus 10–20mcg/kg. Lockout 30 minutes.
  - **Patient-controlled analgesia**. Background 5mcg/kg/h; bolus 20mcg/kg; Lockout 5 minutes.

Other intravenous drugs

- **Fentanyl**. 1mcg/kg (maximum 50mcg) is a useful alternative to morphine if there are concerns about hypotension, renal insufficiency, or histamine release.
- **Paracetamol**. Infuse over 15 minutes. 10–50kg: 15mg/kg 4–6 hourly, maximum 60mg/kg/d. >50kg: 1g 4–6 hourly, maximum 4g/d.

Sedation

Sedation may be light or deep, or general anaesthetic. It is an unpredictable continuum, so sedation should only be commenced where suitably experienced staff and continuous cardiorespiratory monitoring is available. As protective reflexes may be compromised, it is advisable that the child has fasted for at least an hour before sedation is administered.

- Light sedation:
  - minimum depression of consciousness;
  - retains ability to fully control airway;
  - may respond to surroundings.
- Deep sedation:
  - reduced conscious level, or unconscious;
  - partial or complete loss of protective reflexes.
- General anaesthetic. State of hypnosis, muscle relaxation, and analgesia.

General guidelines for sedation include the following.
- Suitably experienced staff are available.
- Non-pharmacological strategies and local anaesthetics are in place, but are inadequate.
- Continuous monitoring of heart and respiratory rate and oximetry possible.
- Titratable doses—increasing as needed.
- Availability of antagonist—naloxone for opiates, flumazenil for benzodiazepines.

Inhaled

- **'Entonox'**—50:50 mixture of nitrous oxide and oxygen. Inhaled through mask/mouthpiece held by patient. Good analgesia in those over 6 who can tolerate. Will cause nausea if inhalation over 20 minutes.

Oral

Excellent for painless procedures, e.g. sedation prior to CT scan.
- **Chloral hydrate:** 30–100mg/kg 45 minutes before procedure; maximum 2000mg (respiratory monitoring at higher end). Contraindicated in cardiac disease, gastritis, porphyria.
- **Triclofos:** 30–100mg/kg; maximum 2000mg (respiratory monitoring at higher end). Less gastric irritation than chloral.
- **Alimemazine** (trimeprazine, Vallergan): 2mg/kg; maximum 90mg. 1–2 hours to full effect. (N.B. Paradoxical stimulation in some; headache; anti-muscarinic effects. Contraindicated in hepatic impairment and can interact with other medications.)
- **Midazolam sublingual:** 1mg/kg (maximum 15mg) 30–60 minutes prior to procedure. Caution in cardiac disease, hepatic impairment and lower dose in renal impairment. Contraindicated in myasthenia and respiratory depression.

Intravenous

Often used in conjunction with IV analgesics. Only to be administered when equipment for resuscitation is available and continuous monitoring available. Advisable to have child fasted for 2 hours before use.

Remember that when noxious stimulus removed, e.g. dislocation relocated, child at risk of respiratory depression.

- **Midazolam** IV over 2–3 minutes.
  - 1 month–6 years: 100mcg/kg, increase in steps to maximum total 6mg.
  - 6–12 years: 50mcg/kg, increase in steps to maximum total 10mg.
  - >12 years: 2–2.5mg, increase in steps to maximum total 7.5mg. N.B. less than for younger children.
  - Excellent anxiolytic and amnestic. Side-effects include: hypotension; GI disturbance; jaundice; respiratory depression (especially in rapid bolus).
- **Ketamine**: 1mg/kg ***plus*** midazolam 0.05mg/kg (maximum 2.5mg). Although an anaesthetic agent, ketamine is analgesic at low doses. Must be administered with midazolam to reduce risk of emergent hallucinations/nightmares.

Antidotes

- **Naloxone**. Half-life shorter than that of morphine, so may need to repeat dose or transfer to PICU for naloxone infusion. Side-effects include nausea and vomiting.
  - Neonate: 10mcg/kg, repeat every 2–3 minutes.
  - 1 month–12 years: 10mcg/kg, then subsequent dose 100mcg/kg.
  - 12–18 years: 1.5–3mcg/kg, then increase in increments of 100mcg every 2 minutes.
- **Flumazenil**: 10mcg/kg repeated at 1 minute intervals until effect. Maximum 250mcg/dose and total 1mg/d (2mg on PICU).
  - Infusion 2–10mcg/kg/h, up to 400mcg/h until response.
  - Side-effects include GI disturbances, agitation on wakening.

Chapter 3

Neonatal emergencies

Introduction

A comprehensive neonatology vade-mecum is beyond the scope of this book. Only neonatal conditions that may present to the emergency department (ED) are covered.

With 6 hour discharges becoming ever more prevalent, ED staff must be able to deal with the acutely unwell newborn. In addition, there are several life-threatening conditions that arise in the first 8 weeks of life that ED staff should be able to recognize.

Delivery

Occasionally, you will get advance warning, whether from the ambulance crew or from the parents as they drive to hospital. If possible, summon staff with midwifery and neonatology experience.

It may be possible to be certain of the gestation before a baby is born. Although extremely premature babies are at greater risk of long-term deficits, many will survive unaffected.

If in any doubt, the baby should be resuscitated and transferred to the neonatal unit, where decisions about further management can be made.

Management

Assemble equipment

- Ideally, obtain a resuscitaire. Otherwise use an overhead radiant heat source.
- Delivery pack.
- Warmed towels.
- Airway equipment. Laerdal bag with a selection of masks (sizes 00 and 0/1), oropharyngeal (Guedel) airways (sizes 000 and 00) and a straight blade laryngoscope, ETT sizes 2.5–3.5, and suction equipment with paediatric Yankauer ('Yanker') sucker or a 12 or 14 gauge suction catheter.

Obtain antenatal history when possible. Salient facts include:

- What is the estimated gestation?
- Any significant obstetric or medical history?
  - Note any history of neonatal problems, e.g. prematurity, SIDS, cardiac conditions.
  - Does the mother know her blood group and group B Streptococcus status?
- Was the mother well during pregnancy?
  - Note hypertension, gestational diabetes.
  - Any drugs taken, prescribed, e.g. steroids, methadone, or recreational?
  - Did she smoke or drink alcohol?
- Any pregnancy complications?
  - Antepartum haemorrhage, febrile illness.
  - N.B. Premature rupture of membranes not only increases the risk of the baby being septic, but also the risk that the lungs may be hypoplastic.
- What screening tests were performed?
  - Antenatal USS, blood tests ± amniocentesis.

After delivery When the cord is clamped, check the time or start clock on resuscitaire.

Thermal care

The temperature of all newborn infants should be maintained at 36–37°C.

Babies delivered at 30 weeks gestational age or above: 'drying and wrapping'
- Newly born babies who require resuscitation at birth, should be dried in a pre-warmed towel and the wet towel removed.
- The baby should then be wrapped in warm dry towels under a radiant heat source.

Babies delivered at less than 30 weeks gestational age: 'occlusive wrapping'
- Infants should be placed immediately into a plastic bag without drying.
- The open end of the bag should be drawn loosely around the baby's neck.
- The baby's head should be dried and wrapped in a towel or knitted cap.
- Assessment of the baby, resuscitation, and stabilization should proceed while the baby remains within occlusive wrapping and under a radiant heat source.
- A hole can be made in the bag if additional access to the baby is required.

Assessment

There are four features to note in the initial assessment of the baby:
- colour: pink, blue, or white?
- breathing: regular, irregular, gasping, or apnoeic?
- heart rate: fast (>100/min), slow (<60/min), or asystolic?
- tone: active, or floppy?

At delivery most infants fall into one of four groups.
- **Healthy**—pink, crying lustily
- **Primary apnoea**—blue, inadequate respirations, pulse rate ~100
- **Terminal apnoea**—pale, limp, apnoeic, pulse less than 60
- **Stillborn**—white, asystolic, apnoeic, limp (may be resuscitatable)

Primary and terminal apnoea cannot be distinguished at the time of delivery. Therefore, for all babies who are breathing inadequately on first assessment, start ABCD of resuscitation (📖 p.22).

Resuscitation of the newborn

This follows the ABC principles of basic life support (p.50). Note that the differences for neonates include:
- head position;
- position of hands for chest compressions;
- early reassessment after intervention;
- different drug doses for treatment of asystole.

Remember to keep the baby warm!

Air versus oxygen in resuscitation of the newborn

Traditionally, newborn infants have been resuscitated in 100% oxygen. More recently, there have been meta-analyses indicating that mortality might be reduced in those infants resuscitated in air. Guidance from local departmental policies is advised.

Airway and breathing

- Control the airway—head in the neutral position.
- Support breathing—deliver **inflation breaths**. Bag and mask ventilation will be adequate for almost all newborns. Tracheal intubation can be performed at any stage of resuscitation.

- Five breaths.
- 30cm water—but 25cm water may suffice for preterms.
- Inspiratory time of 2–3 seconds (count 1000, 2000, 3000!)

- Watch carefully to see ***chest moving***. If ***no*** chest movement, consider:
  - re-positioning to open airway—consider jaw thrust and/or a Guedel airway. A second person to hold mask in position whilst providing jaw thrust may also help;
  - airway obstruction—direct inspection of oropharynx and suction with a wide-bore catheter or Yankauer under direct vision;
  - 'stiff lungs', e.g. pneumothorax, diaphragmatic hernia (scaphoid abdomen), lung hypoplasia. May need to increase pressure to 40cm water;
  - misplaced tracheal tube.

Reassess

- If chest still not moving, repeat above manoeuvres and consider intubation.
- If, in response to lung aeration, the chest is moving and the heart rate has increased ***but*** the baby fails to establish regular breathing, continue ventilation breaths for a further 30 seconds and reassess.
- If opiates have been given within an hour of delivery, the baby may require IM naloxone 0.1mg/kg. ***Make certain*** that mother is not an opiate addict; otherwise naloxone will precipitate acute withdrawal in the child (p.47).

If heart rate under 60bpm and not increasing after 10–20 seconds of adequate lung aeration, commence chest compressions.

Circulation

- Do not start **chest compressions** until the chest is moving adequately.
- Grip chest in both hands. Place thumbs on sternum just below an imaginary line joining nipples, and fingers over the spine. If no assistant, then use two fingers and keep other hand holding mask over mouth.

- Aim to depress chest half the distance between sternum and spine
- 3 chest compressions to one breath
- Continue for 30 seconds

Reassess If no improvement, repeat chest compressions for further 30 seconds then reassess. If still inadequate heart rate, proceed to 'Drugs'.

Drugs

If there is no response to adequate cardiac compression combined with effective lung inflation, drugs are required. Most neonates will suffer asystolic arrests and require the sequence of drugs in Table 3.1.

Remember that hypoglycaemia in a neonate can resemble shock.

N.B. Drugs need to be administered via an intraosseous needle or centrally via an **umbilical venous catheter** (📖 p.464).

Following resuscitation

Pay careful attention to optimizing temperature control during transfer to neonatal unit. Without allowing baby to get cold, allow parents to see their baby before transfer. Explain the events of the resuscitation, the infant's current clinical status, and anticipated plans for the care of their baby.

Table 3.1 Neonatal resuscitation drug doses

	Drug dose (estimate birth weight)
Adrenaline (epinephrine) 1st dose (1 in 10,000)	0.1ml/kg (10mcg/kg)
Adrenaline 2nd dose (1 in 10,000)	0.3ml/kg (30mcg/kg)
Sodium bicarbonate (4.2%)	4ml/kg (2mmol/kg base)
Volume Blood or N/saline 0.9%	10–20ml/kg
Glucose (10%)	2.5ml/kg

Special cases

Meconium stained liquor

If the baby is vigorous, no intervention is necessary, however thick the meconium. Suction on the perineum is no longer recommended, as it does not improve outcome and may delay the time to first assessment.

However, if the baby is ***not*** vigorous and there is any meconium:

- intubate and aspirate meconium from trachea, or suction above and below the cords with a wide bore Yankauer sucker;
- after removing as much meconium as possible, continue normal resuscitation measures;
- aspirate stomach contents;
- refer to neonatal unit as baby is at risk of respiratory compromise, including persistent pulmonary hypertension of the newborn (p.36).

Diaphragmatic hernia

These are usually diagnosed antenatally—the earlier the defect was noted, the greater the probability of pulmonary hypoplasia, which complicates resuscitation.

Typically, the baby has respiratory distress with a scaphoid abdomen. Bowel usually enters the left hemithorax, reducing air entry.

- Bag and mask inflation is to be avoided.
- Intubate as soon as possible after delivery.
- Insert a large bore nasogastric tube and place on free drainage.
- Obtain venous access and administer paralysing agent, e.g. pancuronium 100mcg/kg to prevent air swallowing.
- Perform CXR to confirm position of NGT and diagnosis.
- Refer to paediatric surgeon.

Hydrops fetalis

In this rare condition, the baby is grossly oedematous and ventilation is impaired because of pulmonary fluid.

- If there is tense ascites limiting inflation of lungs, check the position of the liver and spleen, then insert a cannula into the left iliac fossa laterally and slowly aspirate fluid.
- Apply pressures of up to 40cm water to achieve lung inflation.
- If this is unsuccessful, consider aspirating pleural effusions via a three-way tap attached to a cannula inserted in 4th intercostal space mid-axillary line.

Extreme prematurity

Communication before delivery

- Good communication between parents, obstetricians, and neonatologists is optimal.
- A management plan should be clearly recorded in the notes.
- Counselling should be accurate, reflecting local and national survival and morbidity statistics.
- Factors taken into account will include: gestational age, predicted birth weight, severity of pathology, and parental wishes.

Delivery

- An experienced paediatrician, who is attending the delivery will assess whether active resuscitation is considered appropriate depending on the condition of the baby at birth.
- Factors to consider will include maturity of infant, evidence of perinatal asphyxia, extensive bruising, and heart rate at the time of delivery.

If in any doubt, the baby should be resuscitated and transferred to the neonatal unit where decisions about further management can be made.

Discontinuing resuscitation

If the baby fails to respond to resuscitation, discuss the case with a senior paediatrician. If there is no cardiac output by 15 minutes of age, further efforts are unlikely to be successful.

However, if the baby has a spontaneous heart rate, yet is making no respiratory effort, assisted ventilation should continue until a senior paediatrician is available to review the baby.

Documentation

- All events of resuscitation should be carefully documented.
- The record should include:
  - time you were called, to where, and why;
  - time you arrived and condition of baby on your arrival;
  - the mode of, and initial response to resuscitation;
  - time of first adequate chest inflation;
  - time of tracheal intubation and duration of ventilation;
  - air or oxygen concentration used;
  - drugs given, route, and dosage;
  - time to first gasp, regular respirations, and heart rate;
  - umbilical cord pH, blood gases, and base deficit;
  - names and designation of personnel present at resuscitation;
  - time and named member of staff making decision to discontinue resuscitation (if appropriate);
  - reasons for delay in resuscitation;
  - information given to parents.
- The entry should be clearly timed, dated, and legibly signed.

Physiological changes after birth

After the trauma of birth, the newborn has to function independently and cope with physiological changes, which may unmask congenital problems.

Respiratory

In utero, the lungs are fluid-filled and pulmonary blood flow is minimized. Blood flows through the foramen ovale (between the atria), thereby bypassing the right ventricle; and is also diverted via the patent ductus arteriosus (PDA) between the pulmonary artery and the aorta. These usually close as the lungs fill with air, dropping pulmonary pressure. If this does not happen, **persistent pulmonary hypertension of the newborn** (PPHN) ensues, ultimately compromising blood flow to the lungs and resulting in cyanosis (📖 p.36).

Cardiovascular

A PDA provides a link between the systemic and pulmonary circulations. Congenital cardiac conditions with impaired pulmonary blood flow, e.g. pulmonary atresia, require an ASD or a VSD with a PDA for blood to circulate around the heart and flow down the PDA into the pulmonary artery. Cyanosis will develop as the duct closes.

Similarly, left outflow tract obstructions, e.g. critical aortic stenosis, coarctation, need a PDA to provide blood flow beyond the aortic narrowing. Such **duct-dependent lesions** will manifest by 5 days of age.

Gastrointestinal

A newborn has only limited reserves to provide its energy requirements. Provision of a source of glucose soon after birth is important. The glucose may be from breast milk, formula, dextrose infusion, or total parenteral nutrition, depending on the circumstances.

Hypoglycaemia is also likely to arise if the baby is cold as glucose is consumed by thermogenesis. There is debate about the definition of hypoglycaemia and finger-prick levels are inaccurate at low levels. It is important to confirm there is indeed hypoglycaemia, but also to ensure it is immediately corrected as cerebral metabolism swiftly deteriorates. This can usually be done orally (see box).

The fetus does not require a functioning gastrointestinal tract. Thus ***gut atresias*** may not be detected until after birth when the child develops bilious vomiting ± delayed passage of meconium.

Jaundice is common in newborn babies as the liver struggles to cope with the breakdown of fetal haemoglobin. But this is not a benign condition as unconjugated bilirubin can cross the blood–brain barrier resulting in developmental delay, seizures, blindness, and deafness ('kernicterus'). High levels of unconjugated hyperbilirubinaemia or jaundice that persists longer than 14 days of age also warrant investigation (📖 p.42).

Premature babies

Ex-utero life is even harder for the premmie. They may not manage such physiological changes, e.g. failure of PDA closure, or be less able to

Management of hypoglycaemia

- If **asymptomatic** and finger-prick glucose <2.5mmol/l, give additional oral/NG milk and repeat finger-prick glucose post-feed and again before the next feed, until consistently above 3mmol/L
- If asymptomatic, but finger-prick glucose <2mmol/l, obtain venous sample to confirm; feed and repeat sugar level
- If twitchy, reduced level of consciousness, floppy, apnoeic or fitting and finger-prick glucose <2.5mmol/l:
  - obtain IV access and give 2ml/kg 10% dextrose;
  - followed by infusion of 10% dextrose at full maintenance;
  - repeat sugar 10 minutes after bolus given.
  - If no IV access, use buccal Glucogel® or IM glucagon (200mcg/kg; maximum 1mg)
- If no symptomatic improvement, further bolus of 2ml/kg 10% dextrose and infuse at full maintenance to maintain glucose above 3mmol/l

N.B. If glucose still low, dextrose over 12.5% is required. This needs central access (📖 p.464) as well as detailed investigation of hypoglycaemia (📖 p.413). IV hydrocortisone 3–5mg/kg may also be necessary

tolerate the sequelae, e.g. unconjugated hyperbilirubinaemia. In addition, their immaturity increases the likelihood of developing:

- hypothermia;
- hypoglycaemia (see box).

Respiratory

Hyaline membrane disease Lung surfactant levels are usually adequate by 30–32 weeks gestation, especially if mum has had antenatal steroids. However, as surfactant production in sick babies may cease, HMD can present at any gestation.

Gastrointestinal

Feeding difficulties

- Suck reflex develops around 32 weeks; thus premmies may require NG feeds.
- Intolerance—secondary to prematurity, sepsis, or necrotizing enterocolitis (NEC).

Sepsis

May precipitate premature labour and immature immune systems mean premmies are more vulnerable. Treatment should cover urogenital pathogens, e.g. *Escherichia coli*, group B streptococci, enterococcus, listeria.

N.B. Babies delivered by Caesarean section will be at risk if there has been prolonged rupture of membranes.

- Low threshold for treatment with antibiotics in an unwell premmie.

Neurological

Intracranial bleeds

Germinal matrix and choroid plexus remain well vascularized in the premature infant. Abrupt changes in blood flow to the brain may precipitate intracranial haemorrhage. This is often clinically silent, but may present with a metabolic acidosis, sudden collapse, or seizure.

Postnatal assessment

A full antenatal history must be taken, along with a history of the presenting complaint, as conditions such as group B streptococcus sepsis or NEC can emerge long after delivery. Manifestations of drug withdrawal tend to present within the first 5 days of life.

History

Antenatal

- Obtain the mother's obstetric and medical history.
  - Note any history of neonatal problems, e.g. prematurity, SIDS, cardiac conditions.
  - Note the mother's blood group, including rhesus and whether she was screened for group B streptococcus during pregnancy.
- Was mum well during pregnancy?
  - Note hypertension, gestational diabetes.
  - Any drugs, prescribed, e.g. steroids or recreational?
  - Did she smoke or drink alcohol?
- Was the pregnancy uneventful?
  - Antepartum haemorrhage, febrile illness, premature rupture of membranes.
- What was the estimated gestation?
- What screening tests were performed?
  - Antenatal USS, blood tests ± amniocentesis.

Delivery Any CTG changes or abnormal fetal scalp pH or cord gases? What was the mode of delivery and was any resuscitation needed?

Postnatal course

- Is the baby feeding well?
  - Any breathlessness or cyanosis?
- When was meconium passed?
  - This sticky black poo should be passed in first 24 hours of life.
- Is the baby gaining weight?
  - Normal to lose up to 10% of body weight, but to regain birth weight by 2 weeks.
- Has the child been jaundiced?
- Any vomiting?
  - Small milky possets normal; bile suggests obstruction until proven otherwise.
- Has there been any twitching or abnormal movements?
  - Newborns have an exaggerated startle reaction, which can resemble tonic movements.
- Has the neonatal screening been done?
  - Usually includes PKU, TSH, IRT, and some inborn errors of metabolism.

Examination

If in extremis, treat as collapsed neonate (📖 p.32).

Otherwise perform a full examination of baby—removing nappy is mandatory! Auscultate and feel for femoral pulses first, whilst baby quiet—can do prior to undressing fully. If the baby opens eyes, immediately check for red reflex. Unpleasant tests such as 'the hip test' are performed last.

General

- Weight, length, and head circumference.
- Skin colour/rash.
  - Is the child pink, blue, yellow, or white?
  - Erythema toxicum is red macular rash, sometimes with white/yellow central puncti with a distribution that can alter before your eyes.
  - Are there any birth marks?
- Face—is the baby dysmorphic?
  - Look at eyes, ears, mouth, chin, noting any asymmetry.
  - Does the tongue protrude (Down's)?
  - Is there a cleft palate or blocked nose (choanal atresia)?
- Respiratory.
  - Rate and work of breathing.
  - Added sounds, e.g. diaphragmatic hernia.
  - Symmetry—exclude pneumothorax.
- Circulation.
  - Pulse rate, rhythm, and character—SVT, shock.
  - Assess central perfusion. Should be <3s.
  - Palpate femoral pulses. N.B. difficult/absent suggests coarctation/shock; easy to feel may be PDA.
  - Assess heart—palpate apex. N.B. Dextrocardia. Is there an active precordium? Any murmur, thrill, or heaves?
  - Any heart failure, e.g. hepatomegaly, basal crackles?
- Abdomen.
  - Assess shape—scaphoid in diaphragmatic hernia and some atresia; distended if obstructed.
  - Any masses, e.g. palpable kidneys, suggest hydronephrosis.
  - Examine genitalia—if ambiguous, consider CAH in girl.
  - Check anus is normally positioned.
- Musculoskeletal.
  - Check limbs, spine, digits.
  - May be associated with abnormalities of other systems and syndromes (cardio-velo-facial, Turner's, Down's, Noonan's, VACTERL, Pierre–Robin).
- Neurological.
  - Assess fontanelle—soft, depressed, or bulging?
  - Note eye movements and assess red reflex (📖 p.342). N.B. White = retinoblastoma; loss of red reflex/hazy = congenital cataracts.
- Finally perform Barlow and Ortolani tests for dislocatable hips—note any clunks/clicks in the hips when manipulated (see 📖 p.326 for technique).

The collapsed neonate

This is one of the most frightening presentations seen in children. The differential diagnosis is wide, but commonly will be due to a duct-dependent heart lesion or sepsis (pp.34, 44). Regardless of aetiology, the initial resuscitation and further management is the same (Fig. 3.1):

- Summon senior assistance.
- ABC ***plus*** **DEFG** (Don't Ever Forget Glucose).
  - Have a low threshold for ventilatory and inotropic support.
  - Exclude neonatal SVT.
  - Perform BP in both arms and, ideally, all 4 limbs.

Remember to keep the baby warm!

- Obtain IV/IO access.

IO access is easy to obtain (p.469). Do not waste precious time with repeated cannulation attempts.

  - Take blood for blood cultures, FBC, CRP, UEC, LFT, venous gas, bedside glucose.
- Give broad-spectrum antibiotics, e.g. IV ampicillin and gentamicin.
- If signs of heart failure, give IV frusemide 1mg/kg. Otherwise resuscitate with saline 20ml/kg.
- Perform CXR.
  - Note if heart is enlarged—cardiac failure.
  - Note if lungs plethoric or oligaemic, i.e. right-sided obstructive cardiac lesion.
- Perform hyperoxia test. Provide highest possible FiO_2, e.g. via headbox, and then obtain arterial gas. Ideally, from right radial artery as pre-ductal.
  - If respiratory pathology, saturations to increase into 90s.
  - If cyanotic heart disease, O_2 saturation will not go above 90% (nor PaO_2 over 90mmHg).
- Correct metabolic abnormalities, particularly sugar and calcium.
- Discuss with PICU/NICU and paediatric cardiologist.
  - Consider Prostin®, 10ng/kg/min.
  - Prostin® infusion: dilute 0.3ml [150mcg]/kg protaglandin E1 with normal saline to make a 150mcg/kg/50ml solution. 1ml/hr = 0.05mcg/kg/min. Increase by 0.05mcg/kg/min up to 0.2mcg/kg/min. If duct completely shut, may need 1mcg/kg/min.

If Prostin® infusion started, elective intubation advised as increased chance of apnoea. Blood pressure support may also be necessary.

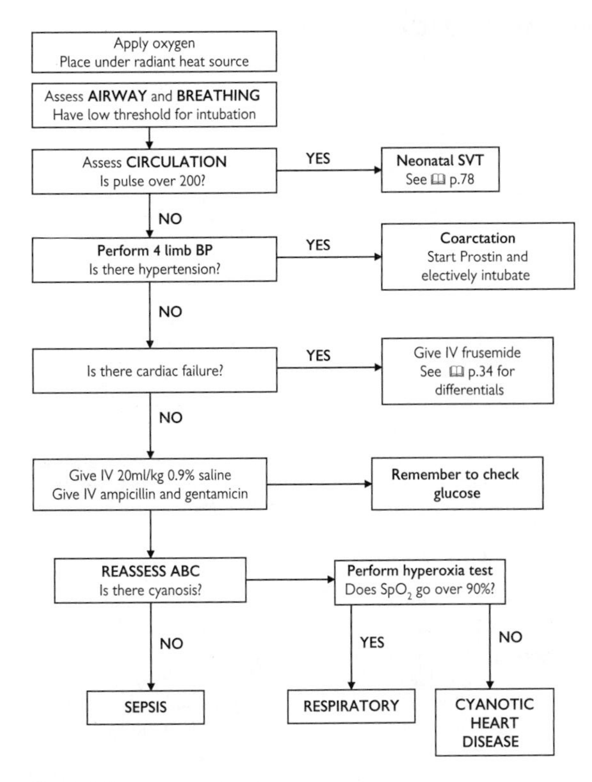

Fig. 3.1 Management of the collapsed neonate.

Neonatal cardiac conditions

The four major presentations are:
- murmur;
- shock;
- heart failure;
- cyanosis.

ⓘ Murmur

Diagnosis is discussed on 📖 p.184. PDA is a common finding in neonates:
- continuous murmur ± thrill under left clavicle, which may be heard throughout the precordium and to the back;
- bounding pulses.

If there is associated respiratory distress, admission is warranted.
- Perform oximetry—if cyanosis, exclude PPHN (📖 p.36).
- Perform CXR looking for failure.
- Discuss fluid restriction with cardiologist.

If a PDA is still present after the first week of life, arrange follow-up with cardiologist as it is a potential endocarditis risk.

Shock Usually secondary to left ventricle outflow tract obstruction, i.e. coarctation of aorta, aortic stenosis, hypoplastic left ventricle. These are all duct-dependent so require Prostin and elective intubation until definitive surgery.

Heart failure The commonest are the conditions causing left ventricular outflow tract obstruction. If there is cyanosis, it could be truncus arteriosus or atrioventricular septal defect. ***Do not forget*** large AV fistula—auscultate the head! Management is covered on 📖 p.182.

Cyanosis The vast majority of congenital cyanotic heart conditions will be diagnosed antenatally or at the postnatal baby check. Cyanosis may evolve after birth (see below). Those marked with an asterisk have duct-dependent pulmonary circulation so the cyanosis may get worse if the hyperoxia test is performed!

Under 2 days of age
- TGA.
- Pulmonary atresia or stenosis* (± VSD).
- Tricuspid atresia*.
- Ebstein's anomaly*.
- Obstructed TAPVD.

Over 2 days of age
- Fallot's tetralogy.
- AV canal defect (common in Down's).
- Truncus arteriosus.
- TAPVD.

To clarify the diagnosis
- Note the distribution of murmur (📖 p.184). N.B. May be quiet if flow diminishing.
- Perform CXR, ECG ± hyperoxia test if diagnosis uncertain.
- Arrange urgent cardiology review.

Persistent pulmonary hypertension

Persistent pulmonary hypertension is a potentially life-threatening cause of cyanosis. Hypoxia and right-to-left shunting compromise ventricular function resulting in cardiovascular collapse.

PPHN may be primary (normal CXR), or secondary to a number of causes, mainly lung pathology.

- Respiratory.
  - Limited lung inflation, e.g. meconium aspiration, hyaline membrane disease.
  - Congenital lung abnormality, e.g. diaphragmatic hernia, cystic lesions, e.g. congenital cystic adenomatoid malformation.
- Other: post-birth asphyxia, anaemia, polycythaemia; sepsis.

Examination

The child will be:

- cyanosed yet little respiratory distress—cyanosis disproportionate to respiratory effort clinches diagnosis;
- normal cardiac examination—occasionally tricuspid regurgitation.

Management

- Summon senior assistance.
- Consider ventilation—obtain senior advice before intubation as a term baby may handle this very badly and spiral out of control. If ventilated, keep PCO_2 to 35–40.
- Keep warm—hypothermia will exacerbate pulmonary vasoconstriction.
- Presume septic—take cultures and start IV antibiotics (📖 p.491).
- Maintain BP—inotropes, e.g. dopamine ± dobutamine often necessary.
- Correct any anaemia, hypoglycaemia (📖 p.29), hypercalcaemia (📖 p.448).
- Arrange urgent cardiology review ± ECHO.
- Admit to NICU.

Apnoea

Babies commonly have **periodic breathing** with pauses of 5–10 seconds between breaths. It becomes an apnoea if the pause in breathing:
- is accompanied by a bradycardia (<100/minute);
- lasts for 20 seconds.

Apnoea does occur in term babies but is most common in premmies—'apnoea of prematurity'. There are two principal causes:
- central hypoventilation;
- obstructive apnoea.

Central hypoventilation

Due to impaired neurological control of breathing. No breathing movement seen.
- Apnoea of prematurity.
- Sepsis, e.g. RSV bronchiolitis.
- Vagal stimulation, e.g. prolonged intubation attempts, pharyngeal suction.
- Nasogastric feeds.
- Gastro-oesophageal reflux (GOR).

Obstructive apnoea

Breathing movements, but no airflow due to upper airway obstruction.
- Choanal atresia, e.g. CHARGE association.
- Macroglossia, e.g. Down's, Beckwith–Wiedemann. N.B. Persistent neonatal hypoglycaemia.
- Micrognathia, e.g. Pierre–Robin sequence.
- Thick neck, e.g. obesity.
- Narrow airway, e.g. tracheomalacia, laryngeal oedema post-extubation.

Infants may have a combination, with initial central apnoea followed by obstruction, e.g. GOR aggravates the laryngeal chemoreceptors causing central apnoea, followed by laryngospasm which is obstructive.

Other factors In addition, there are aggravating factors that are particularly relevant in premature babies.

Perinatal

- Birth asphyxia.
- Birth trauma.
- IVH.

Postnatal

- Metabolic: hypoglycaemia, hypocalcaemia, hyponatraemia, acidosis.
- Thermal: hypo- or hyperthermia.
- Sepsis: any infection; NEC.
- Drugs:
  - maternal opiates, beta-blockers;
  - baby sedatives, narcotics.
- GOR.
- Cardiac insufficiency, e.g. PDA (📖 p.34).

Management

Treatment is aimed at resuscitation, followed by correction of any precipitating or aggravating factors.

- ABC with continuous cardiac monitoring
  - If apnoeic, gentle stimulation may suffice. If not, give oxygen by mask or bag/mask.
  - Ventilation (CPAP or endotracheal) may be required if recurrent apnoea.
- Check electrolytes, glucose, and calcium and correct if necessary (📖 pp.29, 448).
  - Consider need for FBC, blood culture, and IV antibiotics (📖 p.44).
- NPA for RSV and pertussis culture.
- If ill or GOR, stop feeds and start IV fluids.
- If apnoea of prematurity, methyl xanthines are used for babies under 34 weeks gestation.
  - **Caffeine:** 20mg/kg PO/IV; then, after 12 hours, 5mg/kg PO/IV daily. No need to measure levels as a wide therapeutic index.
  - **Theophylline/aminophylline:** 6mg/kg; then, after 12 hours (>1kg baby) or 24 hours (<1 kg), 2.5mg/kg bd. Increase to 3mg/kg after one week and to 4mg/kg in the third week.

Stimulants can be stopped when baby is apnoea-free for a few days or else reaches the equivalent of 34 weeks. Monitor for 48 hours after stopping.

- Admit to NICU or HDU.
- Parents can be reassured that, despite transient episodes of hypoxaemia, there are no neurological sequelae. Moreover, apnoea is not a risk factor for SIDS.

ⓘ Vomiting

All babies bring up milk, so it is important to distinguish posseting from pathological vomiting. Vomiting can be the first manifestation of metabolic illness, e.g. congenital adrenal hyperplasia (📖 p.412), hyperammonaemia (📖 p.452). If vomiting is bilious, then the child has a bowel obstruction until proven otherwise.

The commonest cause of bowel obstruction in the neonatal period is Hirschsprung's, but gut atresias and inguinal herniae also need to be excluded. Obstructed bowel swiftly becomes ischaemic, putting the baby at risk of overwhelming Gram-negative sepsis. Early involvement of surgeons is mandatory.

History

- Is the child vomiting milk? Are any vomits green?
  - Milk vomits + child under 6 weeks of age; consider pyloric stenosis.
  - Bilious vomits + child under 2 days of age = atresia, Hirschsprung's.
  - Bilious vomits + child under 6 weeks of age = malrotation.
- How frequently is the child feeding?
  - Babies with pyloric stenosis remain desperate to feed.
  - If the child is bottle fed, check that they are not receiving over 150ml/kg/day.
- Has the baby ever fed normally?
- What colour are the stools?
  - Breast fed = bright yellow; inadequate intake = green.
  - Bloody diarrhoea—exclude NEC, haemorrhagic disease of newborn.
- Is there any difficulty in passing stool?
  - Constipation is common in bottle fed babies.
  - Those with Hirschsprung's pass explosive stools intermittently. Occasionally, the stool can be ribbon-like.
- Was meconium passed within the first 24 hours of life?
  - A delay is suggestive of Hirschsprung's.
- Does the abdomen appear bigger than usual?
- Check risk factors for sepsis, especially UTI.

Examination

- Assess ABC—if shock, start resuscitation.
- Assess hydration (📖 p.239).
- Is the child febrile?
- Is the abdomen distended (obstruction) or scaphoid (atresia)?
  - If distended, check hernial orifices.
- Auscultate for bowel sounds.
- Is the anus in the normal position?
  - If abdomen distended, insert rectal thermometer—a gush of flatus and poo suggests Hirschsprung's.
- Are the genitalia normal? Exclude CAH (📖 p.412).

Investigation

- Abdominal x-ray (AXR)—should see air in stomach and down to rectum.
  - Obstruction or atresia will cause fluid levels. If malrotation, the dilated bowel will not cross the midline.
  - Perforation will result in free air, under diaphragm or in portal system (black lines 'behind' the liver). If uncertain, perform lateral decubitus AXR.
- Perform UEC, glucose.
  - If child tachypnoeic but not acidotic, think ammonia (📖 p.452)
  - If metabolic alkalosis with low sodium and potassium, CAH distinguished from pyloric stenosis by hypoglycaemia (📖 p.412).
- If bowel obstruction, perform FBC, cross-match, blood cultures, CRP.
- If diagnosis still uncertain, check urine via SPA to immediately exclude UTI.

Management

Pyloric stenosis (see 📖 p.276).

UTI (see 📖 p.254)

If obstruction confirmed:

- resuscitate as necessary;
- keep NBM. Insert largest NGT possible and place on free drainage;
- rehydration is with N/2 +2.5% dextrose—neonates will require glucose supplementation up to 10% dextrose (📖 p.506);
  - in addition, replace NG losses ml for ml with 0.9% saline;
- start broad spectrum antibiotics, e.g. 3rd generation cephalosporin ***plus*** gentamicin ***plus*** metronidazole;
- request urgent surgical review.

Necrotizing enterocolitis

Usually affects premature or ill newborns. But can arise at any time in the first 8 weeks after birth.

Classical symptoms of feed intolerance with vomiting, which may be bile-stained, with bloody diarrhoea. The abdomen will be tender and distended. Signs of shock with peritonism = bowel perforation.

- On AXR look for:
  - dilated bowel loops ± free air. Look in flanks if baby prone;
  - air in portal system (black lines 'behind' the liver);
  - pneumotosis coli—bubbles of gas within the bowel wall.
- Manage as for bowel obstruction.
- Intravenous analgesia likely to be needed.
- TPN will be required—request assistance before attempting long line insertion.
- Consider repeating AXR if any deterioration.

Hirschsprung's disease Congenital aganglionosis of the colon. Commonest cause of bowel obstruction in the neonate. Usually has delayed passage of meconium and then passes stools infrequently. Stools are usually loose and explosive, but may be thin and ribbon-like. AXR may not show gas in the rectum. Diagnosis is confirmed by rectal biopsy.

ⓘ Jaundice

Unconjugated hyperbilirubinaemia is common in the first few days of life. The breakdown of fetal haemoglobin overwhelms the neonate's liver, which may be further compromised by dehydration before feeding is established; or bruising from a traumatic delivery. Investigation is necessary to exclude haemolysis—ABO incompatibility is the commonest cause in the UK.

Kernicterus (📖 p.28) can result if unconjugated levels get too high, but the level at which intervention is necessary depends on the baby's gestation and postnatal age. For example, term infants can tolerate levels up to 300μmol/l at day 1 of life, whereas premmies require intervention at far lower levels.

Unconjugated hyperbilirubinaemia that persists beyond 14 days of age in the term infant and 21 days in the premmie also warrants investigation. Such prolonged jaundice may be due to UTI, hypothyroidism, and galactosaemia.

Conjugated hyperbilirubinaemia is always pathological and may reflect metabolic liver disease, e.g. cystic fibrosis, organic acidosis, or congenital infection. It is also important to exclude post-hepatic obstruction so ask whether the baby's poo has changed colour.

History

- Ask when baby first appeared jaundiced—unconjugated day 1 = haemolysis, sepsis.
- If possible, obtain mother's antenatal health card. Check her blood group and hepatitis B and C status.
- Ask whether family history of jaundice, e.g. Crigler–Najjar, or whether anyone in the family has had a splenectomy—spherocytosis.
- Ask about family's ethnic background—G6PD prevalent amongst those from Mediterranean, West Africa, Middle East, and South-east Asia.

Examination

- ABC—the jaundiced neonate may be septic (📖 p.44).
- Skin colour—unconjugated jaundice is lemon yellow; conjugated jaundice is nearer green.
  - If unconjugated confirmed, check for signs of trauma, e.g. bruising, caput post-suction extraction.
- Assess for hepatomegaly—congenital infections, *E. coli* UTI, post-hepatic obstruction.
- Look in nappy—obstructive jaundice causes white poo and dark urine.

Investigations and management are covered in Table 3.2.

- If not provided by the lab, the unconjugated bilirubin level is total bilirubin ***minus*** conjugated fraction.
- Galactosaemia is a congenital deficiency of galactose-1-phosphate-uridyltransferase (Gal-1-P-UT) that will rapidly progress to liver failure unless a lactose-free diet is started.

Table 3.2 Investigation and management of neonatal jaundice

	Investigations	Interpretation	Management
Unconjugated			
Neonatal	• Total and unconjugated bilirubin		Plot on phototherapy chart If above the line, refer to NICU for phototherapy
	• FBC, blood group and Coombs' test	Coombs' +ve = IgG-mediated haemolysis e.g. ABO or rhesus incompatibility	
	plus if family history suggestive:	Crigler–Najjar (📖 p.244)	
	• Blood film	Spherocytosis	
	• G6PD screen		
Prolonged	• Total and conjugated bilirubin		
	• TSH, T4	Hypothyroidism	Needs urgent thyroxine supplemen-tation. Discuss with endocrinology
	• Bag urine for urine-reducing sugars	Galactosaemia	If positive, admit under gastroenterology and measure Gal-1-P-UT
	• Urine for culture	UTI (📖 p.254)	
Conjugated	• Total and conjugated bilirubin, LFTs, TORCH serology	Congenital hepatitis	Admit under gastro-enterology for further investigation
	• IRT if under 4 days of age	Cystic fibrosis	
	• Urinary metabolic screen	Amino or organic acidoses	
	• Liver ultrasound	Choledochal cyst Biliary atresia, Alagille's (📖 p.247)	

Sepsis

Commoner in small or premature babies, or those with other medical problems. Higher risk if maternal fever antenatally or prolonged rupture of membranes. Most septic babies will present within the first week of life, but some perinatally acquired infections can present up to 3 months of age, e.g. group B streptococcus, listeria.

In neonates, the manifestations of sepsis are non-specific, so have a low threshold of suspicion:

- poor feeding, vomiting, or abdominal distension;
- temperature—high or low, with poor perfusion;
- apnoea, bradycardia;
- tachypnoea with desaturations;
- floppy, lethargic;
- abnormal movements, seizures;
- skin—blue, grey, or pale or persistent jaundice. Rarely, petechiae or purpura.

Investigations

- FBC, CRP—raised inflammatory markers with neutrophilia or leucopenia or thrombocytopenia.
- Glucose.
- Culture—blood, urine, CSF.
  - LP may be deferred if baby too unstable. PCR can be performed on CSF to aid bacterial identification post-antibiotics.
- CXR ± AXR if at risk of NEC (📖 p.41).

Management

- ABC. If abnormal, resuscitate—oxygen, IV bolus 20ml/kg 0.9% saline.
- Correct any hypoglycaemia and start maintenance fluids with 10% dextrose.
- IV gentamicin and 3rd generation cephalosporin.
- Add ampicillin if concerned about listeria (meconium-stained liquor).
- Consider acyclovir if delivered vaginally and mother has history of herpes infection.

Seizures

Babies tolerate fits remarkably well and most will not suffer any long-term sequelae. However, that is dependent on the primary cause, so no guesses at long-term prognosis should be made. The development of an encephalopathy is a poor prognostic indicator. This often follows hypoxic insult, sepsis/meningitis, metabolic derangement, or intracranial bleed.

Causes

- Post-hypoxia: hypoxic–ischaemic encephalopathy.
- Meningitis.
- Metabolic:
  - hypoglycaemia;
  - hypocalcaemia;
  - inborn errors of metabolism.
- Intracranial bleed.
- Structural brain lesions.
- Neonatal abstinence syndrome.

Management

- Apply facial oxygen.
- ABC. Consider elective intubation if recurrent apnoeas or bradycardias.
- IV access— FBC, EUC, glucose, calcium, and phosphate; blood cultures even if afebrile. Check pyridoxine if baby under 48 hours of age.
- Give IV phenobarbitone.
- Give IV antibiotics until cultures known to be negative. CSF can be obtained when baby is stable and sent for PCR for bacterial antigens.

Neonatal abstinence syndrome

The baby can present with seizures and be febrile so may also resemble neonatal sepsis (📖 p.44). Other clinical features include:

- restless, e.g. sucking fists yet unwilling to feed, insomnia;
- autonomic hyperactivity—sweating, snuffly, tachycardic, hypertensive, vomiting ± diarrhoea.

Management

If fitting, manage as above ***plus***:

- give IV morphine 0.1mg/kg;
- obtain neonatal abstinence assessment forms from NICU;
- monitor pulse, temperature, and alertness to determine need for further opiates.

Hypoxic–ischaemic encephalopathy (HIE)

Any cause of perinatal ischaemia may result in hypoxia within the brain and may lead to HIE. The severity defines the long-term outcome.

Grade 1 Irritable, with poor suck and abnormal tone (floppy or stiff). Hyperalert and staring eyes. 95% normal at follow-up.

Grade 2 Lethargic, hypotonic. 70% have seizures. NG feeds required.

Grade 3 Hypertonic with seizures and reduced level of consciousness, requiring respiratory support. 20% normal at follow-up, but 50% die in neonatal period.

Intracranial bleed

Commoner in premature and low birth weight babies. Most bleeds are asymptomatic—a significant number of normal babies will be found to have intracranial blood if a cranial USS is performed. But some bleeds are associated with poor feeding, irritability, or seizures.

The long-term outlook is dependent on the degree of bleeding. Large intraventricular bleeds can extend into white matter, and compression from the subsequent clot results in venous thrombosis, leading to parenchymal damage.

Chapter 4

Resuscitation

The arrest protocols in this book are reproduced with permission from the UK APLS guidelines 2005. There may be differences between countries; and modifications introduced over time. Readers are advised to follow the current protocol applicable in their own country, and update the ones in this book accordingly.

Cardiopulmonary assessment of a seriously ill child

Cardiopulmonary arrest is a rare event in hospital (1 per 5000 paediatric admissions). Typically, cardiac arrest is the result of protracted hypoxia, impairing myocardial function. Whereas an isolated respiratory arrest is associated with a survival rate of 80%, the outcome for cardiac arrest is poor, particularly if the arrest occurs outside of hospital.

Thus, it is important that clinical signs that may herald an arrest are recognized early. Rapid intervention may limit respiratory and, ultimately, cardiac compromise.

Children with any of the following features warrant urgent medical review:
- threatened airway obstruction;
- tachypnoea or hypopnoea (Table 4.1);
- bradycardia or tachycardia (Table 4.2);
- hypotension (Table 4.3);
- altered mental state or convulsion;
- low pulse oximetry values: <92% in any oxygen (<60% if cyanotic heart disease).

Assessment

Cardiopulmonary assessment should take less than 1 minute. If intervention is necessary, summon help; then restart ABC assessment to review any effect.

Do not proceed from A to B, until satisfied that the airway is safe. Do not proceed from B to C until there is adequate spontaneous or supported ventilation.

Airway
- **Is it patent?**
  - Look for obstruction, e.g. vomit, swelling. Remove any foreign matter, under direct vision.
  - Listen for stridor, wheeze, hoarse cry.
- If the airway is maintained adequately, leave well alone.
- If there is compromise, summon assistance and start ***basic life support*** (BLS) (📖 p.52).

Breathing
- **What is the skin colour?** Are the lips/tongue pink or blue?
- **What is the effort and work of breathing?** Is there recession, nasal flaring, grunting, use of accessory muscles, stridor, or wheeze?
- **What is the respiratory rate?** Fast or inappropriately slow, suggesting impending respiratory collapse? (see Table 4.1).
- **Assess air entry.** If there is compromise, apply oxygen and summon assistance. Consider airway manoeuvres and ventilatory assistance as described in BLS (📖 p.52).

Circulation
- **Feel for pulse. What is the heart rate** (see Table 4.2)?
  - Carotid or femoral pulse in child.
  - Brachial or femoral pulse in infant/baby.

- **What is the central systemic perfusion?**
  - Check capillary refill. Press on sternum for 5 seconds, colour should return in <2 seconds.
  - Other indices include pulse volume, level of consciousness, urine output, and skin temperature.
  - N.B. Toe-core gap—more than 2°C difference between skin and central temperature suggests reduced perfusion.
- **What is the blood pressure?** ***Low BP is a late and ominous sign*** (see Table 4.3).

If there is compromise, apply oxygen and summon assistance. Obtain IV/IO access and give bolus of 10–20ml/kg 0.9% saline and review effect.

If pulse rate is <60 and patient is unresponsive, start CPR (📖 p.52).

Disability

- **What is the level of consciousness?** GCS can be used but AVPU is easiest, i.e.
  - **A**lert;
  - responsive to **V**oice;
  - responsive to **P**ain;
  - **U**nresponsive.
- **Assess pupillary response**. What is their size and reaction to light? If only responsive to pain (GCS < 8), intubate (📖 p.474) Remember to assess reflexes before muscle relaxant given.

Table 4.1 Respiratory rates by age

Age (years)	Respiratory rate (breaths/minute)
Under 1	30–40
1 to 2	25–35
2 to 5	25–30
5 to 12	20–25
Above 12	15–20

Table 4.2 Heart rate by age

Age (years)	Heart rate (beats/minute)
Under 1	110–160
1 to 2	100–150
2 to 5	95–140
5 to 12	80–120
Above 12 years	60–100

Table 4.3 Blood pressure by age

Age (years)	Systolic pressure (mmHg)	Hypertension
Under 1	70–90	115/75
1 to 2	80–95	115/75
2 to 5	80–100	115/75
5 to 12	90–110	125/80
Above 12 years	100–120	135/85

Basic life support (BLS)

In the event of an arrest, whether respiratory or cardiac, basic life support must be started (Fig. 4.1). Good technique will limit the effects of hypoxia, so this protocol is described in detail.

For the purposes of BLS, an infant is <1 year of age, and a child is 1 year to puberty.

Use SAFE approach: Check for hazards, e.g. ensure rescuers will not be electrocuted.

- **S**hout for help;
- **A**pproach with caution;
- **F**ree from danger;
- **E**valuate ABC.

Check for response; call for help Try to get a response from the patient. Call out to them as you approach, then place one hand gently on the patient's head to stabilize it while gently tapping them with your other hand and calling to them. If the patient does not respond, shout loudly for help, remembering to state your location. Use the emergency call bell. Proceed with the resuscitation while waiting for assistance.

Assess airway

- Inspect. Look in the mouth and nose for anything that may cause a blockage, and remove what you can reach. ***Never*** prod blindly in the airway with a finger or with suction—you may push the object further down the respiratory tract.
- Open airway. Place one hand on the patient's forehead and the finger-tips of your other hand under their chin. Gently tilt the head and at the same time raise the patient's chin to lift the floppy tongue upwards, away from the posterior pharynx. Chin-lift is the more important aspect of this manoeuvre. As the patient's age increases, greater head-tilt is required to open the airway.
  - Infants—neutral position.
  - Small child—sniffing.
  - Bigger child—gargling.

Assess breathing While holding the patient's airway in their open position, take up to 10 seconds to assess for breathing by looking, listening, and feeling. If the patient is not breathing effectively then they require immediate assistance with ventilation.

When assistance arrives, tell them to summon the paediatric emergency team, to state your location, and to return to help immediately.

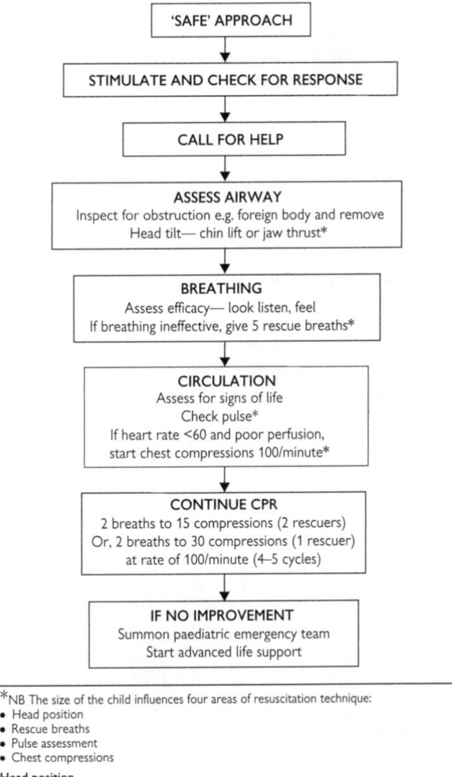

*NB The size of the child influences four areas of resuscitation technique:
- Head position
- Rescue breaths
- Pulse assessment
- Chest compressions

Head position
Infants—neutral
Small child—sniffing
Bigger child—gargling

Rescue breaths
Five breaths. Watch for chest movement
Infant: Mouth over mouth and nose
Child: Mouth to mouth

Pulse assessment
Infant: at the brachial or femoral artery
Child: at the carotid or femoral artery

Chest compressions
Infant: use two fingers a finger's breadth above xiphisternum. Alternatively, if you have an assistant providing ventilatory support, use both hands to encircle the chest and compress with thumbs.
Child: 1–2 hands positioned a finger's breadth above xiphisternum

Fig. 4.1 Basic life support algorithm, (adapted with permission from Advanced Life Support Group (2005). *Advanced paediatric life support—the practical approach*, 4th edn, BMJ Publishing Group, London).

Give 5 rescue breaths

- Ideally, use a paediatric or adult pocket mask with one-way valve to protect yourself and the patient from infection. If not available, start mouth-to-mouth ventilation. N.B. Under 1 year, mouth-to-mouth-and-nose is necessary.
- Attach the mask to oxygen if available.
- Use both your thumbs and index fingers to press the mask firmly down to form a good seal over the patient's mouth and nose.
- Use your remaining fingers to position the patient's airway in their open airway position.
- Breathe into the valve slowly and gently, over 1–1.5 seconds, and watch for chest movement. Aim to make the chest rise like a normal breath, and avoid over-inflating. Give five rescue breaths.
- If the chest does not rise, then it is most likely that the airway is not in an open position. Reposition the head between each attempt, and consider a jaw-thrust manoeuvre. Also check mouth and nose again to exclude foreign body airway obstruction. Remove any foreign material that you can easily reach.
- If all 5 attempts to make the chest rise are ineffective, then treat for presumed foreign body airway obstruction (📖 p.58).

After delivering rescue breaths proceed to circulation.

Assess circulation Take up to 10 seconds to assess adequacy of circulation.

- All ages—look for any signs of life (breathing, moving, swallowing).
- Infants—feel for a brachial or femoral pulse.
- Children—feel for a carotid or femoral pulse.

If there are signs of circulation, then treat as respiratory arrest (📖 p.56).

If you are unsure about the presence of a pulse and the patient has no signs of life, commence chest compressions. Any child with a pulse of less than 60 beats per minute and no signs of life should receive chest compressions.

Give chest compressions

- Give 15 compressions at the rate of 100/minute.
- The chest should be compressed to one-third of its depth.
- The compression and relaxation phases should be of equal duration.
- Chest compression technique depends on the size of the child.

Infant The single rescuer uses the tips of 2 fingers to compress the chest one finger-width above the xiphisternum. If an assistant is available to provide ventilatory support, the hand-encircling technique is preferable: place tips of thumbs on the sternum. Slide the fingers of both hands under the infant's back to provide a firm surface against which to compress the sternum with the thumb tips.

Child Identify the xiphoid process and place the heel of one hand a finger-width above it. The rescuer should position themselves such that their shoulder is directly above their hand when their arm is straight, so that their body weight can be used to help compress the chest. If the chest cannot be effectively depressed using one hand then the rescuer should place their second hand on top of the first, interlocking fingers, both arms straight, and perform two-handed compressions.

Continue CPR

- Continue with the resuscitation at a ratio of 2 breaths to 15 compressions for a minute at a rate of 100/minute; that is 4–5 cycles/minute. (If single rescuer, the ratio is 2 to 30).
- After a minute of CPR, ensure that help is on its way, and then continue with the resuscitation until further assistance is available.

When assistance is available, the priorities are:

- ensure that the paediatric emergency team has been called;
- optimize oxygen intake using a bag and mask with reservoir;
- for infants, change the method of chest compressions to hand encircling technique as soon as an assistant is available to do so;
- attach monitor and determine rhythm;
- initiate appropriate treatment protocol (see 'Advanced life support' 📖 p.64).

Management of respiratory arrest

- Provide breaths for the patient using bag-mask ventilation ± oropharyngeal (Guedel) airway, with high concentration oxygen.

There is no necessity to intubate—adequate ventilation can be achieved with good quality bag-mask ventilation

- Ventilate at 12–20 breaths/min, aiming to make the chest rise as in a normal inspiration.
- Avoid over-inflating the chest.
- After one minute, reassess ABC.
- Ensure that assistance is on the way.
- Proceed with resuscitation as required.

The choking child

The algorithm to follow depends on whether the child is conscious. If the child becomes unconscious after a witnessed choking episode, start basic life support (Fig. 4.1), ***regardless*** of whether the foreign body has been removed.

Conscious child

After SAFE approach, ask patient whether they are choking—they may be aphonic. Encourage patient to cough. If patient is unable to vocalize or is no longer able to cough effectively, then proceed with algorithm (Fig. 4.2).

Airway Inspect airway: if there is anything in the mouth or in the nose that you can easily remove, then do so. ***Never*** prod blindly in the airway with a finger or with suction—you may push the foreign body further in. If nothing can be safely removed, then proceed.

Back blows

Infant Place one hand under the infant's chin to support their head and airway. Position them safely along your arm or over your knee, face downward, with their head lower than their bottom.

Using the heel of one hand apply a sharp blow between their scapulae.

Child Lean the patient forward over your extended arm so that their head is lower than their chest. Tell the patient what you are going to do before using the heel of one hand to apply a sharp blow between their scapulae.

Check whether this manoeuvre has dislodged the obstruction before repeating the back blows up to five times as necessary.

> If back blows are unsuccessful and the airway remains obstructed, ensure that assistance is on the way before proceeding to thrusts.

Thrusts

Infant Perform chest thrusts.
- Support the patient's head and turn them face upwards.
- Place two fingers on the infant's chest, as for chest compressions.
- Press slowly and deliberately on the chest to mimic its movement as when the infant coughs.
- Check whether this manoeuvre has been effective in relieving the obstruction. If not, repeat up to five times as necessary.

Child Perform abdominal thrusts.
- Tell the patient what you are going to do.
- Kneel behind the small child or stand behind the bigger child.

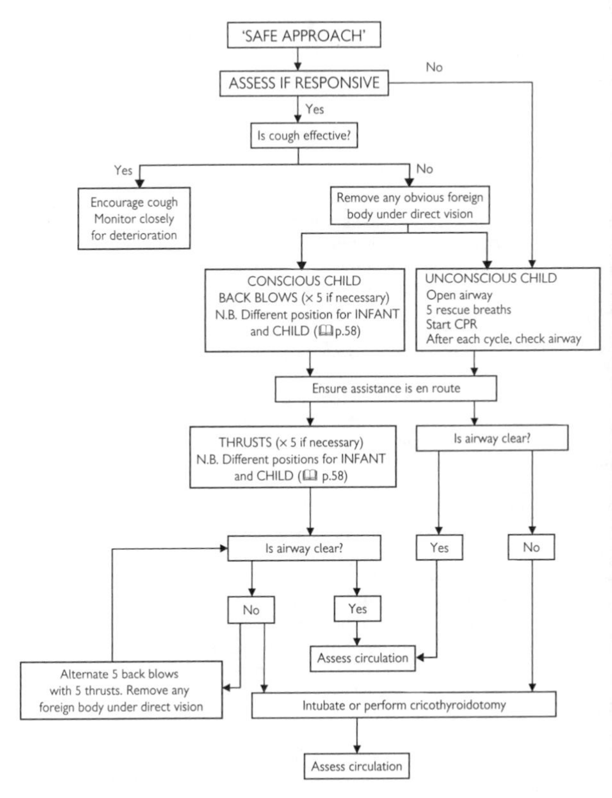

Fig. 4.2 Management of choking, (adapted with permission from Advanced Life Support Group (2005). *Advanced paediatric life support—the practical approach*, 4th edn, BMJ Publishing Group, London).

- Place your fist just above their umbilicus; then place your other hand over your fist.
- Stabilize yourself against the patient's back before pulling your fist inwards and upwards under the patient's diaphragm to mimic its action during a cough.
- Check whether this manoeuvre has been effective before repeating the abdominal thrusts up to five times as necessary.

Continue procedure While the patient remains obstructed but conscious:

- infant—alternate 5 back blows with 5 chest thrusts;
- child—alternate 5 back blows with 5 abdominal thrusts.

If the patient loses consciousness, then ensure that assistance has been called and proceed to the next section, 'Unconscious child'.

Unconscious child

Once the patient loses consciousness after a choking episode, basic life support is initiated, even if the foreign body is still *in situ*.

- Inspect airway. Look in the mouth and nose for anything that may cause a blockage, and remove what you can see. Do not prod blindly in the airway with a finger or with suction.
- Open airway: head-tilt chin-lift.
- Assess breathing.
- Attempt rescue breaths: try to deliver 5 rescue breaths; reposition the head between each attempt as necessary.

If successful, proceed with assessment of circulation and proceed with basic life support as necessary.

If the rescue breaths are unsuccessful, then proceed with basic life support by delivering chest compressions at the rate of 100/minute.

- After each cycle of compressions, look in the patient's mouth to see if the compressions have been effective in moving the obstruction. One attempt may be made to retrieve object if possible.
- Ensure assistance is summoned: paediatric emergency team/ENT surgeon/anaesthetist.
- Advanced life support interventions will include:
  - direct visualization with laryngoscope and removal with Magill's forceps or suction.
  - ventilatory management with bag and mask to displace object into one bronchus.
  - attempt intubation and ventilation (📖 p.474).
  - emergency needle cricothyroidotomy while preparing for urgent bronchoscopy (📖 p.476).
  - emergency tracheotomy only in children over 12 years.

Anaphylaxis

Allergens may be inhaled or ingested. The reaction may rapidly become life-threatening with the development of severe bronchospasm, complicated by laryngeal oedema and circulatory shock secondary to acute vasodilatation and increased capillary permeability.

N.B. If the allergen has been ingested, urticaria is less prominent and GI manifestations such as profuse vomiting and diarrhoea may precede peripheral signs of angioedema.

Assessment Perform rapid cardiopulmonary assessment—ABC. Any compromise necessitates admission as reactions can be biphasic with a delayed deterioration.

Airway

- Look for signs of obstruction, e.g. swelling, vomit.
- Listen for airway compromise, e.g. stridor, wheeze.
- If stridor present:
  - give adrenaline (epinephrine) 10mcg/kg IM;
  - apply oxygen;
  - summon anaesthetist ± ENT. If intubation is necessary, expertise will be required;
  - Consider nebulized adrenaline 3–5mg (3–5ml 1 in 1000).

Breathing

- Is respiratory rate normal for age?
- Assess respiratory effort, i.e. nasal flaring, intercostal recession, head bobbing.
- Assess for hypoxia—colour, level of consciousness.
- Auscultate for wheeze, stridor.

If respiratory compromise:

- give IM adrenaline and apply oxygen if you have not already done so.
- if stridulous, in addition give nebulized adrenaline with oxygen (rapid effect), ± nebulized steroids (delayed effect).
- summon anaesthetist ± ENT. If intubation is necessary, expertise will be required.
- consider nebulized salbutamol 2.5–5mg for wheeze and IV hydrocortisone 1mg/kg. Chlorpheniramine may help itch but has no acute benefit.
- if wheeze is persistent, infusions of salbutamol or aminophylline may be necessary.
- provide bag/mask ventilation if required.
- start continuous cardiac monitoring.

Circulation

- Is pulse character normal and rate appropriate?
- Compare central and peripheral perfusion.
- Check BP (preserved until late).

If circulatory compromise:
- manage as for respiratory compromise;
- give IV 0.9% saline 20ml/kg bolus and review ABC;
- if in shock, intubate and continue IM adrenaline every 5 minutes with boluses of fluid;
- if no improvement after 40ml/kg of fluid, give IV adrenaline 10mcg/kg and start advanced life support (📖 p.64);
- arrange PICU admission.

Table 4.4 lists drugs used in treating anaphylaxis.

Table 4.4 Drugs used in treatment of anaphylaxis

Drug	Route	Dose	Notes
Adrenaline* (1:1000 solution)	IM	10mcg/kg or: <6 months: 50mcg (0.05ml) 6 months–6yrs: 120mcg (0.12ml) 6–12yrs: 250mcg (0.25ml) >12yrs: 500mcg (0.5ml)	IM Adrenaline can be repeated after 5 minutes if required
	Nebulized	3–5mg 3–5ml of 1:1000 solution with O_2 at 10–15l/min	Treatment of stridor
Adrenaline* (1:10 000 solution)	IV or IO	10mcg/kg	*Only* for treatment of cardiopulmonary arrest secondary to anaphylaxis
Chlorpheniramine	IV	1–6yrs: 2.5–5mg 6–12yrs: 5–10mg >12yrs: 10–20mg	IM absorption similar to oral
Hydrocortisone	IM or slow IV	1–6yrs: 50mg 6–12yrs: 100mg >12yrs: 100–500mg	For all severe or recurrent reactions or if wheezy
Salbutamol	Nebulized	1.25–5mg	Treatment of bronchospasm
0.9% saline	IV or IO	20ml/kg	Treatment of shock

* Also called epinephrine.

Advanced life support (ALS)

When basic life support is not expediting recovery, continue CPR but proceed to advanced life support. (Fig. 4.3).

- It is prudent to write down the size of equipment and doses that may be required (Table 4.5).
- Nominate a resuscitation leader to coordinate efforts.

ALS follows the ABC principle.

- Airway and breathing—optimize ventilation and oxygenation.
- Circulation—check for arrhythmia.
- If problems arise, review ABC. There are 8 causes of arrest that are reversible ('4Hs and 4Ts')—if any are found, they must be treated before proceeding (see Table 4.6).
- The effect of any intervention necessitates review of ABC.
- Attach monitors if you have not already done so and note time.

Table 4.5 Resuscitation formulae and drug doses.

	Formula or dose	Notes
Estimation of weight	Newborn = 3.5kg; 6 months = 7.0kg, 1 year = 10kg Aged 1–10 years: Weight in kg = (Age in years + 4) x 2	
Endotracheal tube:	Size = 4 + (age in years ÷ 4) Length in cm for oral tube = 12 + (age in years ÷ 2) cm Length in cm for nasal tube = 15 + (age in years ÷ 2) cm	
DC shock	4J/kg	
Bolus of fluids	20ml/kg 0.9% saline	Give warmed unless contraindicated
Adrenaline*	0.1ml/kg 1 in 10 000 (10mcg/kg)	
10% dextrose	5ml/kg	
Amiodarone	5mg/kg	Flush line with 5% dextrose
Atropine	20mcg/kg	Minimum dose 100mcg, maximum single 600mcg
10% calcium chloride	0.2ml/kg	
Lignocaine	1mg/kg	
Sodium bicarbonate 8.4% (1mmol/ml)	1mmol/kg	Dilute to 4.2% for infants, OR if administered via peripheral line

* Also called epinephrine.

Table 4.6 Reversible causes of arrest

Hypoxia	Tension pneumothorax
Hypovolaemia	Tamponade
Hypothermia	Toxic/therapeutic disturbance
Hyper/hypokalaemia, hypocalcaemia (metabolic)	Thromboembolic

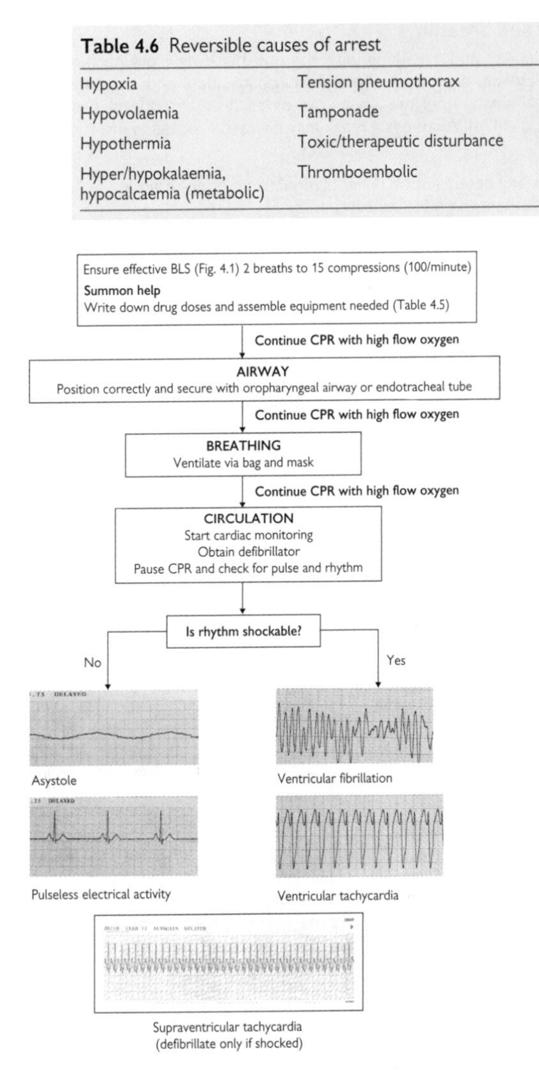

Fig. 4.3 Advanced life support, (adapted with permission from Advanced Life Support Group (2005). *Advanced paediatric life support—the practical approach*, 4th edn, BMJ Publishing Group, London).

Airway and breathing

Manage airway and breathing with bag and mask device with high-flow oxygen. Ensure oropharnyx free from obstruction and consider oro-pharyngeal airway until the airway can be secured by endotracheal intubation (📖 p.474). A laryngeal mask may be used if skilled in insertion.

Troubleshoot

If there is any deterioration in ventilation, remember DOPES.

- **D**isplacement of endotracheal tube.
- **O**bstruction of endotracheal tube or upper airway.
- **P**neumothorax.
- **E**quipment failure, e.g. oxygen not attached, not plugged in.
- **S**plinting of diaphragm by air—insert NG tube.

Circulation

- Establish cardiac monitoring.
- Pause compressions to check rhythm and feel for pulse.
- Determine whether defibrillation is necessary—VF or pulseless VT are shockable. Most arrests will be asystolic (📖 p.70).
- Obtain vascular access, whether by IV or IO (📖 p.469), so that fluids and medications can be given.
- If time permits, take bloods for glucose, FBC, UEC, blood cultures ± clotting studies and insert second line.

Troubleshoot

Vascular access lost If vascular access is lost during resuscitation, certain drugs can be given via the endotracheal tube:

- **A**drenaline 100mcg/kg (0.1ml/kg of 1 in 1000 adrenaline);
- **L**ignocaine 2mg/kg;
- **A**tropine 40mcg/kg;
- **N**aloxone.

N.B. This method is suboptimal and vascular access must be restored as soon as possible.

Hypoglycaemia If fingerprick glucose is under 4mmol/l, treat with 5ml/kg of 10% dextrose.

Drugs

Before giving any medication, ensure that it is compatible with the means of vascular access and the fluids running through it, e.g. amiodarone is not compatible with saline, so flush line before and after administration with 5% dextrose.

During resuscitation, ensure that one member of staff records all drugs used, the dose, route of administration, and time drug given.

Troubleshoot

Circulatory collapse If no response to the initial dose of adrenaline and there is dilated circulation (warm shock 📖 p.92), discuss the use of a vasopressor agent with senior doctor/PICU.

Persisting arrhythmia

1. Consider anti-arrhythmics.
   - Amiodarone used most often, but is contraindicated in long QT syndrome where lignocaine should be used.
   - Atropine is not routinely used, but should be considered if there is a suspicion of vagal overactivity, e.g. post-intubation bradycardia. Atropine is also used when there is bradycardia resistant to adrenaline and oxygen. IV atropine: 20mcg/kg (minimum, 100mcg; maximum, 600mcg).

2. Consider alkalizing agents. If serum pH < 7, adrenaline's efficacy is reduced. Thus, if no response to CPR and documented acidosis, try sodium bicarbonate 8.4% 1mmol/kg.

N.B. In infants or if via peripheral IV, must be diluted to 4.2% ***and*** flush line thoroughly before and after administration.

Rhythm disturbances: introduction

- Confirm effective basic life support is being provided with high concentration oxygen.
- Summon further assistance.
- Attach monitor and note the time.
- Pause chest compressions; then palpate for a central pulse and look for any signs of life. Confirm the rhythm (Fig. 4.3) as either:
  - shockable: ventricular fibrillation (VF)/pulseless ventricular tachycardia (VT); supraventricular tachycardia (SVT) with collapse, shock;
  - non-shockable: asystole/pulseless electrical activity (PEA); supraventricular tachycardia (if not in shock).

If it is a shockable rhythm, familiarize yourself with defibrillator technique (📖 p.72).

Asystole and pulseless electrical activity

60% of paediatric arrests are asystolic, secondary to hypoxia ± acidosis. Confirm rhythm whilst continuing CPR with high flow oxygen. If asystole is shown on the monitor, confirm on other leads in case the lead has become dislodged.

See protocol (Fig. 4.4).

Deliver CPR in 2 minute cycles. A new rescuer should take over delivery of chest compressions each cycle or sooner as necessary to ensure consistently effective compressions.

- Give adrenaline (epinephrine) as soon as vascular access is available, whether IV or IO. Adrenaline must be followed by a generous flush of 0.9% saline.
  - 10mcg/kg is 0.1ml/kg of 1:10 000 solution.
- Give adrenaline every 3–5 minutes. Reassess rhythm and pulse after every cycle and respond.
- If in PEA, give a fluid bolus of 20ml/kg 0.9% saline. Give warmed fluids unless contraindicated.

During the resuscitation do as follows.

- Intubate as soon as possible, then provide continuous chest compressions at 100/min with asynchronous ventilation.
- Secure additional vascular access and obtain blood for analysis (Glucose, UEC, FBC, culture, cross-match, ± clotting).
- Obtain patient history.
- Consider and treat any reversible causes (4Hs and 4Ts).
  - Treat glucose <4mmol/l with 5ml/kg 10% dextrose.

Checklist
- Intubate as soon as possible
- Secure vascular access (IV/IO)
- Take bloods
- Obtain fingerprick glucose
- Obtain history

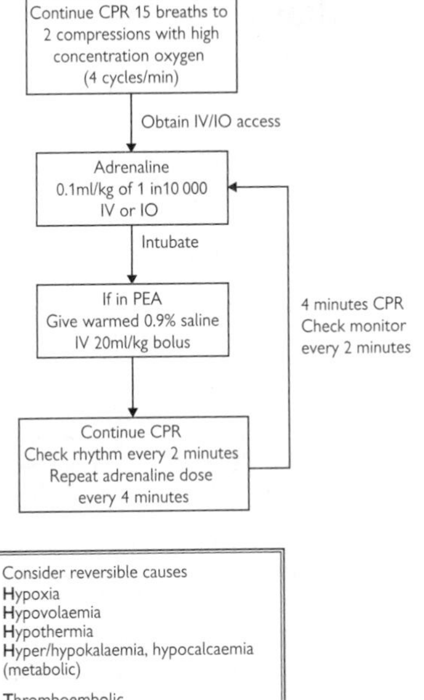

Consider reversible causes
Hypoxia
Hypovolaemia
Hypothermia
Hyper/hypokalaemia, hypocalcaemia (metabolic)

Thromboembolic
Tension pneumothorax
Tamponade
Toxic/therapeutic disturbance

Consider alkalizing agents
e.g. 1ml/kg 8.4% sodium bicarbonate. N.B. dilute in equal volume water if administered peripherally or to infants

Fig. 4.4 Management of asystole and pulseless electrical activity, (adapted with permission from Advanced Life Support Group (2005). *Advanced paediatric life support—the practical approach*, 4th edn, BMJ Publishing Group, London).

Defibrillator technique

Although early defibrillation is the first priority in shockable rhythms, do not rush. Defibrillating a colleague makes a bad situation worse!

Continue with resuscitation while preparing for defibrillation, but do not delay defibrillation to perform other interventions

Choice of defibrillator

An automated external defibrillator (AED) that delivers a fixed energy level of 150 joules or more (depending on manufacturer) can be used in children over 8 years of age. Follow the voice prompts given by the machine.

Some AEDs have attenuated paediatric pads that reduce the shock to 50–75J. These devices can be used on children aged 1 to 8 years. If no attenuated pads are available and a child aged 1 to 8 years is in a shockable rhythm, then the adult dose should be used if using AED. In this situation, not giving a shock is more likely to be fatal than the injury associated with a high dose of energy.

The use of AEDs, with or without attenuated pads, is not currently recommended for infants. This is because some AEDs cannot distinguish between infant tachycardia and life-threatening tachyarrhythmias.

Manual defibrillator technique

It is essential to be familiar with the manual defibrillator prior to using it in an emergency situation. Be aware of:

- whether it uses hands-free pads or paddles;
- how to access the paediatric pads/paddles, and what age-range they should be used for;
- how to select energy levels, and how to charge and discharge the shock;
- how to disarm the machine when charged;
- how to adjust the size of the ECG trace and change the lead view;
- how to give 'asynchronous' shocks. Synchronous setting is only used for reversion of VT if pulse present and SVT (📖 pp.76, 78).

Never hold both paddles in one hand.

Technique for hands-free pads

- Apply hands-free pads, avoiding any metal on or in the patient's chest.
- Select energy level—round up if exact dose cannot be given.
- Call 'Everybody clear' whilst doing visual sweep up and down the bed.
- Ensure oxygen is removed (disconnect circuit from ET tube).
- When all standing back call 'Clear!', reconfirm that the rhythm is shockable, then defibrillate by pressing the shock button(s) on the machine.
- Resume CPR as soon as shock delivered and continue for 2 minutes, before checking rhythm.

Technique for paddles

- Place gel pads on child's chest; pads should be cut but not folded to ensure they do not touch each other.
- Select energy level. If exact dose cannot be given, round up to nearest.
- Press paddles firmly on chest.
- Call 'Everybody clear' whilst doing visual sweep up and down the bed.
- Ensure oxygen is removed (disconnect circuit from ET tube).
- When all standing back, step back from bed yourself and call 'Clear!'
- Reconfirm that the rhythm is shockable; then defibrillate by pressing the buttons on both paddles simultaneously.
- After shock delivered, replace paddles and resume CPR for 2 minutes, before checking rhythm.

N.B. The paddles should either be on the patient's chest or in the machine, ***never*** held in mid-air or in the same hand!

☠ Ventricular fibrillation and pulseless ventricular tachycardia

Aim to defibrillate as quickly but as safely as possible. Continue with resuscitation whilst preparing for defibrillation, but do not delay; intubation and venous access can be obtained between shocks. Confirm a shockable rhythm then defibrillate immediately, noting the time.

1. Give 1 shock of 4J/kg.
2. Resume CPR without reassessing the pulse or monitor. Deliver CPR for 2 minutes; then check the monitor.
3. If still in a shockable rhythm, continue algorithm (Fig. 4.5).
4. If in non-shockable rhythm, e.g. asystole, see 📖 p.70 (Fig. 4.4).
5. If organized electrical activity obtained, check pulse. If not palpable, treat as pulseless electrical activity, see 📖 p.70 (Fig. 4.4).
6. If pulse present, commence post-resuscitation stabilization (📖 p.80).

During the resuscitation:

- intubate, if not already done. This allows asynchronous ventilation at 20 breaths/minute with continuing chest compressions at 100/minute;
- secure additional vascular access and obtain blood for glucose, UEC, FBC, blood culture, cross match, ± clotting;
- obtain fingerprick glucose and treat glucose <4mmol/l with 5ml/kg of 10% dextrose;
- obtain patient history;
- consider and treat any reversible causes (4Hs and 4Ts).

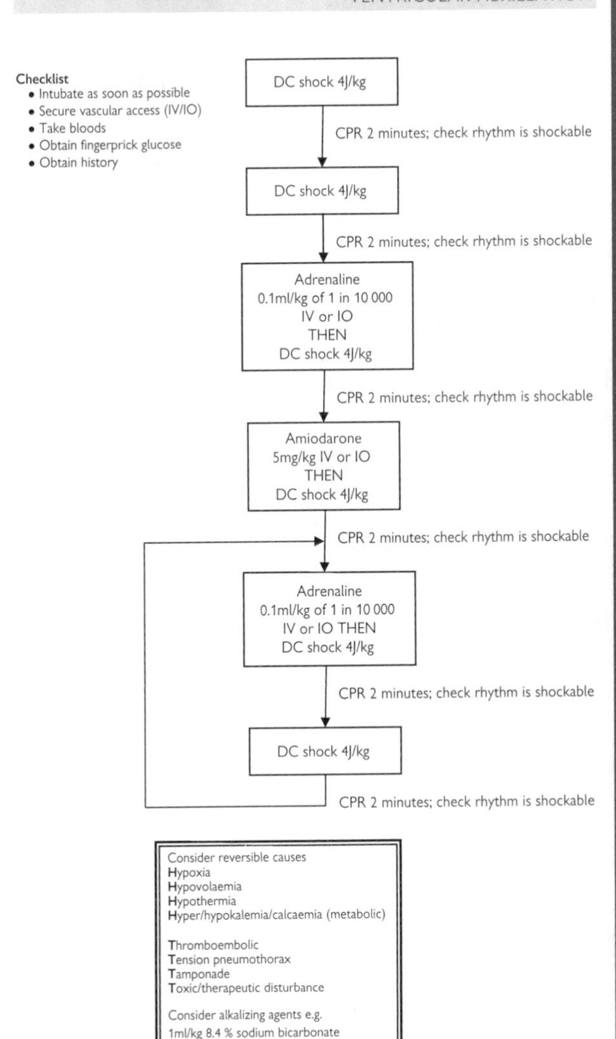

Fig. 4.5 Management of ventricular fibrillation and pulseless ventricular tachycardia, (adapted with permission from Advanced Life Support Group (2005). *Advanced paediatric life support—the practical approach*, 4th edn, BMJ Publishing Group, London).

Ventricular tachycardia with pulse

This is rare in children and usually reflects an underlying cardiac problem or else a poisoning, e.g. tricyclics (p.165). The heart rate is between 120 and 250 per minute, with an almost regular rhythm, but QRS is wide (>2 small squares). If there is shock, **synchronous** defibrillation (i.e. cardioversion) is required (Fig. 4.6). If the child is not shocked, act quickly as they may deteriorate to pulseless VT or VF.

- Urgent consultation with cardiologist. Treatments include amiodarone or procainamide.
- If unable to contact cardiologist treat with IV amiodarone 5mg/kg. N.B. Volume support likely to be needed.
- Consider following immediately with synchronized shock (1J/kg)
  - Short anaesthetic required—ketamine 2mg/kg plus midazolam 100mcg/kg may preserve cardiac output better than an opiate with midazolam.

If resistant to synchronous shock and amiodarone, treat as pulseless VT (p.74)

Torsades de pointes ventricular tachycardia

This rare form of VT has QRS complexes that change in appearance. It is precipitated by:

- long QT (p.181);
- medications such as amiodarone, digoxin, tricyclics.

Treatment is by IV magnesium sulphate 25–50mg/kg (up to 2g).

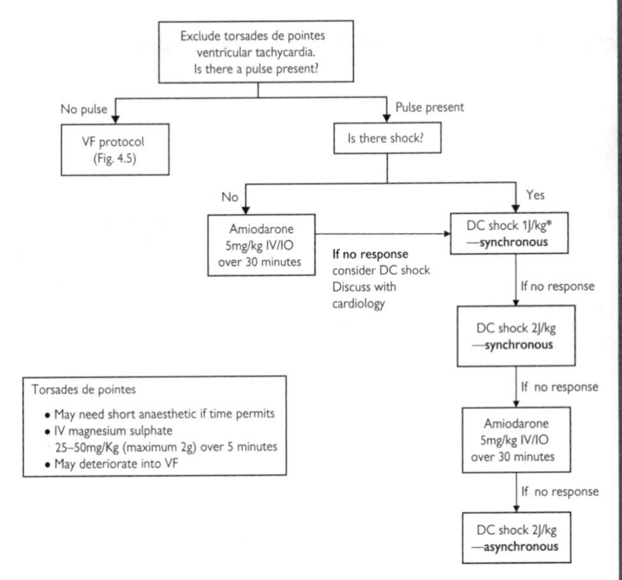

Fig. 4.6 Management of ventricular tachycardia, (adapted with permission from Advanced Life Support Group (2005). *Advanced paediatric life support—the practical approach*, 4th edn, BMJ Publishing Group, London).

Supraventricular tachycardia

SVT is the commonest arrhythmia and usually presents in infancy. Causes include febrile illness or drug exposure (20%) and congenital heart disease including Wolff–Parkinson–White (30%), and 50% have no known aetiology.

Presentations include poor feeding, irritability, or pallor, with the older children being able to describe dizziness, chest pain, or palpitations. The pulse rate is over 180 beats per minute (over 220 beats per minute in infants) and, unlike sinus tachycardia, there is no beat-to-beat variation.

Treatment can cause asystole or bradycardia and necessary drugs should be to hand. Continuous rhythm strip printout during treatment is recommended as the aberrant pacemaker can be unmasked transiently.

Management

- Move the child to resuscitation room.
- Reassess ABC—check BP and assess for cardiac failure.
- Perform 12 lead ECG. N.B. P waves may not be visible.
- Start continuous cardiac monitoring.
- Ensure rhythm strip can be printed out from monitor.
- Follow algorithm (Fig. 4.7).

If shocked, summon senior assistance.

- Have airway equipment available.
- Sedation or short anaesthetic, if time permits.

If stable

- Vagal manoeuvres include immersing face in iced water, ice on the face, unilateral carotid massage. Warn parents before attempting!
- Obtain IV access in large vein with 3-way tap.
- Prepare all doses of adenosine in advance, with 5ml normal saline flushes.
- Warn parents and child about possible side-effects—flushing, shortness of breath, chest pain, headache, nausea.
- Push dose of adenosine and then flush; repeat at 2 minute intervals in increasing doses.
  - Adenosine has a half-life of 10 seconds, so must be administered rapidly. This is best done by having both adenosine and a 5ml flush attached to a 3-way tap and pushing adenosine, then saline.

If successful, perform 12 lead ECG and admit for cardiac monitoring. Refer to cardiologist.

If unsuccessful, increase dose of adenosine and discuss ongoing treatment with cardiologist. Check UEC ± thyroid function tests before starting digoxin or flecanide. N.B. Digoxin is contraindicated for use in Wolff–Parkinson–White.

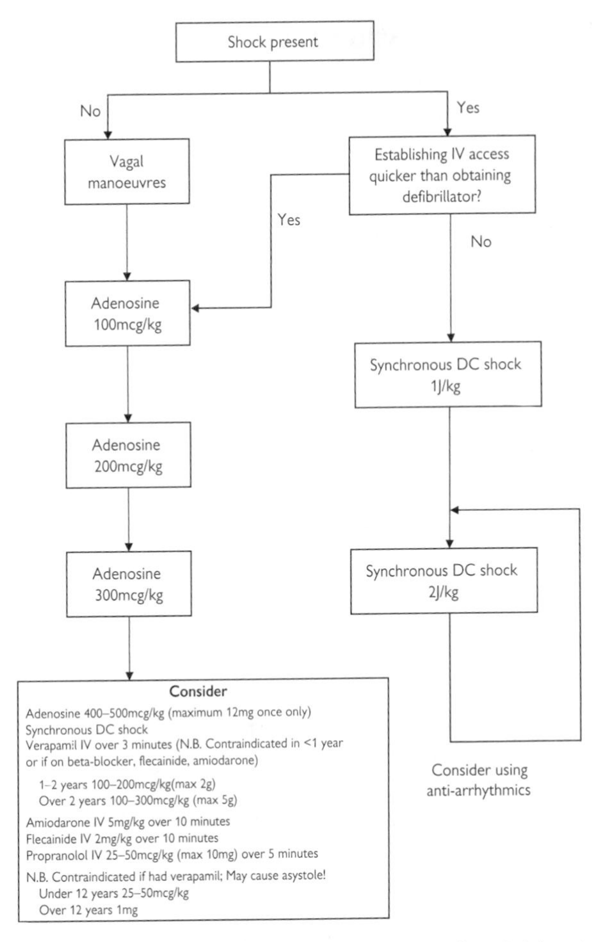

Fig. 4.7 Algorithm for the management of supraventricular tachycardia (adapted with permission from Advanced Life Support Group (2005). *Advanced paediatric life support—the practical approach*, 4th edn, BMJ Publishing Group, London).

Post-resuscitation care

The objectives of post-resuscitation care are to stabilize the child and avoid deterioration. It is also important to explain fully to the family what has happened and the plans for ongoing care.

Immediate management

- Establish comprehensive monitoring so that any changes in condition are rapidly noticed.
  - Continuous cardiac monitoring: pulse, BP, SpO_2.
  - Skin temperature ± core temperature.
  - GCS.
- Obtain specimens to establish baseline parameters.
  - Bloods: glucose, FBC, UEC, LFT, clotting studies, cross-match, arterial blood gas ± blood cultures.
  - 12 lead ECG.
  - CXR.
- Arrange transfer to PICU. If there are no PICU facilities available in your hospital, arrange transfer by a specialist paediatric retrieval team. Your local PICU can give advice on management. An unstable child must not be moved, so you are responsible for optimizing the child's condition until the team's arrival (📖 p.82).
- Communication.
  - Confer with consultants involved in the child's care.
  - Notify PICU of any adverse change in the child's condition.
  - Document the resuscitation in the child's notes.

Key features to document

- Significant medical history and events immediately prior to the emergency call
- The child's condition on presentation—**A**irway, **B**reathing, **C**irculation, and **D**isability
- Events of the arrest, including interventions and drugs given, and what was the clinical response
- Length of time from start of resuscitation to restoration or stabilization of vital functions
- Sizes and sites of all lines and tubes inserted and remaining
- The names and bleep numbers of key resuscitation team members and their roles in the resuscitation attempt
- Attach any ECG recording strips from monitor
- The child's condition on cessation of resuscitation (ABCD)
- Current management, investigations initiated, and treatments given and planned
- Exact information given to parents

Stabilization for interhospital transfer

Your local PICU will advise on its transfer protocol. As a general rule, endotracheal intubation and sedation are necessary to reduce demands of the respiratory and circulatory system. Thereby minimizing potential complications in the back of the ambulance!

Airway and breathing

- Secure airway with endotracheal tube.
- Insert nasogastric tube and place on continuous drainage.
- Confirm tube placement by observation of equal and bilateral chest wall movement, and by auscultation.
- Perform CXR to check position of ETT and NGT.
- Record ETT size, length, and position on CXR in medical notes.
- Monitor nature and quantity of any secretions.
- Monitor effects of respiratory management on SpO_2, $etCO_2$, blood gas values, and heart rate.
- Ensure the child is receiving adequate sedation. Muscle relaxation and analgesia facilitate positive pressure ventilation.

Suggested infusions for transfer

Vecuronium	100–200mcg/kg/h
Morphine	20–40mcg/kg/h
Midazolam	100–200mcg/kg/h

- Prepare ventilator—gases should be humidified and warmed.
- If a choice is available, pressure-limited mechanical ventilation is safest for infants, while volume ventilation is often used for children. Suggested ventilator settings are shown in Table 4.7.

Any deterioration in respiratory status, remember DOPES!

Displayed ETT
Obstructed ETT or airway
Pneumothorax
Equipment failure
Splinting of diaphragm by air in stomach

Table 4.7 Initial ventilator settings

Ventilatory parameter	Setting	Notes
Pressure-limited ventilation	Peak pressure 20–25cm H_2O	Adjust as necessary to obtain reasonable chest movement and provide acceptable blood gas values
Volume-limited ventilation	Tidal volume 5–10ml/kg	
Inspiratory–expiratory (I:E) ratio	1:2	Ti 0.5 in baby to 1s in older child. Increasing Ti may improve oxygenation
Positive end expiratory pressure	4–10cm H_2O	Increase if atelectasis or persistent hypoxia. Low (3–5) if air-trapping e.g. asthma
FiO_2	1.0 then wean as tolerated	To maintain SaO_2 >92%
Respiratory rate (breaths/min)		
<6 months	25–40	Modify according to arterial blood gas values
6 months–2 years	25–30	
2–5 years	20–25	
5–10 years	15–20	
>10 years	12–15	

Circulation

There are 3 aspects to circulatory management.

- Monitor circulatory function.
- Minimize demands on circulatory system.
- Provide support as required to maintain cardiac function and tissue perfusion.

Monitoring

- Continuously monitor: ECG, SpO_2, BP, core and peripheral temperatures. $etCO_2$ provides a good indication of pulmonary perfusion.
- Insert urinary catheter and record hourly urine output.
- Frequently record: GCS, ventilatory parameters, arterial blood gases, blood glucose.

Minimize demands

- Sedation.
- Coordinate care to minimize handling and stress.
- Maintain normothermia.
- Maintain adequate fluid and calorie input.
- Ensure Hb >8g/dl.

Provide support Consider inotropic agents to support cardiac function (Table 4.8). For information on preparing infusions see 📖 p.526

Don't forget

- A copy of your notes, with documentation of the arrest.
- Include copies of all blood results, imaging, and ECGs.
- Communicate with retrieval team leader. They will appreciate updates on changes in the child's condition and, in turn, they can inform you about transportation arrangements. The nursing staff on-site and in PICU should maintain ongoing communication.
- Continue to update parents on progress in their child's condition and the transfer.

Table 4.8 Inotropes and their actions

Drug	Dose mcg/kg/min	Inotrope	Chronotrope	Vasodilator	Vasopressor
Dopamine	1–3	+	+		
	3–10	**++**			
	>10	**++**			**+**
Dobutamine	5–20	++	+	+	
Adrenaline*	<0.3	++	++		
	>0.3	**++**			**+++**
Noradrenaline†	0.1–2.0	++			+++

* Also called epinephrine.
† Also called norepinephrine.

Following unsuccessful resuscitation

Resuscitation is unlikely to be successful if:
- there is no restoration of circulation after 30 minutes;
- ***and*** there is no recurring or refractory VF/VT.

However, exceptions are made in hypothermia (📖 p.122) and in poisonings, which can respond after a prolonged resuscitation.

Discuss case with a consultant before ceasing resuscitative efforts

If the parents are present, explain that the likelihood of their child's survival is small and that withdrawal of care is the kindest thing to do. Many parents appreciate having witnessed the resuscitation so that they know that 'everything possible' was done. Stop chest compressions, then ventilation; then remove monitoring leads. IV lines must be left *in situ*, but ET tubes and IO needles can be removed.

If the parents or carers are not present at the cessation of resuscitation, then arrangements should be made for them to come to the hospital. The family should be seen in private and the events of the resuscitation explained in simple terms. Most parents will want to see and hold their dead child and they should be offered this opportunity.

Involve a senior nurse or hospital social worker to provide support for the family until the child's body is transferred to the mortuary. Offer to contact any member of family, friend, or religious advisors that the parents would like to have with them.

In the UK, the coroner needs to be informed of:
- unexpected deaths (📖 p.88);
- infants brought in dead before arrival in the emergency department;
- children who die soon after arrival in the emergency department;
- deaths where there has been recent surgery or an accident;
- deaths where there are suspicious circumstances.

Some post-mortems can be expedited to conform with religious beliefs. Ask the coroner's officer if this is possible.

Don't forget

- Document fully the events of the arrest (📖 p.80) and the time at which resuscitation ceased (time of death).
- Notify any consultants involved in the child's care.
- Notify the child's general practitioner. It is also important that the practice is informed so that the parents do not receive reminder notices for immunizations.
- Bereavement counselling for the parents, provided either by GP, child's paediatrician, or agencies such as CRUSE.
- Yourself and your colleagues. The death of a child is distressing. The opportunity to debrief should be offered to staff. Many find reliving the arrest is more traumatic, so attendance should not be compulsory.

Sudden unexpected death in an infant

SUDI is often referred to as cot-death or **S**udden **I**nfant **D**eath **S**yndrome (SIDS). In the period 1999–2003, 88% of SIDS were in babies under 1 year of age.

Typically, the child is brought to hospital after resuscitation has ceased. However, if resuscitation is ongoing:

- obtain a brief history of the baby's health and of recent events;
- note any sign of trauma, e.g. bruising or bleeding.

Investigations If possible, obtain:

- bloods, particularly blood gas and serum for toxicology and metabolic screen;
- urine for toxicology and metabolic screen;
- nasopharyngeal aspirate for virology and bacteriology;

Decide when to cease resuscitation in conjunction with the parents and your consultant.

Once death has been declared

The coroner must be informed. At this point, any handling of the child, e.g. cleaning the face, taking clinical specimens, can only be undertaken with approval from the coroner. Even if there is a pre-agreed protocol, confirm with the coroner's officer that you can remove resuscitative equipment and take post-mortem specimens. Even taking a lock of hair as a memento for the parents requires approval!

- Explain to the parents that it is a legal requirement to involve the coroner and that a post-mortem will be performed. Emphasize that it is possible that no cause of death may be found ('unascertained') or that it may be attributed to SIDS or cot death. In addition, explain that it is usual for the police to visit them at home in the next 24 hours.
- Allow the parents to spend as much time as they need with their child.
- Retain the child's clothing and bedding. Place in labelled specimen bags for the coroner.
- Some hospitals have a dedicated SUDI team. Involve them as soon as possible.
- If possible, get a senior paediatrician to examine the child. Document:
  - the baby's general appearance, nutritional status, and cleanliness;
  - the baby's weight, allowing for any clothes or equipment retained at at coroner's request. Plot approximate position on centile chart;
  - rectal temperature;
  - any rashes or birth marks;
  - marks from invasive or vigorous procedures such as venepuncture or cardiac massage;
  - any other marks on the skin, including bruises or abrasions, with an estimate of their age. Nasal blood may be seen in suffocation;
  - appearance of the retinae;
  - any lesions in the mouth (allowing for effects of intubation).
- Check Child Protection Register.

Don't forget

- If the infant was a twin, consider admission of the surviving twin for investigations/observation.
- If mother is breast feeding, arrange lactation suppression.
- Notify:
  - any consultants, e.g. neonatologist, involved in the child's care;
  - the family's general practitioner;
  - police according to your hospital's protocol. Some only wish to be contacted if there are suspicious circumstances.

Follow-up

Arrangements should be made for the family to discuss the results of the coroner's postmortem and, when appropriate, consider its implications for future pregnancies. Genetic counselling may be needed.

Bereavement counselling should be offered: this may be provided by the family practitioner, health professionals within the paediatric team, or from other agencies (e.g. Foundation for the Study of Infant Deaths,[1] Child Death Helpline, and CRUSE).

1 The Foundation for the Study of Infant Deaths produces a leaflet, 'When a baby dies suddenly and unexpectedly', and has a Helpline number 0207 233 2090. (www.sids.org.uk)

Chapter 5

Shock

Pathophysiology

Shock is the inadequate perfusion of the body's vital organs. Perfusion is dependent on:
- cardiac output;
- stroke volume (blood expelled from left ventricle);
- heart rate.

Factors that reduce any of these basic functions may eventually lead to shock. The result is failure to supply oxygen and substrate to cells as well as impaired removal of their waste products. Anaerobic metabolism and tissue acidosis will result. If there is insufficient compensation to reverse these changes, multiple end-organ failure and death will follow.

Shock may be classified by its physiological sequelae (see Table 5.1).

The primary determinant of effective end-organ perfusion is myocardial function. If impaired, children can compensate by:
- reduced blood flow to non-vital organs—decreased capillary refill and cool peripheries;
- increase in heart rate—up to 200bpm for a finite period of time;
- increase in respiratory rate—to improve oxygen delivery.

This is 'compensated shock'. Simultaneous activation of renin–angiotensin system conserves water with reduction in GFR and urine output. There may be agitation and confusion, but the blood pressure is maintained. However, this is costly in terms of substrate and cannot be maintained indefinitely.

Failure to treat the cause at this stage will lead to inevitable decline, i.e. 'uncompensated shock'. Anaerobic metabolism increases, further impairing myocardial function. The resultant reduction in blood flow to the vital organs causes:
- anuria;
- a further reduction of conscious level—GCS <8, only responsive to pain (AVPU);
- respiratory failure;
- hypotension.

An inappropriately normal heart or respiratory rate should not fool you into thinking the child is improving. Only rapid and sustained intervention will now prevent cardiorespiratory failure and arrest.

Shock—cold versus warm

When the body's vital organs are underperfused, blood is diverted from non-vital areas like skin. Such children have cool peripheries and are 'shut down', as they increase systemic vascular resistance (SVR) to improve venous return and cardiac output. This is 'cold shock'.

However in 'warm shock', e.g. Gram-negative sepsis, anaphylaxis, and neurogenic shock, cytokines or neural responses cause vasodilatation and reduce SVR. Such children will be tachycardic, but with inappropriately warm peripheries. ***Always*** consider possibility of warm shock—it must never be missed.

Causes

Table 5.1 Causes of shock

Type of shock	Mechanism	Cause
Cardiogenic	Weak pump	Arrhythmia Heart failure Cardiomyopathy Multi-organ failure Drugs—chemo- or radiotherapy Infiltration—mucopolysaccharidosis, glycogen storage disease
	Increased demands	Pericardial tamponade Obstructed left heart Thyrotoxicosis Phaeochromocytoma
Hypovolaemic	Empty pump a) Water loss	Diarrhoea, vomiting, DKA, burns, gut obstruction, excess diuretics, pancreatitis
	b) Blood loss	Trauma—obvious or occult Fractured pelvis, femur Intracranial bleed Blunt abdominal trauma (spleen, liver)
Distributive	Blood not reaching peripheries ('third spacing')	Sepsis, especially Gram-negative Anaphylaxis Spinal shock Drugs—barbiturates, phenothiazines, antihypertensives
Obstructive	Blood can't get out	Tension pneumothorax Cardiac tamponade Massive pulmonary embolus Critical aortic stenosis Hypoplastic left heart syndrome
Dissociative	Blood doesn't work	Profound anaemia Carbon monoxide poisoning Methaemoglobinaemia
Other		Congenital adrenal hyperplasia

Assessment and treatment

High flow O_2 and ABCs

In children, the commonest forms of shock are:

- septic shock, i.e. distributive;
- hypovolaemic shock secondary to trauma or gastroenteritis.

Oxygen and fluid resuscitation should suffice in most cases.

However, this treatment will worsen cardiogenic shock and conditions with raised intracranial pressure, e.g. traumatic head injury, meningitis. Thus it is imperative to exclude these during your assessment and to review ABC after every intervention, to ensure the child is improving. If the child is requiring more than 40ml/kg, i.e. over half their circulating volume, it is prudent to review your diagnosis and obtain a second opinion from a senior paediatrician.

Take a history focusing on events of the previous 24 hours as you quickly assess the child (Fig. 5.1). Remember to protect the spine if trauma suspected. A detailed examination is deferred until ABC is complete and fluid resuscitation is starting.

History

- Are there underlying medical problems (e.g. asthma, diabetes)?
- Has there been any trauma?
- Is the child on steroids?
- Are there any missing medicines in the home (antihypertensives, antidepressants)?
- Are there any unexplained deaths or illnesses in the family (CAH, inborn errors of metabolism)?

Examination features

- Temperature—hyper- or hypothermia with an increased toe–core gap, i.e. difference between central and peripheral temperature.
- Reduced urine output: >1ml/kg/h is normal.
- Rash—meningococcaemia may present with erythema, purpura, or petechiae, which may progress in front of your eyes. Urticaria is suggestive of anaphylaxis.

Airway and breathing

- Is the airway patent?
- Is the child breathing adequately?

There is usually respiratory compensation, with tachypnoea.

- Always give high flow oxygen and do not proceed until happy with both A and B.

A child who looks septic and has respiratory distress may need ventilatory support. Intubation removes the work of breathing and should precede volume replacement in the critically ill child. This is a clinical decision—blood gas results are seldom helpful.

> Induction of anaesthesia may cause vasodilatation and worsen hypotension, so consider using ketamine, rather than thiopentone, and give fluid simultaneously.

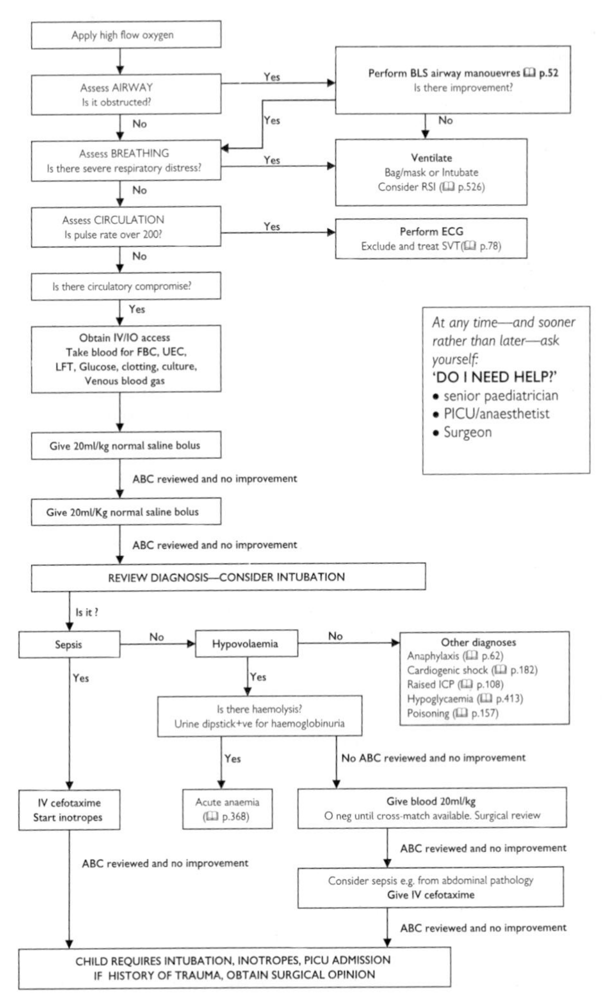

Fig. 5.1 Algorithm for management of shock.

Circulation

- What is the colour?
- What are the rate and character of the pulse?
  - Is it fast, or weak and thready?
  - N.B. Normal rate is worrying.
  - N.B. Bounding pulses of warm shock.
  - Tachycardia over 200/min is SVT (📖 p.78) until proven otherwise.
- What is the central capillary refill time?
  - Press over sternum for 5 seconds; normal <2 seconds in warm child, but longer if cold (peripheral perfusion less informative).
  - N.B. Warm shock is quick capillary refill with low diastolic pressure.
- What is the blood pressure?

> Blood pressure is maintained until very late—hypotension is a pre-terminal sign.

Fluid resuscitation depends on the degree of compromise in the child. If circulation is impaired:

- check A,B are still stable—if not, correct then proceed;
- obtain IV access.

IV access

Access may be difficult in a cold child who is peripherally shut down.

- Peripheral IV cannula (📖 p.462)—antecubital fossae, or long saphenous areas. ***Three attempts maximum.***
- Intraosseous access if child under 6 years (📖 p.469)—***first line in collapsed child under 6 years old.***
- Central access—the femoral route is safe in experienced hands (📖 p.463).

Take blood for:

- fingerprick glucose;
- FBC, UEC ± amylase, LFT, clotting;
- cross match (group-specific, if actively bleeding);
- blood cultures;
- venous gas—for acidosis and ionized calcium.

Fluid resuscitation

Fluid resuscitation involves boluses of normal saline, blood, or colloid. Once fluid is given, reassess ABC and note any changes in pulse or perfusion. If no clinical response, further fluid is required.

- Normal saline bolus of 20ml/kg. NB if trauma, give in aliquots of 10ml/kg.
  - ***Never*** use hypotonic fluid for resuscitation, i.e. no 2.5% or 4% or 5% dextrose solutions.
- Blood loss is best replaced by blood—O negative until cross-matched sample available.
- Colloid use is controversial—most avoid albumin, but Hartmann's or Gelofusin are fine.

Once 40ml/kg has been given without clinical response, blood will be necessary as there will be haemodilution. Septic children may require over 100ml/kg of fluid, so inotropes are used early to minimize fluid overload.

If there is no improvement, further resuscitation involves:

- blood, even when not bleeding;
- broad spectrum antibiotics (ceftriaxone 50mg/kg daily, or cefotaxime 50mg/kg/dose tds IV, plus, in <3 month old, ampicillin 50mg/kg/dose qds);
- rule out hidden bleeding, e.g. long bones, pelvis, or intra-abdominal pathology.

A surgical review is mandatory if any history of trauma and prudent to exclude hidden intra-abdominal pathology.

- Inform the duty anaesthetist and PICU and consider intubation and ventilation, if not done already. Children this ill benefit from removal of the work of breathing—pulmonary oedema from fluid overload is rare.
- Inotropic support is likely to be needed—consider central line insertion (📖 p.463).
- Inform PICU.

Inotropic support

The inotrope used depends on the physiological correction necessary (Table 5.2). See 📖 p.526 for preparation of infusions.

Table 5.2 Inotropic support

	Inotrope of choice	
Type of shock	**Peripheral access**	**Central access**
Cold shock: Low CO, high SVR	Dopamine, or dobutamine	Adrenaline (Epinephrine)
Warm shock: Low CO, low SVR	Dopamine	Noradrenaline (Norepinephrine)
Resistant shock*	Hydrocortisone	Hydrocortisone

* Exclude: on-going blood loss; pneumothorax; pericardial effusion; hypoadrenalism (N.B. chronic steroid use); hypothyroidism; hypopituitarism.

Imaging

Do not move the child to the radiology department until adequately resuscitated. They don't call the CT scanner the 'doughnut of death' for no reason! On-going haemorrhage requires surgery not scans.

On-going management

- Resuscitation continues until there is a definite and sustained improvement in heart rate and perfusion.

Heart rate will increase by 10 beats/minute for every 1°C increase in body temperature.

- Maintain normothermia (i.e. temperature <37.5°C) and correct any metabolic abnormalities, particularly glucose, potassium, and calcium and any coagulopathy.
- Thereafter, treatment is directed by the underlying pathology.
- Shock carries a significant mortality, so early involvement of senior colleagues and PICU is important.

Chapter 6

Trauma

Assessment

This structured approach allows problems to be identified and treated in order of priority. Nominate a team leader at the outset. If time allows, estimate the weight, determine ETT size/length, and chart saline bolus volume and emergency drug doses (📖 p.527).

Outline of assessment

- Primary survey and resuscitation.
- Emergency treatment.
- Secondary survey.
- Transfer to definitive care.

Life-threatening problems should be treated as they are identified in the primary survey. Secondary survey does not begin until:

- the primary survey is completed;
- *and* resuscitative efforts are in progress;
- *and* the patient is demonstrating improved vital functions.

Reassess from A to C whenever there is a change in status or treatment.

> Cervical spine should be assumed unstable until excluded by thorough examination and investigation

Primary survey

Airway with cervical spine control

- Airway management.
  - Oxygen—high flow via mask with re-breathing bag.
  - Jaw thrust. N.B. Head tilt and chin lift contraindicated as possibility of cervical spine injury.
  - Suction/removal of foreign body under direct vision.
  - May require oral airway **or** tracheal intubation, if respiratory support necessary. N.B. Avoid nasal airway in facial trauma.

Breathing If inadequate, requires assistance:

- ventilation;
- chest drain—indications (📖 p.103); technique (📖 p.478).

Circulation Assessment BP, HR, respiratory rate, skin perfusion, temperature, urinary output, mental state. Start continuous ECG monitoring. If shock:

- 2 large bore IV cannulae;
- 10ml/kg saline bolus, if no improvement, repeat until a maximum of 40ml/kg saline has been given;
- if no improvement—20ml/kg blood + surgical opinion.

Disability Glasgow Coma Scale, AVPU, pupil assessment.

Exposure/environment Expose patient. N.B. Hypothermia.

> Repeat primary survey until vital signs improving

Secondary survey

'AMPLE' history as a minimum:

- **A**llergy;
- **M**edications;
- **P**ast medical history;
- **L**ast meal;
- **E**vents/environment.

Obtain a full description of mechanism of injury, e.g. speed at impact, wearing seatbelt/helmet, followed by examination of the whole of the body. Assess pelvic integrity by pressing on iliac crests and symphysis; then rock whilst holding on to the iliac crests. Log roll the patient to fully examine the back and spine. Palpate vertebral bodies noting any tenderness or steps in integrity. Rectal examination to assess anal tone should be performed by senior staff.

Investigations

Blood

FBC, UEC, LFT, glucose, cross-match plus:

- amylase if abdominal trauma;
- coagulation screen if hepatic trauma or need for multiple blood transfusions anticipated.

Imaging

- Cervical-spine AP and lateral ± peg view.
- CXR—AP.
- Pelvic x-ray—AP.

Further imaging, e.g. x-ray of suspected fractured limb, CT head as clinically indicated. Review x-rays and, if able, 'clear the spine' (🕮 p.110).

Transfer to definitive care If ICU care needed and is not available, arrange retrieval and transfer.

Log roll technique

- Have at least three assistants, who control the **head**, **chest**, and **pelvis**, respectively. In older children, a further assistant is necessary to control the patient's legs
- Explain to the patient what you are going to do and ask them to cross their arms over their chest, placing their hands near their shoulders
- **Head**—stands at the head of the bed and holds either side of the patient's head. Responsible for maintaining spinal alignment and controlling when the roll begins
- **Chest**—reaches over the child and holds the patient at the shoulder and just above the elbow. Responsible for supporting the chest and ensuring that it rotates at the same speed as the head
- **Pelvis and legs**—holds child at the iliac crest and under the knee, supporting the upper leg on their forearm. If the legs cannot be held securely, obtain another assistant
- The assistant holding the head states 'ready–steady–roll' and the others commence slowly rolling the patient towards them. All assistants watch the head so that all parts roll at the same rate
- The assistant holding the head rotates the head **maintaining spinal alignment**
- After the back and spine are examined, the assistant holding the head states 'ready–steady–back' and the patient is rolled back

Chest trauma

Substantial amounts of energy can be transferred through the relatively elastic chest wall with significant intrathoracic visceral disruption and limited external signs. Thoracic trauma is a marker of serious injury and is associated with extrathoracic injury in 70% of cases.

Assessment

- ABC with oxygen. Once airway is secure, assess breathing:
- Inspect. Alarming signs include: abnormal chest movements; bruising (= high impact injury); distended neck veins (= pericardial tamponade); tension pneumothorax.
- Palpate. Check tracheal and apex beat position; palpate clavicles and ribs for tenderness. Percuss noting hyperresonance (pneumothorax) or dullness (haemothorax).
- Auscultate. Absence of breath sounds = pneumo/haemothorax; muffling of heart sounds = pericardial effusion.

☠ Cardiac tamponade

Can occur after blunt or penetrating trauma. Blood accumulates in the fibrous pericardial sac and progressively compromises cardiac output.

Signs

- Shock.
- Distended neck veins; muffled heart sounds.

Treatment

- High flow oxygen through reservoir mask.
- Rapid fluid resuscitation to temporarily increase filling pressures.
- Emergency needle pericardiocentesis and referral for cardiac surgery.

Emergency needle pericardiocentesis

- Obtain: 20ml syringe and 16G cannula; surgical drapes and skin cleansing solution ± local anaesthetic; three-way tap and tapes for securing
- Palpate trachea and apex beat to exclude mediastinal shift
- Start continuous ECG monitoring
- Clean xiphoid and subxiphoid area and apply drapes; infiltrate cannula insertion site with local anaesthetic if patient conscious
- Secure cannula to syringe
- Insert cannula 1–2cm below and to the left of the xiphisternum at an angle of 45°
- Ask assistant to notify you of any ECG changes
- Aim for tip of left scapula and advance needle whilst aspirating continuously. If myocardium struck = ST segment changes
- Once fluid is aspirated, draw off as much as possible. N.B. If over 100ml aspirated, probably in ventricle. Withdraw cannula and review ABC
- If improved cardiac output, remove needle but keep cannula *in situ*. Tape into position and apply three-way tap. This permits further aspiration if tamponade recurs

Tension pneumothorax

Air under pressure builds up in the pleural space, thereby decreasing venous return to the heart and reducing cardiac output. The diagnosis is clinical and should be made prior to x-ray.

Signs

- Hypoxic and shocked.
- Decreased air entry, hyperresonance on side of pneumothorax.
- Distended neck veins.
- Trachea deviated away from the side of the pneumothorax.

Treatment

- High flow oxygen through reservoir mask.
- Immediate needle thoracocentesis to relieve tension, using large bore cannula in 2nd intercostal space in mid-clavicular line. Should hear a hiss, followed by clinical improvement.
- Chest drain should be inserted immediately to prevent recurrence (p.478) and to treat the simple pneumothorax that you have now created.

Open pneumothorax

Seen with penetrating chest wall injury with pneumothorax. Examine the back to ensure no additional sites of injury.

Signs

- Air sucking and blowing through wound.
- Decreased air entry with hyperresonance on affected side.

Treatment

- High flow oxygen through reservoir mask.
- Occlusion of the wound on three sides to create a valve, allowing air to escape but not be sucked back in.
- Urgent chest drain (p.478).

Haemothorax

Accumulation of blood in the pleural space.

Signs

- Shock if substantial proportion of circulating blood volume lost.
- Decreased chest movement, decreased air entry, dull percussion note on side of haemothorax.
- CXR will show white-out on the affected side.

Treatment

- Oxygen.
- Fluid replacement.
- Large bore chest drain before definitive surgery (p.478).

Flail chest

Sequential rib fractures cause a section of the chest to move paradoxically, i.e. inwards on inspiration. It signifies a major injury as the chest wall is relatively resistant to fractures. Rib fractures are difficult to diagnose on plain x-rays and these should not be relied on for a diagnosis.

Signs

- Hypoxic.
- Paradoxical chest movements with rib crepitus.
- Initial reflex splinting may mask flail segments on first examination.

Treatment

- High flow oxygen. May need ventilation
- Analgesia, consider intercostal nerve blocks.

Pulmonary contusion

Usually follows significant blunt trauma; relatively more common in the child because of the mobility of the chest wall. Hypoxic as pulmonary capillaries rupture, filling alveoli. Crepitations ± loss of resonance may be elicited. Initial CXR may be normal but subsequently will show diffuse interstitial shadowing and eventually consolidation. Treat with high flow oxygen and consider ventilation.

Ruptured diaphragm

Can occur following blunt trauma and is more common on the left due to the protection of the liver on the right side. Pulmonary compression can occur, and abdominal visceral injury should be excluded. Reduced air entry with dullness to percussion on affected side. Bowel sounds may even be audible in the thorax! Insert NGT to decompress stomach.
CXR shows eventration of diaphragm ± abdominal contents in the chest cavity. Urgent surgical referral should be made for repair.

Simple pneumothorax

Self-limiting leak of air into the pleural space causing partial lung collapse. If hypoxia or signs of distress present, a chest drain should be inserted (p.478). If the patient is to be ventilated, a chest drain is mandatory as a simple pneumothorax will become a tension pneumothorax. Otherwise, gradual re-inflation possible with the application of high flow oxygen.

Abdominal trauma

The abdomen is the third commonest site of injury after head and isolated limb injuries. Pre-adolescents are very susceptible as the diaphragm lies flatter, the rib cage is more elastic, and the abdominal wall is thin. A precise description of mechanism of injury can guide the examination, e.g. flexion/extension injury over lap sash seatbelt is associated with small bowel injury and lumbar vertebral fractures.

Assessment

Abdominal injury should be considered in the shocked patient with no obvious site of haemorrhage. Examine abdomen for bruising, lacerations, and penetrating wounds.

- ABC especially BP, HR, respiratory rate, temperature, urinary output.
- Check external urethral meatus for blood. If blood present, ***DO NOT*** catheterize.
- Repeat examination frequently.
- Ensure child has stable vital signs before being moved for imaging.

Investigations

- FBC, UEC, LFT, amylase, cross-match. Consider coagulation screen if large volume loss or if hepatic injury.
- Radiographs—erect CXR looking for free air under the diaphragm (= bowel perforation).
- USS—free fluid, lacerations in liver, spleen, and kidney.
- CT—double contrast is method of choice for defining visceral injury.

Treatment

Urgent referral to general surgery on clinical grounds or if high suspicion, because of mechanism of injury. The majority of solid-organ injuries can be treated conservatively with careful fluid management and frequent monitoring and assessment. Ensure adequate analgesia.

Intestinal perforations require urgent surgery.

Pelvic trauma

Only occurs after major trauma. Pelvic disruption causes major haemorrhage as well as bowel and bladder disturbances. If the pelvis is fractured, there will be tenderness ± crepitus on palpation and one-half will move differently from the other.

- X-ray pelvis shows disruption of contour from ischium–ilium–pubis.
- Haematomas may displace bladder laterally.

Treatment

- Fluid resuscitation until improvement of vital signs.
- Stabilization of the unstable pelvis—a pelvic binder is applied, which requires three people. The binder (or sheet) is passed under and around the pelvis, compressing the sacroiliac wings medially, and the third person secures the binder. This is a life-saving manoeuvre as it limits blood loss by decreasing the volume of the pelvis.
- All open pelvic injuries require general surgery referral to perform a de-functioning colostomy.

Head injury[1]

Head injury is the most common single cause of trauma death in children. Severe injury is associated with NAI, road traffic accidents, and falls from more than twice the child's height. The mechanism of injury needs to be documented thoroughly to exclude risk factors for severe injury.

Despite this, over 85% of head injuries will be mild (GCS 13–15) on initial presentation. However, intracerebral bleeding can manifest after a lucid period, necessitating observation in hospital and at home.

Assessment ABC with cervical spine control if GCS <13 (📖 p.526). Head injuries are often associated with cervical spine injuries.

History

- Mechanism of injury, with time and place that injury sustained.
- Loss of consciousness, or any fluctuations in consciousness.
- Period of amnesia following head injury.
- Any seizures?
- Has there been any vomiting or diplopia?
- Pre-existing factors affecting assessment, e.g. cerebral palsy.

Examination

- Level of consciousness using AVPU/Glasgow coma scale (📖 p.526).
- Record vital signs—respiratory rate, heart rate, blood pressure.
- Pupil—size and reactivity. Note any nystagmus.
- Is there symmetry of limb movements, reflexes?
- Palpate skull for fracture. Bruising behind ear (Battle's sign) is suggestive of base of skull fracture.
- Examine tympanic membrane for haemotympanum or CSF leak.

Fractures may be felt as a boggy swelling or as a skull depression. A firm lump is indicative of a haematoma, overlying an intact skull. CSF leaks, e.g. rhinorrhoea, otorrhoea, will be positive for glucose on dipstick and, if mixed with blood, will have a halo effect on fabric.

Skull x-rays are seldom performed as they are difficult to interpret. However, they are indicated if the mechanism of injury is unclear or if there is evidence of a focal impact to the head. Skull x-rays are unnecessary if a CT head is going to be performed.

☠ Severe head injury (GCS 3–8)

- Intubate with cervical spine protection.
    - Aim for an end-tidal $PaCO_2$ of 35–40 mmHg to optimize cerebral perfusion. Hyperventilation to lower $PaCO_2$ <35 mmHg may lead to ischaemia.
- Monitor for hypotension and hypoxaemia. Consider inotropic support to maintain blood pressure—cerebral perfusion will be compromised if blood pressure is low when ICP is raised.
- Notify neurosurgeon and ICU.

1 Children's Hospital at Westmead guidelines reproduced with permission.

- Take blood for FBC, cross-match, clotting studies, UEC, glucose.
- If signs of raised ICP, give IV mannitol 250mg/kg.
- Obtain urgent CT scan once vital signs are stable.

ⓘ Moderate head injury (GCS 9–12)

CT scan necessary, along with cervical spine x-rays. If the child requires sedation for the scan, electively intubate. All children will require admission for observation in high dependency or intensive care unit.

ⓘ Mild head injury (GCS 13–15)

No imaging is required, if there are no neurological signs and no evidence of a skull fracture.

It is common policy to observe the child for 4 hours after the time of injury, with hourly neurological observations. The child can be discharged home if they have attained GCS of 15 at the end of the observation period.

Parents should be given a card advising them to return for review if, in the following 24 hours, the child:

- loses consciousness;
- has a seizure;
- has a persistent headache that is not relieved by paracetamol;
- has recurrent vomiting. (N.B. Most will have at least one vomit.)

Indications for CT scan

- Neurological deterioration or failure to improve to GCS of 15.
- Focal neurological deficit, e.g. pupillary asymmetry.
- Skull fracture and abnormal GCS.
- Possible penetrating skull injury.
- Possible base of skull fracture, e.g. CSF leak, haemotympanum.

Indications for admission if child is neurologically normal with GCS of 15

- Any history of loss of consciousness.
- Post-traumatic seizure.
- Persistent headache, nausea, or vomiting.
- Children who are difficult to assess, e.g. the very young, those with pre-existing neurological deficit.
- Suspected child abuse.
- Skull fracture or other abnormality on CT scan.
- Absence of a suitable caretaker to observe child at home, or child unable to return for further care if needed.

Spinal trauma

Spinal injuries are uncommon in children. However every severely injured child should be treated as though they have an unstable spinal injury until excluded by examination and investigation.

Spinal injuries in children tend to be high (C1, 2, or 3) or at C7/T1, because of the flexion/extension of the relatively large head on a flexible spine. The movement may be severe enough to cause spinal cord damage, yet the flexible vertebrae do not fracture. This entity is called SCIWORA—Spinal Cord Injury WithOut Radiological Abnormality—so neck pain must be taken seriously, even if the x-rays are 'normal'.

Assessment

- Triple cervical immobilization (hard collar, sand bags, head taped).
- Neurological examination.
- Log roll to assess for spinal and paraspinal tenderness.
- PR to assess anal tone—only by senior medical staff after full explanation.
- Trauma x-rays—cervical spine AP + lateral x-rays (± peg view). Look for any disruption of kyphosis or any retropharyngeal swelling. (N.B. Pseudo-subluxation of C2/C3 and of C3/C4 occurs in 9% of children.)
  - Cervical spine x-rays must cover C7/T1 junction. If inadequate view, repeat x-rays with assistant pulling down on the patient's arms.
  - Further imaging of vertebral spines often required—CT/MRI.

'Clearing the spine' If the examination is normal and no abnormality is seen on x-rays, the cervical spine is then assessed. This can only be performed if the child is conscious and there are no distracting injuries, e.g. limb fracture. If the child is requiring ventilation or opiate analgesia, further spinal imaging by CT or MRI is recommended.

- Explain to the child that they must keep still during the examination with no head movements. Ask the child to tell you if any of the examination hurts.
- Ask an assistant to hold the child's head steady.
- Loosen the cervical collar—remind child not to move!
- Palpate spine and paraspinal muscles for tenderness. Remind child to tell you if it hurts.
- If no pain, remove collar—the spine is cleared.
- If tenderness, secure the collar.
  - Explain to the child and parents that there is an injury, either musculoskeletal or to the spinal cord.
  - Arrange CT/MRI of cervical spine.
  - Replace cervical collar with Philadelphia collar if child will be in cervical collar for several hours.
- All children with spinal injuries require orthopaedic review.

Limb trauma

Skeletal injury accounts for 10–15% of all childhood injuries. It is uncommon for limb injuries to be life-threatening. Injuries to the immature skeleton differ from these in adults, e.g. fractures arise at growth plates as they are weaker than other skeletal structures including ligaments. Moreover, immature bone can absorb more force, but has a greater remodelling potential. Life-threatening injuries include those covered in the rest of this section.

Traumatic amputation of an extremity

Complete amputation

- ABC with fluid resuscitation.
- Control haemorrhage with local pressure.
  - If this is insufficient, apply a proximal wide tourniquet. Time of application must be documented.
- Obtain amputated limb.
  - Clean with 0.9% saline, place in sterile towel within occlusive bag, and pack in ice. Warm survival time is 8h; cold survival time is 18h.
- Refer patient to specialist for consideration of re-implantation. The patient must be stabilized prior to transfer. The amputated limb should travel in the same vehicle as the patient.

Partial amputations can result in increased blood loss as completely transected vessels go into spasm proximally.

Massive open long-bone fractures

Blood loss from long bones can be significant, e.g. 40% of circulating volume can be exsanguinated from open femoral shaft fractures. 30% of children with open fractures have other life-threatening injuries.

Treatment

- ABC.
- IV antibiotics, cefuroxime, penicillin (and metronidazole if wound contaminated). Check tetanus status.
- Clean wound with 0.9% saline.
- Photograph injury to document pre-operative state of limb.
- Dress wound with iodine packing and do not disturb until theatre.
- Splint fracture.
- Referral to orthopaedic team and maintain nil by mouth.

Compartment syndrome

A surgical emergency—increased pressure within soft tissue compartments results in irreversible muscle and nerve damage. Compartment syndrome can occur after crush injuries and in open fractures. Common sites are the forearm and lower leg.

Note:

- pain out of proportion to the injury;
- pain with passive stretch.

Remove any compression, e.g. bandages, plaster of Paris. Request immediate surgical review. Monitor compartmental pressure by attaching an IV cannula to sphygmomanometer tubing and inserting cannula into tissue. Proceed to fasciotomy if compartmental pressure within 30mmHg of diastolic pressure, or if there is clinical suspicion and monitoring is unavailable.

Fractures

Are described according to:

- appearance (Fig 6.1);
- plane of displacement of distal fragment relative to anatomical position (medial versus lateral; dorsal versus volar);
- degree of angulation of distal fragment (Fig. 6.2)
- % of displacement where 100% = off-ended (Fig. 6.2);

Neurovascular status must be assessed and documented (📖 p.299).

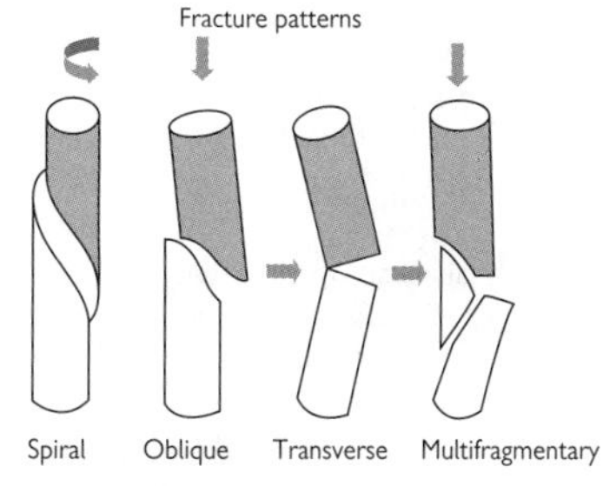

Fig. 6.1 Fracture patterns.

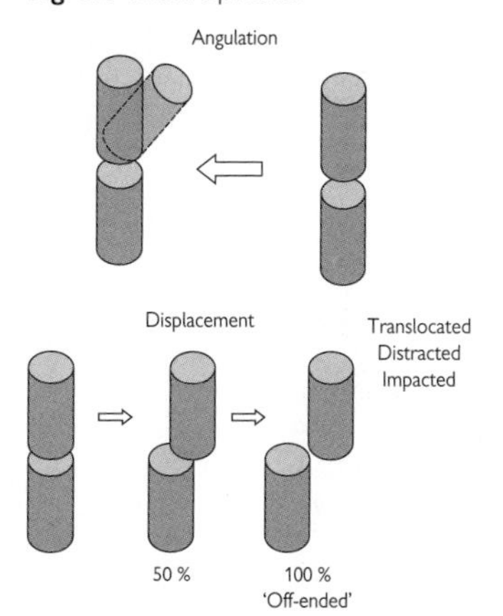

Fig. 6.2 Diagram comparing angulation and displacement.

The aim of treatment is to:

- reduce the fracture to restore anatomical alignment;
- maintain position until union;
- rehabilitate.

This is usually done using plaster of Paris or splints. Most fractures will heal within 6 weeks.

Never describe a fracture as 'simple'—growth plate damage may be innocuous on first presentation, yet will require operative correction as the child grows.

Urgent referral should be made for:

- open fractures;
- high energy/multiple trauma;
- intra-articular fractures;
- fractures associated with neurovascular deficit;
- supra-condylar elbow;
- femoral shaft fractures.

Physeal fracture (growth plate fracture)

Physeal fractures are commonly classified according to the Salter–Harris system (Fig. 6.3). The higher the grade of fracture, the increased incidence of growth disturbance.

Always consider the possibility of physical abuse when dealing with a child with a fracture. The following merit discussion with a senior colleague.

- Fractures in children under the age of 12 months
- Fractures inconsistent with mechanism of injury described
- Spiral fractures
- 'Chip' fractures of distal radius or ulna
- Transverse midshaft fracture of radius and ulna
- Fractures with a delayed presentation

Risk factors for child abuse are covered on 📖 p.434

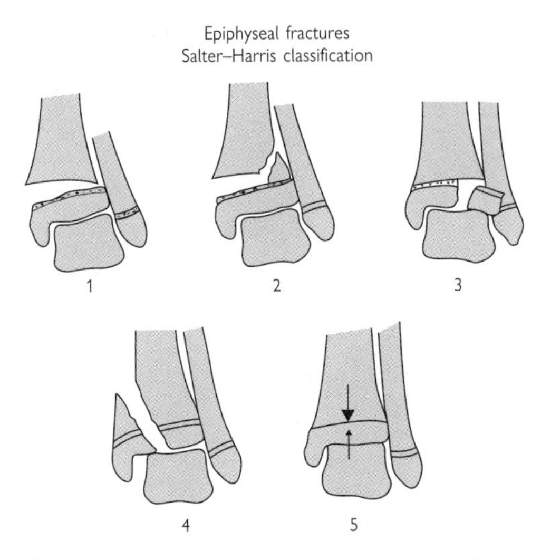

Fig. 6.3 Salter–Harris classification of epiphyseal fractures. (Modified with permission from Salter, R. B. and Harris, W. R. (1963) Injuries involving the epiphyseal plate (AAOS Instructional Course Lecture), in *J. Bone Joint Surg.* volume 45A, American Academy of Orthopedic Surgeons.)

Chapter 7

Environmental conditions

Burns

Burns can be thermal, chemical, or electrical (p.128). The majority are thermal from hot surfaces, fire, or scalding.

Tissue damage from thermal burns is limited by **first aid:** 30 minutes application of cold water within 2 hours of the burn. Treatment with ice is not advised as it exacerbates any skin damage.

A major concern is the possibility of inhalational injury, which increases the risk of mortality. Steam tends to affect the lower airway, whereas smoke can aggravate the upper airway, resulting in obstruction from oedema within minutes. Consequently, special attention must be paid to victims of fires within enclosed spaces, particularly if they are intoxicated or have suffered head injuries.

Do not attempt to distinguish between 1st and 2nd degree burns. The full depth of injury will only become apparent in 72 hours. 3rd degree burns are easily identified as they are painless and the skin is pale and leathery.

Sadly, a further consideration is whether the burn was inflicted, e.g. punitive scalding after failed toilet training. Take a precise history of what happened and note any possible family stressors (p.434).

Management

- ABC with oximetry. Apply oxygen if shocked or SpO_2 <95%.
- Airway is at risk if perioral burns, particles in sputum, loss of vibrissae.
  - Ask to count to 10—progressive dysphonia suggestive of oedema. ***If concern, electively intubate.***
- If shocked, IV access and 20ml/kg normal saline.
  - Bloods: FBC, cross-match, UEC.
  - Try to avoid burnt areas—intraosseous access if necessary.
- Minimize exposure as child will lose heat rapidly through damaged skin, especially after water application. Apply warming blankets and overhead heating lamps if necessary.
- When stable, give adequate analgesia, oral or IV. Catheterize if perineal burns.
- Is further **first aid** necessary?
- Quantify percentage of body surface area (BSA) involved in burn. Do not include erythema. BSA affected by growth—use age-appropriate charts; or compare child's palm and fingers = 1% to area affected.

> Children's fluid requirements increase with burns:
> Maintenance ***plus*** (% BSA x weight (kg) x 4)

- 50% of fluid requirements is given in first 8 hours; the remainder over 16 hours. Cannulate if child cannot drink required amount.
- If burn over 10% BSA:
  - obtain IV access;
  - insert urethral catheter—urine output should be 1ml/kg/h;
  - consider morphine infusion.
- Depict burn on Lund and Browder charts.

Treatment Discuss case with local burns unit. In some units, silver sulphadiazine is being superceded by products that do not require such frequent dressing changes.

Children who require immediate transfer to a burns unit are those with:

- burns over 10% BSA;
- full thickness burns of 5% BSA;
- circumferential burns.

If child is to be followed up at the burns unit, explain to parents that some burns can take several weeks to heal fully, and may require repeated visits to the burns unit. Transport difficulties may require social work involvement.

Before discharge, make sure that there are no child protection issues and provide parents with advice ± medication should further analgesia be required.

Chemical burns Chemical burns are rare and the caustic substance should be brushed off. Water should not be applied in case this exacerbates the reaction with skin. However, if there is eye involvement, irrigation is recommended along with urgent ophthalmology review (📖 p.344).

Bites and stings

Dogs are the usual culprits, but occasionally bites can be from venomous creatures such as insects and snakes (📖 p.121 Envenomation). Human bites can be from a jealous sibling, but can also be a sign of abuse by an adult. Human bites are distinguished as they are semicircular, with an adult bite being over 3cm in diameter (📖 p.434).

Bite wounds are often infected with aerobes and anaerobes. Wounds that are prone to infection, e.g. on hand, are not sutured but are allowed to heal by secondary intention. Many EDs have their own protocols for when to prescribe prophylactic antibiotics. A booster dose of tetanus may be required if there is soil contamination. In addition, certain animals, e.g. bats, carry rabies and prophylactic immunization is warranted.

⑦ Dog bites

Typically with dog bites, the dog has mistaken the child's play for an aggressive act, e.g. bone taken away, face placed near the dog's. Generally, bites are isolated but, occasionally, dogs attack in a frenzy.

Most dogs can puncture skin and the bigger breeds, e.g. rottweiler, can fracture human bones as well.

Management

- Irrigate wound thoroughly—200ml normal saline in 10 or 20ml syringe, with cannula (without needle) mounted on end.
- Lacerations of the hands or feet should not be sutured as there is a high risk of infection. Lacerations of the scalp, neck, or trunk are safe to suture in the ED.
- Surgical review for irrigation ± suturing under GA is necessary if:
  - the child cannot tolerate the above procedures;
  - the wound is deep;
  - there are facial lacerations requiring cosmesis.
- Check tetanus status.
- Bites to the hand require antibiotic treatment. If no ED protocol, seek advice from microbiology, e.g. clindamycin with ciprofloxacin.
- Advise parents about signs of infection and arrange GP review in the next 24 to 48 hours.

Envenomation

Clinicians should know the venomous animals in their area and be familiar with their presentations. Recognition of the snake or spider responsible may be difficult, and antivenom kits exist to facilitate identification.

ⓘ *Bee and wasp stings*

Both venoms can cause irritating local reactions—inflammation with pain and swelling—but are also capable of triggering an anaphylactic reaction (📖 p.62). There is also the toxic reaction—vomiting and diarrhoea followed by fainting. There is no urticaria or bronchospasm, but victims can suddenly suffer respiratory arrest. Observation for several hours is necessary to ensure that deterioration does not occur.

Management

- Remove any barbs.
- Clean sting site to minimize infection.
- Apply ice packs to limit swelling.
- Oral NSAIDS for analgesia and antihistamines for pruritis.

☼ *Poisonous bites*

First aid is crucial: apply a pressure bandage over the bite; wind a bandage proximally to distally to limit systemic spread of the toxin. Occlusion should restrict venous and lymphatic flow, but still enable distal perfusion. Immobilize the limb in a splint and transfer the victim to hospital.

Management

- ABC with IV access. Bloods: FBC, UEC, clotting studies.
- If identification necessary, obtain antivenom kit. Cut hole in pressure bandage above bite site, swab bite, and replace bandage. Perform test without distraction—very easy to get all wells same colour as control!
- Discuss with poisons information service about whether to give anti-venom and what dose is appropriate.
- Antivenom can provoke anaphylactic reactions—adrenaline should be to hand (📖 p.62).

Hypothermia

Babies and young children lose heat rapidly as they have a large surface area compared to their weight. The possibility of hypothermia should be borne in mind during resuscitation, when a child may be unclothed for a prolonged period of time. Septic babies or children suffering near-drowning are particularly at risk.

Hypothermia is defined as a core temperature below 35°C. As the temperature falls further, cerebral metabolism slows so the patient becomes confused then comatose. Ventricular arrhythmias arise when the temperature is below 30°C, but most arrhythmias will revert spontaneously when the patient is rewarmed.

Blood gas machines will warm the sample so that pH is falsely lowered and gas partial pressures are spuriously elevated. However, 'normal' values for hypothermia are not known, so it is easier to use sequential uncorrected blood gas results to assess the response to resuscitation.

Treatment

Temperature above 33°C

- Take core temperature, e.g. rectal.
- Remove cold clothing.
- Wrap in warm blankets ± heating blanket.
- Apply overhead radiant heaters.

Temperature below 33°C Core rewarming necessary as external warming will drive cold peripheral blood centrally resulting in further cooling.

- Use warmed IV fluids ± heated ventilator gases.
- Start bladder or peritoneal lavage with warmed saline.
- Use blood rewarmer.

If asystole or ventricular fibrillation:

- start CPR.
- give one shock.
- if no response, rewarm to over 30°C before delivering further shock.
- most drugs are ineffective—lignocaine may be helpful.

Hyperthermia

Hyperthermia is defined as a core temperature above 41°C. Adolescents are the most susceptible as they may exercise excessively in humid conditions or else overdose on medications such as SSRIs or ecstacy. Sadly, young children who have been left in cars on hot days may also present.

ⓘ Heat exhaustion

The patient feels weak and dizzy and may vomit or faint. On examination, the temperature is 39–41°C and the child is very sweaty. There is no altered level of consciousness.

Management

- Ask what fluids have been taken:
  - if none = water depletion ± hypernatraemia;
  - if water = salt depletion ± hyponatraemia.
- Place in a cool environment.
- IV access: UEC.
- Rehydrate with normal saline. Rehydrate over 24 hours if hypernatraemia (📖 p.444).

Heat stroke

Heat stroke is hyperthermia with altered mentation. The skin may be sweaty or dry as thermoregulation fails. Heat stroke may be life-threatening because of rhabdomyolysis, renal and hepatic failure, and DIC.

Management

- ABC with regular assessment of core temperature.
- Continuous cardiac monitoring and ECG.
- Start active cooling, e.g. ice packs in axilla and groin, spray water on the skin, place patient on cooling blanket.
- IV access: UEC, LFT, CK, FBC, clotting studies, blood cultures.
- Rehydrate starting with 20ml/kg bolus of normal saline. Monitor sodium and potassium.
- Urinary catheterization. Check urine for myoglobin (positive for blood on dipstick, negative on microscopy).
- Consider using benzodiazepines to stop shivering.
- Admit to PICU.

Hyperthermia secondary to medications

Hyperthermia can be found with:

- malignant hyperthermia—succinyl choline. Usually family history of GA reactions. Avoid using suxamethonium in myopathies;
- neuroleptic malignant syndrome—chlorpromazine, respiridone;
- serotonin syndrome—SSRIs, ecstacy (📖 p.164, 📖 p.170);
- anticholinergic overdose—tricyclic antidepressants, antihistamines (📖 p.162, 📖 p.166).

The first three have fever with muscle rigidity and may progress to heat stroke.

Drowning

By the time of presentation at hospital, children have usually received basic life support. If resuscitation is still required, many children will survive neurologically intact so try not to despair!

Cold water may result in hypothermia, which complicates resuscitation, e.g. increases chances of arrhythmias, but, paradoxically, increases the chances of intact survival by slowing physiological processes and thus preserving organ function.

From witnesses and ambulance crew:

- estimate period of immersion;
- determine whether immersion in salt or fresh water;
- find out whether child has responded to resuscitation attempts, e.g. gasp.

Management

If immersion transient and child well, check oxygen saturations. If OK, consider discharge. If child well despite significant immersion, observe for 4 hours. Discharge if saturations fine and parents able to return if deterioration at home.

If child is hypoxic, apply oxygen until saturations improve. Most children will diurese any inhaled water, but some will require admission because of pneumonitis from inhaled particulate matter.

If child unwell on presentation

- ABC with cervical spine precautions if diving accident.
  - If intubation necessary, apply cricoid pressure to reduce chance of aspiration. Once ETT *in situ*, insert NG tube and aspirate stomach contents.
- Apply 100% oxygen.
- IV access: FBC, UEC, glucose, blood gas, blood cultures.
  - Rarely, freshwater immersion causes electrolyte anomalies and haemolysis, which require correction.
- Consider starting IV antibiotics, e.g. cefotaxime.
- Obtain rectal temperature.
- Check for trauma, e.g. head injuries.
- When stable, obtain CXR ± cervical spine films.
- If symptomatic after 4 hours, repeat CXR.

Treatment

If hypothermic, see 📖 p.122.

CPR is only discontinued if ***all*** of the following criteria apply:

- no response after 40 minutes of full resuscitation ***and***
- core temperature is over 33°C ***and***
- blood pH <7 ***and***
- consultant and parents agree to withdrawal of care

Electrocution

Fortunately, low voltage electrocutions (under 600V) are declining since the introduction of circuit breakers to domestic supply (220V). However, injuries from high voltage still occur, e.g. lightning strike, playing near substations. The type of current influences the injuries seen: direct current such as lightning expels the victim from the source, with possible resultant trauma such as fractures; alternating current, e.g. domestic supply can cause muscular tetany, increasing the duration of exposure to the current.

Skin has moderate resistance to electricity but this is lowered if the skin is broken or moist. Once through the skin, electricity is conducted primarily along nerves and blood vessels. The power of the current generates heat, causing burns to surrounding structures. The intensity of the burn is heightened if heat dissipates through a small cross-sectional area, e.g. digit. The current will head to earth so all organs along its route may be damaged.

Long-term sequelae, e.g. contractures, paralysis, neuralgia, are secondary to the ischaemic effect of the burn. These potential complications necessitate that all children with electrical injuries are followed up.

Management

- Determine whether high or low voltage, i.e. over or under 600V.
- Determine type of current: AC or DC.
- Determine pathway of current.

Treatment

- If high voltage, ABC with cervical spine precautions if indicated.
- ECG then continuous cardiac monitoring if:
  - high voltage injury;
  - concerning symptoms or signs, e.g. loss of consciousness, palpitations, chest pain, confusion;
  - transthoracic pathway.
- IV access if:
  - high voltage injury;
  - trauma;
  - extensive burns.

Avoid siting IV in extremity with burn as there may be vascular damage, limiting fluid resuscitation. N.B. Fluid requirement in major electrical burns is higher than in thermal burns. (📖 p.118).

- Take blood for FBC, UEC, LFT, CK ± amylase.
- Check urine for myoglobinuria—positive dipstick for blood; negative on microscopy.
- Look for current's entry and exit points.
  - Circular greyish burn with black punctum in centre.
  - Assess for neurovascular compromise of surrounding tissue.

Admit if

- Cardiac monitoring required for over 24 hours.
  - high voltage injury;
  - vertical pathway;
  - unconscious at scene, palpitations;
  - abnormal ECG.
- Cutaneous burn requiring circulation observations.
- Home still unsafe.

All burns should be discussed with the surgical team before discharge home, and the appropriate follow-up arranged.

Children with oral burns can be discharged as long as they can drink. Parents should be warned that the wound may bleed and that pressure should be applied. The wound should be reviewed within 24 hours and follow-up with plastics arranged, as strictures can develop.

The majority of children will be fit for discharge home. Arrange follow-up with their GP or paediatrician.

Altitude

Paediatricians who live near mountains should be familiar with the manifestations of high altitude illnesses. As most resolve with descent, they are seldom seen elsewhere. Children are particularly vulnerable to the effects of altitude.

Altitude acclimatization is necessary for all climbs above 8000ft (2480m), when arterial oxygen saturations will be below 90%. It is recommended that one should only climb 1000ft (305m) a day, falling to 500ft (150m) a day after 14 000ft (4265m). Acetazolamide (Diamox®) 5mg/kg/dose bd can facilitate acclimatization.

ⓘ Acute mountain sickness

The key symptoms are due to hypoxia:
- throbbing headache—particularly on waking, at night or after exertion;
- lassitude, weakness;
- sleep disturbance with sleep apnoea;
- shortness of breath;
- dizziness and vomiting.

If the patient rests, the symptoms should resolve within days. However, if this does not occur or if there is worsening mentation, descent to 3000ft (915m) must occur. If this is not immediately possible, supplementary oxygen will be required. Headaches can be treated with paracetamol and any vomiting with prochlorperazine, which may also be beneficial by increasing respiratory drive.

High altitude pulmonary oedema

Pulmonary hypertension secondary to hypoxia, in combination with altitude-induced fluid retention, results in pulmonary oedema. Children are particularly prone to this illness, exacerbated by their difficulty in acclimatization and susceptibility to viral URTIs.

The symptoms include a dry cough, fatiguability, and shortness of breath on exertion. Overlooking the innocuous initial symptoms may be fatal. If the child remains at altitude, there is increasing respiratory compromise with confusion as hypoxia and cerebral oedema worsen.

Treatment involves descent with minimal exertion and supplemental oxygen. Ventilatory support may be required.

High altitude cerebral odema

Initially, this may appear similar to acute mountain sickness, but it progresses to confusion, and ataxia, especially truncal. Diplopia may also be reported as ocular nerve palsies develop. Treatment should not be delayed.
- Begin descent.
- Apply oxygen.
- Give IV dexamethasone 4mg qds.
- Intubation and hyperventilation may be required to reduce ICP. IV mannitol and frusemide can help.

Diving

Few children are certified scuba divers so such presentations are rare.

? Barotrauma

Gases in the body's air-filled spaces, e.g. sinuses, GI tract, increase in volume as the diver descends, and resume their usual volume on ascent. To prevent damage, equalization, e.g. swallowing to clear Eustachian tube, burping, or passing flatus, should be performed during the dive. The common areas affected are the following.

- Middle ear—pain in the ear ± disorientation, transient hearing loss. Tympanic membrane may rupture.
  - Treatment—analgesics and decongestants. If tympanic membrane ruptured, treat with oral augmentin for 10 days and no further diving until ENT review to confirm that membrane healed.
- Sinuses—usually the frontal and maxillary sinus affected. Very painful with possible bloody nasal discharge.
  - Treatment—analgesia and augmentin for at least 2 weeks.

Air embolism

Air may enter the systemic circulation from the pulmonary veins. The patient is symptomatic within 20 minutes of surfacing. The brain is affected most frequently with resultant stroke-like manifestations.

Treatment 100% oxygen, IV fluids, and hyperbaric treatment. N.B. Before placing in hyperbaric chamber, perform CXR to exclude pneumothorax, pneumopericardium as source of embolus. If present, insert drainage catheters. If urinary catheter inserted, ensure balloon inflated with water.

Decompression sickness

As the dive progresses, inhaled nitrogen is absorbed into the blood and then into body fat. A gradual ascent will ensure that the nitrogen dissolves back into the blood and is thence exhaled. If this equilibration does not occur, then the nitrogen forms bubbles in the blood during the ascent. The complications include:

- 'the bends'—throbbing pain around joints with possible paraesthesiae within 12 hours of resurfacing. Classically involves knees, shoulders, and elbows.
- 'the chokes'—a feeling of suffocation, chest pain worsened on inspiration, paroxysmal cough. There is no radiation to the neck or arms so is not to be confused with a cardiac event.
- cerebral—may resemble air embolism but present 1–6 hours after surfacing. Children may report headaches—usually unilateral; visual disturbances, e.g. lines—usually contralateral to headaches. Parents may notice that the child is confused and has memory loss.
- spinal—back pain with weakness and paralysis in distal extremities.

Treatment 100% oxygen, IV fluids, hyperbaric treatment.

Chapter 8

Febrile illness

Assessment

The majority of paediatric infections are self-limiting viral illnesses. However, serious bacterial infections may resemble viral illness, e.g. pneumococcal sepsis presenting with fever, vomiting, and diarrhoea. Distinguishing viral from serious bacterial infection requires clinical acumen and judicious use of investigations.

When assessing a febrile child, take into account the age of the child and their immune status as these influence the child's susceptibility to particular infective agents. The examination is to assess whether there is:
- shock;
- a focus for the infection.

History

From when the child was last completely well. Allow parent/child to describe the symptoms, but ensure you ask about the following.
- Fever—duration, any rigors (📖 p.137)?
- Cough or breathlessness—is the cough paroxysmal (whooping cough)? Is there recession?
- Diarrhoea—is there blood or mucus?
- Vomiting—is there blood or bile?
- Rash—how long has it been there, where did it start, and where did it spread to?
- Headache—worse when supine; early morning or night-time is worrying (raised ICP).
- Photophobia—or just prefers a dark room?
- Neck stiffness—sore or stiff?
- Fluid intake—less than a third of normal is worrying.
- Urine output—no wet nappies for >8 hours is suggestive of dehydration (but nappies are very absorptive and small amounts easily missed).
- Alertness—does the baby watch mum? Any smiles? Any altered level of consciousness?
- Colour—blue around mouth and pallor are common and may not be significant. Blue lips are.

Other relevant questions include:
- Anyone else ill at home or play group/school?
- Any exotic travel?
- Any contact with animals, e.g. pets, farm.

Risk factors

- Age—infants under 3 months, especially if premature.
- Immune status—steroid use, parents at risk of HIV infection, chronic illness, e.g. diabetes, asthma, eczema.
- Functional asplenia, e.g. splenectomy or sickle cell disease.
- Deficiencies in complement factors, e.g. properdin.

Examination

- ABC—exclude warm shock (📖 p.92). Record BP.
- Full examination, including skin and joints. Palpate spine (discitis).
- Exclude meningitis—palpate fontanelle in infants under 18 months. Otherwise try to elicit Kernig's sign—flex the hip and knee to 90°. Any attempt to straighten leg produces severe pain as sciatic nerve stretched. Brudzinski's sign is positive when flexion of child's neck causes them to flex leg. Both are suggestive of meningeal inflammation.

Investigations

Only do tests that will alter management. For example, looking for bugs in the stool of most children with diarrhoea is only relevant if the child is to be admitted or if you suspect a notifiable disease. If there is no obvious focus on examination, then investigation is mandatory.

- Blood—FBC, blood cultures must be obtained before IV antibiotics given.
  - Blood film—thick/thin if considering malaria.
  - UEC, LFT, if underlying disease or prior to starting IV antibiotics such as gentamicin or flucloxacillin.
  - Glucose—particularly in babies
  - Acute phase proteins (CRP ± ESR and, in near future, pro-calcitonin). Absolute number is not indicative of severity of infection and there may be a lag. A rising APP suggests worsening inflammation and is of most use in surveillance of chronic infections, e.g. osteomyelitis, septic arthritis, as well as in chronic inflammatory conditions, e.g. JIA.
- Urine—dipstick for leucocytes and nitrites; culture if positive for either, but not if negative. N.B. Method of collection is critical (📖 p.254). (Mild proteinuria or haematuria in a febrile child is unlikely to be significant.)
- Radiology—CXR if focal respiratory signs or if febrile with no focus, yet tachypnoeic. Generalized wheeze is more suggestive (but not diagnostic) of a viral infection.
- Lumbar puncture—can be delayed in the very sick, but must be considered whenever there is no focus of infection. Obligatory in those under 3 months with an unexplained fever.

Management

- If there is shock, summon senior assistance.
- Apply oxygen and obtain immediate IV access.
- Take blood for cultures before giving IV antibiotics.
- Give bolus of 20ml/kg 0.9% saline and start IV antibiotics (Table 8.1).
- Review response; a further bolus may be required.
- Arrange admission in HDU/PICU.

If a focus is evident, see relevant section:

- meningitis (📖 p.138);
- encephalitis (📖 p.142);
- pneumonia (📖 p.224);
- UTI (📖 p.330);
- ENT (📖 pp.308, 312, 318);
- septic arthritis/osteomyelitis (📖 p.330);
- periorbital cellulitis (📖 p.349).

If no focus is evident, see 📖 p.144

Table 8.1 Suggested empirical antibiotic therapy according to age

Age of child	**Common causes**	**Empirical antibiotic choice (📖 p.496)**
<1mo	Group B Streptococcus *Escherichia coli* *Listeria monocytogenes*	Cefotaxime or ceftriaxone ***plus*** ampicillin ± gentamicin
1–3mo	*Neisseria meningitidis* *Haemophilus influenzae* *Streptococcus pneumoniae* Group B Streptococcus *Escherichia coli* *Listeria monocytogenes*	Cefotaxime or ceftriaxone ***plus*** ampicillin
3mo–5y	*Neisseria meningitidis* *Streptococcus pneumoniae* *Haemophilus influenzae*	Ceftriaxone or cefotaxime
>5y	*Neisseria meningitidis* *Streptococcus pneumoniae*	Ceftriaxone or cefotaxime

Rigors

Violent shivering associated with fever secondary to bacteraemia or viraemia. Seen in:

- UTI with pyelonephritis;
- lower lobe pneumonia;
- ascending cholangitis;
- central venous (Hickman) line infection—often following line being flushed;
- malaria.

Ensure that the carer/child is describing the shivering of a rigor, rather than a (febrile) fit, i.e. no incontinence, alert when the rigor ceases. Rigors will cease if hand is laid on the limb; seizures will not.

Manage according to the focus of the infection. If none evident, treat as fever without focus (📖 p.144).

Meningitis

The typical presentation in older children is neck stiffness, photophobia, headache, ± reduced consciousness. However, not all of these symptoms may be present and the diagnosis should always be considered if there is no focus for the child's fever. Babies may have non-specific symptoms, e.g. reluctance to feed, lethargy, and may be hypothermic rather than febrile. Viral meningitis has a more gradual onset and is seldom associated with shock.

History

As described on p.134—particularly note the speed of onset, any symptoms suggestive of photophobia, raised ICP, or altered consciousness, and whether any rash is present. It is also useful to know if there has been any preceding antibiotic therapy, e.g. IM penicillin, oral Augmentin which may influence LP results.

Examination

- ABC including BP—document vital signs; exclude shock.
- Assess the level of consciousness (AVPU p.520).
- Note any rash. Petechiae can arise with viruses (e.g. enterovirus). Meningococcaemia typically causes petechiae or purpura, but can also be macular.
- Assess fontanelle in children under 18 months and neck stiffness in older children. Is Kernig's sign positive? (p.135)
- Fundoscopy to exclude raised ICP.

Investigations

Blood—FBC, blood culture, UEC, glucose, LFT, acute phase proteins (CRP or ESR), clotting, meningococcal PCR, and pneumococcal antigen (± virology).

- Lumbar puncture (p.470)—***not*** if GCS <13 or coagulopathy or platelets <50 × 10^9/l.
  - CSF for Gram stain, cell count, protein, and glucose; PCR for meningococcus and herpes ± opening pressure.
- Gram stain of swab from skin lesion.
- Throat swab—will grow meningococcus in 40% even after antibiotics.

See Table 8.2 for CSF findings.

Treatment

- ABC—intubate if GCS <8 or unresponsive to pain.
- If shocked ± rash, apply oxygen and give IV 0.9% saline 20ml/kg bolus. Summon senior help.
  - Children with meningococcaemia may require massive volumes (100ml/kg) and can deteriorate rapidly. Ventilatory ± inotropic support is often necessary. Admit to HDU or PICU until child improving.
- If signs of meningitis, but no rash, consider steroids prior to antibiotics to improve CSF penetration—IV dexamethasone 0.2mg/kg/dose qds for 2 days or 0.4mg/kg/dose bd (no difference in efficacy).
- Start antibiotics promptly (see Table 8.1)
  - Consider adding vancomycin if *S. pneumoniae* likely.
  - IM ceftriaxone 50mg/kg daily is useful if IV access difficult.
  - Once *Neisseria* confirmed, change to penicillin and await sensitivities (resistance very rare).
- Consider acyclovir if the history is less acute (see encephalitis 📖 p.142).
- Notifiable disease (📖 p.156).
- Don't forget the rest of the family—public health arrange prophylaxis for close contacts, but may ask you to prescribe (see box).

Meningococcal prophylaxis to prevent secondary cases

- Rifampicin
  - Neonate–1 year: 5mg/kg bd for 2 days
  - 1–12 years: 10mg/kg (maximum 600mg) bd for 2 days PO
  - 12–18 years: 600mg bd for 2 days PO

Or

- Ciprofloxacin (unlicensed indication)
  - 5–12 years: 250mg once PO
  - 12–18 years: 500mg once PO

If pregnant, use

- Ceftriaxone (unlicensed indication)
  - 12–18 years: 250mg once **IM**

Table 8.2 CSF values

	Normal		Bacterial meningitis			
	Child	**Newborn**	**Untreated**	**Partially treated**	**Viral meningitis**	**Tuberculous meningitis**
Appearance	'Gin' clear	'Gin' clear	Turbid	Clear or turbid	Often clear	Cloudy
Polymorphs (cells/ml)[*]	0	0–10[†]	>10–10 000	10–1000	5–500 in early stages	>10–10 000
Lymphocytes (cells/ml)[*]	0–6	0–30	0–20	10–1000	10–1000	10–1000
Gram stain	Absent	Absent	Often see organism	Rarely see organism	No organisms	May see AAFB on ZN stain
Glucose (mmol/l)	2.5–4	>1[‡]	<2/3 blood level	Low or normal	>2/3 of blood level	Very low
Protein (g/l)	0.15–0.5	0.61–2.0[§]	0.5–4	0.15–0.5	<1.0	1–6

* May be up to 100/ml if intracranial haemorrhage. Will be associated with CSF glucose <1mmol/l.

† If traumatic tap, calculate from peripheral blood ratio of red to white cells. Approximately 1:500 white to red cells. If in doubt, treat as significant. Xanthochromia suggests old intracranial haemorrhage.

‡ Must compare to blood sugar.

§ Up to 3 in pre-term infant.

Encephalitis

Clinical manifestations can range from mild lethargy to acute changes in personality or behaviour to altered consciousness and seizures. The child may not be febrile, e.g. reactivation of latent herpes, and may have generalized or focal neurological signs, which can even fluctuate! Viral infections are the principal cause, but the possibility of bacterial infection, e.g. *Mycoplasma*, or drug ingestion, e.g. antihistamines, should be considered.

Other relevant sections: altered level of consciousness (📖 p.290); acute confusional state (📖 p.424).

History

Key factors in the history include:

- meningeal irritation—vomiting, neck pain/stiffness, photophobia;
- behavioural change—emotional lability, delirium;
- neurological symptoms—seizures that may be focal; loss of bowel and bladder control; altered consciousness, e.g. confusion, coma.

These symptoms may be constant but can fluctuate and also progress. The diagnosis should not be discounted if the child is afebrile.

Risk factors for encephalitis include the following.

- Recent illness, e.g. sore throat, or exposure to ill contacts.
- Ask specifically about previous herpes exposure—cold sores on carers, previous herpes stomatitis.
- Occupation, e.g. agriculture, work involving exposure to toxic chemicals.
- Recent travel, e.g. tick or mosquito bite.
- Medications—taken by patient or other family members, recreational.
- Immunocompromised—note immunization status, chemotherapy or steroid use, risk factors for HIV.

Examination

- ABC with AVPU. Intubate if GCS <8 or unresponsive to pain.
- Exclude raised ICP—Cushing's triad of bradycardia, hypertension, and irregular respiration. Papilloedema is a late sign.
- Are there focal neurological signs?
- Any sign of rash or bites (check behind the ear for tick bites—if the tick still there, remove with tweezers and keep for identification).

Investigations

Blood, urine, CSF must be obtained and cranial imaging is necessary.

- Blood.
  - FBC, film (sickle and malaria), clotting.
  - UEC, LFT, glucose, calcium, magnesium, phosphate ± ammonia, lactate (requires special bottles and lab notification).
  - Cultures and serology—*Mycoplasma* and viral.
  - If possibility of inborn error—amino acids, TFT, biotinidase in fitting infant.
  - If possibility of toxic ingestion—lead level, ethanol (📖 p.166, p.168).
  - If immunocompromised or failure to thrive—HIV test and immunoglobulins.

- Urine.
  - Urinalysis for ketones.
  - Culture. Consider CMV PCR and viral culture.
  - Metabolic screen—organic acids.
  - If possibility of toxic ingestion—specifically request barbiturates, benzodiazepines, tricyclics, salicylates, iron, lead, anticonvulsants, anti-epileptics.
- Lumbar puncture if no contraindications.
  - Opening pressure.
  - CSF for glucose, protein, lactate.
  - Microscopy and stains for bacteria, fungi, AAFB. Prolonged culture may be warranted.
  - PCR for HSV, VZV, enterovirus, CMV, *Mycoplasma*, EBV.
- Stool culture—bacterial, viral.
- Throat swab—bacterial, viral.
- NPA—Influenza A, B.
- Cranial imaging—CT or MRI with contrast.

Treatment

- Start hourly neurological observations until GCS >13.

It is difficult to be certain whether a bacterial or viral illness is responsible, so initially both are treated until cultures are available.

- Cefotaxime or ceftriaxone.
  - Add erythromycin if *Mycoplasma* is likely.
  - Add ampicillin if <3 months and risk of *Listeria*.
  - Add vancomycin where strains of *S. pneumoniae* resistant to penicillin/cephalosporins.
- Acyclovir when HSV encephalitis is suspected.
  - Ganciclovir if CMV is suspected.
- Notifiable disease (📖 p.156).

Most patients completely recover from viral encephalitis. However, the prognosis is poor if:

- the child is under 3 months;
- there is parenchymal involvement on cranial imaging.

Potential deficits include intellectual, motor, psychiatric, epileptic, visual, and auditory abnormalities.

ⓘ Fever without focus

- Fever is defined as axillary temperature over 38°C
- A response to anti-pyretics does not indicate whether the infection is due to a virus or a bacterium
- Antibiotic therapy for fever without focus should ***never*** be instigated without performing investigations

The majority of children with fever without focus have viral illnesses. However, children under the age of 4 years can have a serious bacterial infection without clinical signs. The commonest bacterial pathogen is *S. pneumoniae* and around 2% of children with occult pneumococcal bacteraemia will develop meningitis. Thus, faced with a child with a fever without focus, it is important to distinguish between viral illness and an infection with potentially severe sequelae. This requires a thorough history and examination (📖 p.134) and investigations if necessary.

Under 3 months

Sepsis in infants may have subtle manifestations, e.g. reduced feeds, more sleepy than usual. Even if they appear 'too well', any febrile infant without an obvious focus of infection requires a full septic work-up.
- FBC, blood cultures.
- Urine—a sample obtained by suprapubic aspirate is optimal (📖 p.472).
- Lumbar puncture—this can be deferred if child too unwell, but should not be omitted. Even after antibiotic therapy, CSF can be sent for PCR to identify pathogens.

If very unwell, take a blood culture immediately on presentation then start antibiotics (Table 8.1). If access difficult, give IM ceftriaxone.

No investigation can confirm occult bacteraemia within hours—the role of CRP and pro-calcitonin is still being evaluated. The risk of bacterial sepsis is increased—but still remains low—if the white cell count is >15 000/l. If the WCC is over this threshold, IV antibiotics are started until the results of all cultures are known.

Over 3 months

Older children are more likely to appear toxic with occult bacteraemia. So one can be more confident in not investigating the well-looking child.

If concerns remain, some hospitals have the facilities to observe the children overnight to see if the clinical picture evolves. Where prolonged observation is not possible, investigation may be helpful.
- FBC, blood cultures.
- Urine—a sample obtained by suprapubic aspirate is optimal (📖 p.472).
- Lumbar puncture if clinical suspicion. However, have a low threshold for full septic screen in babies under 6 months.

If WCC >15 000/l, IV antibiotics are started until the results of all cultures are known (Table 8.1).

If there has been no change in the clinical picture ***and*** WCC is under 15 000/l ***and*** urine microscopy is normal, the child can be discharged home. However, any child discharged home must have easy access to medical review if there is any deterioration—it is important to tell the carers what to look out for and document that advice. Moreover, the carers should be advised to have the child reviewed by the GP ***daily*** until the child is improving. If possible, arrange appointment with the GP before the family goes home.

ⓘ Rashes

Exanthems are acute viral rashes and are common in young children. They usually are comprised of pink macules, but can be any shape or size. As a general rule, these eruptions fade as rapidly as they came, and no specific investigation or treatment is necessary.

History

- When rash first started.
- Evolution of rash—where did it start and progress to?
- Any itchiness.
- Any associated symptoms suggestive of systemic illness.
- Any recent contact with infection or travel abroad?
- Are there allergies or pets, i.e. flea bites?
- Is it recurrent, e.g. infected eczema, urticaria?
- Has the child taken any drugs—medicinal or recreational?

Examination

- Describe the lesion (📖 p.394).
- Examine the mouth, fingers, genitalia, and toes for peeling or ulceration.
- Is there hepatosplenomegaly—Glandular fever?
- Are there secondary lesions of lichenification or excoriation?
  A few can be identified on clinical grounds alone.
- **HHV6**—three days of high fever (>38.5°C); then suddenly afebrile with appearance of generalized morbilliform rash. Patient should avoid contact with pregnant women and patients with haematological disorders, as can precipitate miscarriage and aplastic crises, respectively.
- **Coxsackie**—erosions on palms, soles, and palate ('hand, foot, mouth'). Not vesicular and no gum or tongue involvement as in herpes.
- **Measles**—morbilliform rash that appears behind ears, then on face then on trunk. Lesions coalesce and become coppery in colour. Remember the '4 Cs'.
  - Cranky child.
  - Coryzal.
  - Conjunctivitis.
  - Cough.

Koplik spots resemble grains of rice and appear on the inner cheek wall during the first 4 days of the illness. Notifiable disease (📖 p.156).

- **Rubella**—morbilliform rash that migrates like measles but original lesions fade. Often associated with lymph nodes in occipital triangle. Notifiable disease (📖 p.156); patient should avoid contact with pregnant women.
- **Scarlet fever**—caused by erythrogenic toxin from *Streptococcus pyogenes*. Deep red, generalized rash on day 1, which feels like sandpaper. Often circum-oral pallor and a white, furred 'strawberry' tongue. Fever settles after day 2 if treated, or persists for 3–4 days. Tongue changes to red colour, often with petechiae on palate.

Other diagnoses for febrile children with exanthematous rashes include:

- acute rheumatic fever (📖 p.187);
- Kawasaki's disease (📖 p.190);
- Still's disease (📖 p.334).

Immunodeficient child with a fever

Immunodeficiency should be suspected if the child either suffers recurrent infections from mundane pathogens, or else is susceptible to unusual pathogens. Consider too, in failure to thrive. The defect in the immune system influences the susceptibility:

- neutrophil abnormalities, e.g. newly diagnosed ALL (Table 8.3);
- antibody abnormalities, e.g. splenectomy, nephrotic syndrome, protein-losing enteropathies (Table 8.4);
- cell-mediated immune deficiency, e.g. HIV/AIDS (Table 8.5).

Primary immunodeficiencies are rare and tend to present during infancy.

- Defects in specific immunity:
  - lymphocyte function (B-cells and T-cells);
  - antibody production.
- Defects in non-specific immunity:
  - abnormal neutrophil function—delay in shedding umbilical cord, e.g. impaired chemotaxis; generalized pustulosis, e.g. chronic granulomatous disease;
  - complement deficiency—recurrent meningococcaemia, e.g. factor B deficiency.

The other major cause of lowered immunocompetence is medication. The commonest is steroids: >2mg/kg/d for more than a week. Others include:

- carbamazepine, sulphalsalazine, co-trimoxazole, procainamide, phenothiazines;
- rarely, NSAIDS (diclofenac), benzodiazepines, barbiturate, sulphonamides, penicillins, and cephalosporins.

Whenever an immunodeficient state is suspected, remember that signs of infection may be absent or attenuated, so a low threshold for investigation and treatment is necessary,

History

As described on p.134, ask about risk factors in child and parents.

- Age—infants under 3 months, especially if premature.
- Immune status—steroid use, parents at risk of HIV infection, chronic illness, e.g. diabetes, asthma, eczema.
- Family history of unexplained infant death and unusual or recurrent infections.
- Ask specifically about VZV exposure and any contact with an adult with chronic cough (TB).

Examination should include joints, skin, mucous membranes, fundi, and growth.

Investigations

If immunodeficiency suspected:

- blood cultures, FBC, CRP, UEC, LFT;
- as directed by likely pathogens (Tables 8.3–8.5), e.g. NPA, urine, stool, LP—liaise with microbiology;
- start broad spectrum antibiotics without waiting for results.

Table 8.3 Pathogens associated with neutrophil abnormalities

	Pathogens	Empirical therapy
Bacteria	Staphylococci, Gram-negative bacilli (*E. coli*, *Pseudomonas*)	Anti-pseudomonal B-lactam, e.g. piperacillin, or ceftazadime ***plus*** aminoglycoside, or single agent, meropenem
Fungi	*Candida*, *Aspergillus*	Amphotericin, if febrile after 48 hours

Table 8.4 Pathogens associated with antibody abnormalities

	Pathogens	Empirical therapy
Bacteria	Encapsulated organisms, e.g. Streptococci, *Haemophilus*, Gram-negative bacilli	Ceftriaxone or augmentin ± immunoglobulin infusion
Protozoa	*Giardia lamblia*	Metronidazole or tinidazole
Viruses	Enteroviruses	Pleconaril

Table 8.5 Pathogens associated with abnormal cell-mediated immunity

	Pathogens	Empirical therapy
Bacteria	Intracellular organisms—*Salmonella*, *Listeria*, *Mycobacterium*, *Legionella*	If neutropenic, then as per neutrophil abnormalities; if not, as per antibody deficiency
Protozoa	*Cryptosporidium*, *Toxoplasma*	Paramomycin, spiramycin
Viruses	Herpes (HSV, VSV, CMV, EBV) RSV, adenovirus, influenza	Acyclovir, ganciclovir, Foscarnet
Fungi	*Candida*, *Aspergillus*, *Pneumocystis*, *Cryptosporidium*	Co-trimoxazole
Helminths	*Strongyloides*	Thiobendazole

? Protracted fever

The textbook definition is having a temperature above 38°C for 3 weeks, but most parents become anxious if the fever has not resolved after 5 days. The common illnesses are viral, e.g. infectious mononucleosis, but remember to exclude Kawasaki disease (📖 p.190).

Causes of protracted fever include:

- infection, e.g. EBV, endocarditis:
  - Occult abscess—brain, liver, kidney, bone;
- immunodeficiency, especially HIV. (N.B. At risk of fungal infection.);
- inflammatory disease, e.g. Kawasaki's, juvenile idiopathic arthritis (JIA);
- tumour, e.g. lymphoma, atrial myxoma;
- CNS white matter disorders, e.g. Krabbe's;
- complications after surgery:
  - recent, e.g. pus in peritoneal cavity post-appendicectomy;
  - modified anatomy, e.g. ascending cholangitis post-Kasai's.
- medication, e.g. phenytoin;
- rarities—familial Mediterranean fever[1] (FMF), thyroiditis, pulmonary emboli.

Ask about:

- associated features, e.g. cough, diarrhoea;
- any rashes;
- any joint swelling—JIA, lupus, rheumatic fever;
- any weight loss;
- unwell contacts, e.g. glandular fever at school, elderly relatives with chronic cough (tuberculosis);
- overseas travel ***in the past year***, including stopovers—malaria may have a long incubation period;
- family and social history—assess likelihood of HIV, FMF.

Examination Note any rashes, joint swelling, lymphadenopathy. Murmur necessitates investigations to exclude endocarditis (📖 p.188).

> Make certain that you have excluded Kawasaki disease

Investigations If child is known to be immunodeficient, discuss what investigations to perform with child's consultant.

If no cause is evident, check:

- blood—FBC + film, blood culture, ESR, CRP, LFT, TFT, serology for EBV, CMV;
- urine—dipstick and culture and PCR for CMV.

If a diagnosis cannot be made, admission is not obligatory but close follow-up is mandatory, whether by GP or paediatrician.

The following sections cover 3 infectious causes of protracted fever:

- infectious mononucleosis;
- malaria;
- tuberculosis (TB).

1 Familial Mediterranean fever is a hereditary condition, typified by recurrent episodes of fever with serositis, i.e. abdominal or joint pain.

Infectious mononucleosis is included as it is frequently encountered, and malaria and TB are prevalent notifiable diseases not discussed elsewhere in this book.

ⓘ Infectious mononucleosis

Caused by either Epstein–Barr virus or cytomegalovirus. Adolescents more profoundly affected than younger children. Symptoms include:

- pharyngitis, which may be severe;
- malaise;
- lymphadenopathy ± hepatosplenomegaly;
- rash—only in 10%; can be maculo-papular or petechiae. N.B. 90% develop a contiguous rash if started on ampicillin.

  Confirm by:
- FBC—may show lymphocytosis with atypical lymphocytes;
- IgM serology for EBV and CMV;
- monospot test.

Treatment is symptomatic, e.g. local anaesthetic spray/lozenges for throat to encourage oral fluids. Emphazise importance of: minimizing exercise as at risk of developing prolonged post-viral fatigue; complete avoidance of alcohol.

ⓘ Malaria

Should be considered in the febrile traveller. Incubation period can vary from a week to up to a year!

Plasmodium falciparum is responsible for the majority of cases and causes the life-threatening complications such as renal failure, DIC, and cerebral manifestations such as seizure, delirium, and coma.

The symptoms and signs are varied and do not help distinguish the causative species. Symptoms may include: fever, headache, myalgia, cough, diarrhoea, vomiting, jaundice, or abdominal or joint pain. The fever and rigors may be intermittent (especially in *P. vivax/ovale/malariae*), but are rarely the textbook tertian/quartan periodicity.

History Enquire about travel in the past year, including stopovers. Exactly what prophylaxis was taken and for how long? Were any over-the-counter drugs taken? Has there been a change in the level of consciousness?

Examination
- ABC—reduced level of consciousness is an ominous sign.
- Skin—pallor (anaemia); jaundice (haemolysis); bleeding (DIC).
- Massive splenomegaly—tropical splenomegaly syndrome also includes pancytopenia and hyper-IgM with *P. falciparum*.
- Oedema—*P. malariae* can trigger nephrotic syndrome.
- Full neurological exam—focal signs are poor prognostic indicators.

Investigation

Check the blood sugar—malaria and quinine treatment both cause hypoglycaemia, which must be corrected immediately (📖 p.413).
- FBC and thick and thin films. Three films needed to exclude diagnosis, ideally taken as fever rises, i.e. when parasites are shed.
- UEC, LFT, glucose.
- Urgent screen for glucose-6-phosphate dehydrogenase (G6PD) deficiency—primaquine may precipitate haemolysis in deficient individuals.
- Clotting.
- Dipstick urine—exclude haemoglobinuria ('Blackwater fever').

Treatment
- If shock, apply oxygen and give 20ml/kg 0.9% saline.
- If altered level of consciousness, notify PICU. Intubate if GCS <8.
- Consult with local paediatric infectious disease team.
- Sick children should receive IV quinine 10mg/kg (maximum dose 600mg) in 250ml normal saline over 4 hours, every 8–12 hours.
  - Consider loading dose of 20mg/kg over 4 hours in those with any reduction in their level of consciousness.
- Consider exchange transfusion for a parasitaemia >10% or with worrying complications.
- Monitor blood sugar level hourly until levels stable; and LFT daily.
- Uncomplicated *P. falciparum* may be treated with oral quinine 10mg/kg 8–12 hourly for 5 days, followed with sulphadoxine/pyrimethamine (Fansidar).
  - N.B. if G6PD-deficient, only use quinine for 14 days.
- Notifiable disease (📖 p.156).

ⓘ Tuberculosis (TB)

TB is caused by *Mycobacterium tuberculosis* (1.5% *M. bovis*). It is a huge problem worldwide (90 million new cases in the 1990s), particularly in those with HIV infection and immigrants from the Indian subcontinent, as well as the poor. Children usually catch it from prolonged contact with household members who have 'open' pulmonary TB. The BCG provides only 75% protection.

Presentation depends on how the infection spreads.

- Pulmonary (66%)—bronchopneumonia. Hilar lymph nodes may obstruct bronchi leading to atelectasis or hyperinflation of a lobe.
- Lymphatic. Local spread—to cervical and axillary lymph nodes; or rupture resulting in pericarditis.
- Haematological. Results in multiple metastatic foci, e.g. CNS (meningitis), bone, lymphadenitis, renal.
- Other—erythema nodosum, conjunctivitis, pleural effusion. Multisystem involvement ('miliary TB') raises the possibility that the child is immunocompromised.

History

Try to determine the duration of the illness and how the disease was contracted. Ask about:

- the duration of cough;
- weight loss, anorexia, or chronic intermittent fever;
- any changes in conscious level?
- travel and the health of close contacts. Are the parents in a high risk group for HIV?
- immunization status—ask specifically about BCG.

Examination

- Document and plot growth parameters. Note any cachexia.
- Chest signs may be absent.
- Assess for hepatosplenomegaly.
- Exclude meningitis. Examine fundi for choroid tubercles.
- Note any joint swelling.

Investigation

- Acid-fast bacilli are best isolated from early morning gastric lavage. Sputum is seldom useful in children as they rarely have reactivation of primary TB.
- Blood tests are rarely diagnostic (<30%). Screen UEC, LFT as long-term therapy may be necessary.
- CXR—bronchopneumonia with parenchymal changes (Ghon focus) ± hilar lymph nodes (Ghon complex). Lymphadenopathy may be unilateral and there may be calcification in lung, neck, or abdomen. There may be lucencies in bone.

Perform Mantoux test

- Intradermal injection of 10U tuberculin on volar aspect of left forearm. (N.B. only give 1U tuberculin if BCG in last 12 months or erythema nodosum.)

- Do control injection on right forearm with same volume of normal saline.
- After 72 hours, the diameter of the indurated, palpable area (not just erythema) is measured:
  - >5mm is positive, if no previous BCG.
  - >10mm is suggestive, if had previous BCG.

Management

- Consult with infectious disease specialist. Patients usually need 6 months of rifampicin and isoniazide, with pyrazinamide for the first two months. Compliance is difficult.
- Notify public health so they can begin contact tracing (🕮 p.156).
- Exclude relatives with a cough from the ward.

Notifiable diseases

In the UK, if the following diseases are ***suspected***, it is mandatory for the doctor to report the case to a 'proper officer' of the local authority. They are responsible for public health surveillance, as well as arranging contact tracing.

When in doubt about who is the 'proper officer', your microbiology lab will know.

- Acute encephalitis
- Acute poliomyelitis
- Anthrax
- Borrelia (relapsing fever)
- Cholera
- Diphtheria
- Dysentery
- Food poisoning
- Leptospirosis
- Leprosy
- Malaria
- Meningitis
  - Meningococcal
  - Pneumococcal
  - *Haemophilus influenzae*
  - Viral
- Meningococcal septicaemia without meningitis
- Mumps
- Ophthalmia neonatorum
- Paratyphoid fever
- Plague
- Rabies
- Rubella
- Scarlet fever
- Smallpox
- Tetanus
- Tuberculosis
- Typhoid fever
- Typhus fever
- Viral haemorrhagic fever
- Viral hepatitis
  - Hepatitis A
  - Hepatitis B
  - Hepatitis C
  - Other
- Whooping cough
- Yellow fever.

Chapter 9
Ingestion

This chapter is not intended to be comprehensive, as advice for a specific poisoning can be obtained from a poisons information centre or from your hospital's pharmacy. However the chapter does cover the common presentations, as well as the major three toxicities: anticholinergic (📖 p.162); sympathomimetic (📖 p.163); and serotoninergic (📖 p.164).

Assessment

Drug ingestions are common presentations, with the usual age groups being the inquisitive toddler and the risk-taking adolescent. The medications are often over-the-counter preparations or prescription medicines that are within the household. Despite childproof containers, frequently lids are left unsecured, e.g. grandparent with arthritis, sibling with ADD, and within reach of an exploring toddler. Any indication that an adolescent has hoarded medication prior to the overdose is alarming (p.420).

Poisoning must be considered in every child presenting with behavioural change or altered level of consciousness

Try to determine the following.

- The time period over which the medications were consumed.
- What medications were taken.
  - N.B. Combination preparations, e.g. paracetamol and codeine.
  - Slow release preparations necessitate protracted observation.
  - To aid identification, contact GP or dispensing pharmacy.
- How much was consumed.
  - Count remaining tablets in packet or pot.
  - When in doubt, assume the maximum amount was taken.
- Whether other drugs, e.g. alcohol, were taken as well.

On examination, perform ABC and check vital signs.

- If GCS < 8, intubate. Consider ECG or continuous cardiac monitoring.
- Note any odd smells, e.g. garlic (= organophosphates), or signs suggestive of self-harm, e.g. scars at wrist.
- If the child is confused, ensure that they are observed in a place of safety.
- If polypharmacy is suspected, obtain a urine sample for a drug screen.
- Obtain or estimate the child's weight (p.527).

Discuss significant poisonings with a local poisons information centre or else the hospital pharmacy. Refer for assessment by psychiatry and even child protection services if indicated. Before discharge, remind parents to make the house toddler-proof.

Treatment

Certain drugs have specific antidotes (Table 9.1). Activated charcoal can be given for most ingestions, ***except for*** alcohol, concentrated acids, or alkalis or heavy metals. Contraindications include delayed presentation, at risk of aspiration, or ileus. Activated charcoal is not pleasant to drink and can be mixed with ice cream or else administered by NG tube.

There is no role for induced vomiting, e.g. with syrup of ipecac. Gastric lavage should only be undertaken if recommended by poisons information centre.

Table 9.1 Antidotes

Poison	**Antidote**
Benzodiazepines	Flumazenil
Beta blockers	Glucagon
Calcium channel blockers	Calcium
Carbon monoxide	Oxygen
Digoxin	Fab
Iron	Desferrioxamine
Lead	Calcium EDTA
Methanol	Ethanol
Methaemoglobinaemia	Methylene blue
Opiates	Naloxone
Organophosphates	Atropine
Paracetamol	*N*-acetyl cysteine
Tricyclic antidepressants	Sodium bicarbonate

Paracetamol and aspirin

Paracetamol

Toxic levels are thought to be over 140mg/kg. However, hepatotoxic levels may be reached by the cumulative effect of maximal doses of paracetamol (90mg/kg/day) over the preceding days. Moreover, children will be more susceptible to paracetamol if they have:

- pre-existing liver disease, e.g. inborn error of metabolism;
- malnutrition including recent starvation;
- enzyme-inducing medication, e.g. phenytoin, carbamazepine.

Management

If there is any possibility of poisoning, do the following.

- Give activated charcoal 1g/kg (maximum 50g) within 4 hours of acute ingestion.
- Obtain IV access.
- Take paracetamol levels—immediately if massive overdose or chronic ingestion; if acute ingestion, 4 hours after time of ingestion.
- Take LFT, glucose, coagulation studies as baseline.
- If single ingestion and time of ingestion is certain, use nomogram to see if over toxic threshold. Nomogram should be available in your ED or else in packet of *N*-acetyl cysteine.
  - **N.B. Nomogram units may be mcg/ml (mg/l) or micromol/l.** To convert μmol/l to mcg/ml multiply by 0.151, and to convert from mcg/ml to μmol/l multiply by 6.61.
- **N.B. Do not use nomogram** if:
  - chronic ingestion;
  - sustained-release preparation consumed;
  - time of ingestion uncertain.
- If any of the above apply, paracetamol poisoning is likely if transaminases are raised.
- If in doubt, consult with poisons information centre.

Treatment

If levels are toxic or poisoning probable

- Admit.
- IV *N*-acetyl cysteine in 5% glucose. Infuse according to protocol for child's weight.
- Explain that the infusion is to reduce the likelihood of liver damage. The infusion will run over 24 hours and further blood samples will be necessary to monitor liver function.
- Warn about potential side-effects, e.g. nausea; anaphylactoid reactions such as urticaria and bronchospasm, especially in asthmatics; rigors; hypo- or hypertension; and, extremely rarely, cortical blindness.
- Consult with gastroenterologist and psychiatry.

If fit for discharge

- Is psychiatric review necessary?
- How will the parents secure medicine in the future?

Aspirin

Ingestions of over 150mg/kg are concerning. There may be tachypnoea, followed by vomiting, diuresis; then increased agitation and confusion with hyperthermia. Older children may describe tinnitus. The classical picture of respiratory alkalosis preceding metabolic acidosis is not always seen in children. In addition, children need to be monitored for hypoglycaemia.

Management

- ABC.
- Assess for dehydration from insensible losses.
- Activated charcoal 1mg/kg (maximum 50g) if child is alert.
- IV access.
- FBC, UEC, glucose, calcium, venous blood gas, salicylate levels. Changes in sodium, potassium, calcium, and glucose levels may occur. Serial salicylate levels may be required to assess treatment progress.
- Done nomogram has been devised to extrapolate toxicity from a single ingestion. However, the nomogram cannot be used if:
  - the ingestion has been over several hours;
  - a sustained-release preparation has been ingested;
  - the time of ingestion is not known;
  - the patient is acidotic.
- It is safer to judge toxicity from the patient's clinical status and to check salicylate levels every 1 to 2 hours to confirm that levels are falling.

If toxicity is suspected, elimination is hastened by alkalinization. This should be discussed with the poisons information centre.

- An additional sampling cannula and a urinary catheter are advisable.
- IV fluids are given, aiming for a urinary output of 2ml/kg/h.
- IV sodium bicarbonate can be given as a bolus of 1–2meq/kg (sodium bicarbonate 8.4% contains 1meq/ml), aiming for a urinary pH of 7.5–8. Further doses of bicarbonate are adjusted according to the response. Serial blood gases are necessary to monitor blood pH.
- Hypokalaemia is common, especially with urinary alkalinization, and requires correction.
- Dialysis may be necessary if:
  - poor response, particularly if slow-release preparations taken;
  - renal failure;
  - falling GCS;
  - persistent metabolic acidosis.

Antihistamines

Antihistamines are prescribed for allergy, urticaria, and pruritis and are also found in over-the-counter preparations for coughs and colds. They have variable anticholinergic effects, so the typical clinical picture may not always be seen:

- hot as hades (febrile);
- blind as a bat (unreactive dilated pupils);
- dry as a bone;
- red as a beet (flushed, dry skin);
- mad as a hatter (confusion, delirium, or coma).

The key concerns are:

- blood pressure—hypo- or hypertension are possible;
- tachycardia, dysrhythmias;
- seizures, loss of consciousness.

Management

- ABC. Intubate if GCS under 8.
- Continuous cardiac monitoring.
- Activated charcoal 1g/kg (maximum 50g) if child is alert.
- IV access.
- Consult with poisons information centre.

Treatment

- Admit.
- Blood pressure—hypotension is treated with 20ml/kg boluses; hypertension is usually transient.
- Arrhythmia—usual treatment (📖 pp.68, 180). Avoid class Ia drugs, e.g. quinidine. If persistent, consider sodium bicarbonate 1–2meq/kg (sodium bicarbonate 8.4% contains 1meq/ml).
- Seizures—normally self-limiting, but will respond to benzodiazepines (📖 p.286).

ADHD medications

An increasingly common presentation. The drugs have variable sympathomimetic effects: tachycardia and hypertension; hyperthermia; seizures; and pupillary dilatation.

Dexamphetamine, methyl phenidate

Management is complicated by the CNS effects, ranging from agitation to paranoid hallucinations. CVS side-effects include tachyarrhythmias and hypertension, which may even cause strokes.

Management

- Attempt to calm down and place in a quiet area, where the child can still be observed and monitored.
- ABC with cardiac monitoring.
- Sedate if necessary, e.g. haloperidol (📖 p.425).
- Give activated charcoal 1g/kg (maximum 50g) if possible.
- Arrhythmias (📖 pp.68, 180).
- Hypertension may necessitate nitroprusside (📖 p.264). Beta blockers and calcium channel antagonists are contraindicated.
- Seizures respond to benzodiazepines and necessitate cranial imaging.
- External cooling may be required (📖 p.124).

Clonidine (Catapres®)

Principally an alpha 2 agonist, clonidine also affects other receptors, e.g. opiate, resulting in pupillary ***constriction***. The cardinal effects include:

- agitation progressing to drowsiness, coma;
- bradycardia;
- hypotension;
- respiratory depression, apnoea.

Children may also suffer seizures. PICU admission is frequently required for ventilatory support when consciousness is impaired.

Management

- ABC with cardiac monitoring. Intubate if GCS < 8.
- Hypotension usually responds to fluid boluses of 20ml/kg. Rarely, dopamine 2–5mcg/kg/min is necessary (📖 p.526).
- Bradycardia is treated with IV atropine 20mcg/kg.
- Naloxone may be required to distinguish clonidine from opiate poisoning.
- Admit as symptoms can last up to 72 hours.

Selective serotonin re-uptake inhibitors (SSRI)

SSRIs include fluoxetine (Prozac®), sertraline (Zoloft®), paroxetine (Paxil®), fluvoxamine (Luvox®), and citralopram (Celexa®).

As these are a relatively new medication in paediatrics, side-effects are still being determined and their safety in children is currently under review. However, early reports from fluoxetine overdoses show that the majority of children (over 75%) suffer no adverse effects.

However, some patients develop the potentially life-threatening serotonin syndrome:

- **CNS:** confusion, hallucinations, hyperactivity;
- **PNS:** ataxia, hypertonia, and hyperreflexia ± clonus;
- **Other:** tachycardia, hypertension, shivering, sweating, and hyperthermia.

These symptoms usually resolve without intervention. However, the hyperthermia in severe cases can warrant ICU admission for active cooling and correction of rhabdomyolysis and DIC (📖 p.124). The picture may be further complicated by the concurrent ingestion of other medications, e.g. alcohol.

Management

- ABC.
- Ask whether other medications ingested, e.g. antihistamines, potentiate SSRI effects.
- Ask about epilepsy—SSRI may lower seizure threshold.
- Cardiac monitoring—citralopram is associated with long QT (📖 p.181).
- IV access: FBC (possible thrombocytopenia); UEC (reports of SIADH); CK; coagulation studies.
- Activated charcoal 1g/kg (maximum 50g).
- Psychiatric review. Discuss whether medication should be ceased—slow weaning advisable—and whether overdose should be reported as an adverse drug reaction.

Tricyclic antidepressants

Tricyclics include amitriptyline, imipramine and can be prescribed for depression in adults, and bedwetting and even ADD in children. Although their principal action is anticholinergic (p.162), they also potentiate the effect of noradrenaline and act similarly to a class I antiarrhythmic on the heart. The symptoms of poisoning involve the CNS and the CVS:

- **CNS:** agitation to delirium and coma;
- **CVS:** arrhythmias, especially tachycardias; BP instability: cardiac arrest;
- **Other:** hyperthermia, rhabdomyolysis, renal failure (p.124).

If the ingestion is concealed, the delirious febrile child who has a seizure may be misdiagnosed, until the CVS manifestations become apparent.

Management

- ABC. Intubate if GCS < 8.
- Apply oxygen—respiratory acidosis worsens cardiac side-effects.
- Continuous cardiac monitoring.
- ECG: QRS >160ms = probable arrhythmia, seizure.
- IV access.
- UEC, venous blood gas (at risk of hypokalaemia and metabolic and/or respiratory acidosis).

Treatment

- If ventilated, hyperventilate to minimize respiratory acidosis. Aim for a $PaCO_2$ of >35mmHg.
- Activated charcoal 1mg/kg (maximum 50g) if child can maintain airway.
- If hypotensive, give 20ml/kg fluid bolus. If dysrhythmia, correct any hypokalaemia.
- If arrhythmias persist, discuss alkalinization with poisons information centre.
  - Sodium bicarbonate 1–2meq/kg bolus and then infusion to attain serum pH of 7.45–7.5. (Sodium bicarbonate 8.4% contains 1meq/ml.)
- Seizures are usually self-limiting but will respond to benzodiazepines. When stable, admit with cardiology and psychiatry review.

Lead and iron

Lead

Exposure is diminishing with the increased use of unleaded fuel. However, children at risk are those who live in houses being renovated or near smelters or whose parents who work with lead. The risk is potentiated if the child is iron-deficient. Manifestations of toxicity may be non-specific: drowsiness, irritability, anorexia, occasional abdominal pain. But lead poisoning should be a differential diagnosis on children who develop clumsiness, hearing or growth impairment, speech regression, or deteriorate in their cognition or attention.

Management

- Take lead levels, FBC and blood film, iron, ferritin, and TIBC.
- If lead level over 10mcg/dl (0.3μmol/l), discuss with poisons information centre.
  - Over 45mcg/dl (1μmol/l) necessitates treatment. Options include penicillamine or EDTA.
  - 10–45mcg/dl (0.3–1.0μmol/l) requires dietary advice, involvement of environmental services ± treatment as an outpatient. Arrange follow-up with a paediatrician, who ideally has previous experience of children suffering lead toxicity.

Iron

Iron tablets can look very appealing to a toddler. The initial innocuous presentation of nausea, vomiting ± diarrhoea may then be followed by a phase when the child improves. However, 12 hours after ingestion, resultant fluid shifts can cause hypotension and increasing lethargy. There may also be GI haemorrhage, renal and hepatic failure, and, ultimately, coma.

Management

- If child has mild signs of toxicity, e.g. persistent vomiting, start treatment.
- Determine the amount of ***elemental*** iron consumed.
- Calculate the dose/kg, assuming worst case scenario:
  - >40mg/kg: instigate treatment;
  - <40mg/kg: encourage fluids and observe.

Treatment

- AXR to see if tablets are still visible. If present, there is the possibility of delayed absorption.
- Take iron levels 4 hours after ingestion. Further samples may be necessary to be certain that the level has peaked.
- If level over 300mcg/dl (55μmol/l), consult with poisons information centre.
  - Desferrioxamine is given IM (90mg/kg, maximum 1g), although IV doses and PICU admission may be necessary in severe cases.
- If level under 300mcg/dl (55μmol/l) at 4 hours post-ingestion, only discharge if parents know signs of poisoning and can return to hospital easily.

Alcohols

Ethanol is the most frequent cause of poisonings, but other alcohols can be found in the home, e.g. solvent, antifreeze. The clinical concerns are the degree of CNS depression, metabolic acidosis, and hypoglycaemia (Table 9.2). Ataxia is a common feature and the child should be assessed for trauma, especially head injury. With adolescents, the possibility of the consumption of additional medications should be considered.

Management

- Observe closely in a place of safety. ABC with fingerprick glucose.
- Consult with biochemistry before taking levels. Assays for alcohols may require transportation to a specialized laboratory.
- IV access: UEC, LFT, glucose, calcium, venous blood gas and levels.
- Urinary drug screen if polypharmacy is suspected.
- Consult with poisons information centre.
- All adolescents require psychiatric review before discharge.

Treatment

Ethanol poisoning is treated with IV dextrose and hourly GCS assessment with fingerprick glucose, until child sobers up. In adolescents, there is an association between alcohol abuse and early conduct disorder or depression. The episode should not be dismissed as 'part of growing up'.

Methanol ingestion is treated with alcohol, ***before levels are known***. Oral administration is acceptable, but IV may be necessary. GCS and glucose monitoring should be undertaken as for ethanol. IV treatment and the need for folate supplementation should be discussed with the poisons information centre.

Isopropanol ingestion necessitates GCS monitoring, along with BP monitoring. Hypotensive episodes require 20mg/kg saline boluses.

Ethylene glycol The treatment is similar to that for methanol. Hypocalcaemia should be corrected by 10% calcium gluconate 0.3ml/kg (0.07mmol/kg) given slowly IV.

Table 9.2 Alcohols

Type of alcohol (possible sources)	Clinical findings	CNS depression	Odour	Acidosis
Ethanol (drinks, perfumes)	Nausea, vomiting, ataxia, seizures, coma, hypothermia	+	Ethanol	+/–
Methanol (antifreeze, fuel)	Delayed onset of intoxication. Visual symptoms, pancreatitis		None	+++
Isopropanol (solvent in cleaners)	Similar to ethanol, but marked GI irritation, CNS depression	+	Acetone	+
Ethylene glycol (antifreeze)	Similar to ethanol, nystagmus, cardiac and renal failure	+	None	+++

Illicit drugs

Although these presentations are seen more frequently with adults, paediatric trainees should still be familiar with them.

Morphine

CNS and respiratory depression are the principal symptoms. There may also be hypotension and bronchospasm. Pupils are constricted.

Management

- ABC. Intubate if RR less than expected for age or GCS < 8.
- IV naloxone 0.1mg/kg. May need repeat doses ± infusion.
- Check for track marks. Consider screening for HIV, hepatitis B and C.

Ecstacy

Although the symptoms resemble those of sympathomimetics (p.163), hyperthermia and hyponatraemia are potentially life-threatening complications. In addition, the serotoninergic effects will be potentiated if SSRI antidepressants are also being taken (p.164).

Malignant hyperthermia is the greatest concern with the ensuing risk of rhabdomyolysis, acute renal failure, and DIC (p.124).

Management

- ABC with continuous cardiac monitoring. Assess dehydration.
- Activated charcoal 1g/kg (maximum 50g) if patient able to comply.
- IV access: UEC, LFT, CK, clotting studies.
- Fluid resuscitation.
- External cooling methods.
- Hypertension, tachycardia respond to benzodiazepines. Avoid beta blockade. If blood pressure still high, try nitroprusside (p.264).
- Consult with poisons information centre.

LSD

Hallucinations; often unresponsive staring. Sympathomimetic so pupils widely dilated with tachycardia and hypertension. Increased muscle tension with hyperreflexia may also be noted.

Management

- Try to reassure patient and keep calm.
- Agitation may require benzodiazepines oral or IV (p.425).
- Activated charcoal 1g/kg (maximum 50g) if patient able to comply.
- Confirm diagnosis with urinary drug screen. Differentials include hypnotics, anticholinergics, and stimulants.
- Arrange psychiatric follow-up as psychosis can be a long-term sequela.

Marijuana Rare presentation, but occasionally panic reactions or short-lived psychoses. Mild tachycardia, conjunctival injection, and mild ataxia may be noted. Reassurance is usually all that is required.

Slang terms used in drug abuse

The following list of slang terms is taken with permission from pp. 658–9 of Wyatt, J.P., Illingworth, R.N., Clancy, M., *et al.* (1999). *Oxford Handbook of Accident and Emergency Medicine*, 1st edn. Oxford University Press, Oxford.

The following vocabulary may assist in the identification of an agent, but it must be emphasized that these terms are often transient in use and may bear no relation to the actual substance taken.

A	amphetamine
Acid	LSD/MDMA
Adam/AKA	MDMA
Angel dust	phencyclidine
Barbs	barbiturate
Bart Simpson	ecstacy
Base	cocaine free base
Bennies	amphetamine
Bhang	cannabis
Big C or C	cocaine
Big O	opioids
Blotter acid	LSD
Blow	cocaine
Blues	barbiturates
Boy/Brown sugar	heroin
Cadillac	phencyclidine
Candy/Cake/Charlie	cocaine
China white	designer drugs/fentanyl/opioids
Chinese	heroin
CJs	phencyclidine
Clear rocks	amphetamine
Coke	cocaine
Crack	cocaine free base
Crank	amphetamine
Crap	heroin
Crystal	amphetamine/phencyclidine
DCM	2, 5-dimethoxy-4-methylamphetamine
Dead on arrival/DOA	hallucinogens
Denis the menace	MDMA
Dexies	dexamphetamine
Dike	dipipanone
Disco biscuits	MDMA
Doll/dollies	methdone
DOM	dimethoxymethyl-amphetamine

Dome/dots/domes/dots	LSD
Dope	cannabis
Downers	barbiturates
Dust	cocaine/hallucinogens/opioids/phencyclidine
Dynamite	cocaine
E/Ecstasy/X/XTC	MDMA
Elephant/Elephant juice	heroin
Embalming fluid	phencyclidine
EVE	methylenedioxy *n*-ethylamphetamine
Flake	cocaine
Freebase	cocaine free base
Ganja	cannabis
Gas	solvents
GBH/GHB	gamma hydroxybutyric acid
Ghost	LSD
Glue	organic solvents
Gold dust/Happy dust	cocaine
Grass	cannabis
H	cannabis/heroin
Happy sticks	phencyclidine cigarettes/cannabis
Happy trails	cocaine
Hash/Hashish	cannabis resin
Homegrown	marijuana
Hong Kong rocks	opioids
Horse	heroin
Ice	amphetamines/cocaine
Joint	cannabis
Jive sticks	phencyclidine cigarettes/cannbis
Junk	heroin
Kiff	cannabis
KJ	phencyclidine
Laughing gas	nitrous oxide
Liquid X	gamma hydroxybutyric acid
Locker popper/locker room	butyl nitrate
Love drug/love pill	methylene dioxyamphetamine
M	morphine/3, 4-methlene dioxyamphetamine
Magic dust	hallucinogens
Magic mushrooms	psilocybin
Mandies	methqualone
Marijuana	cannabis
MDA	methlene dioxyamphetamine
MDMA	3, 4-methlene dioxyamphetamine

Mesc	mescaline
Microdots	LSD
MMDA	3-methoxy-4, 5-methlene dioxyamphetamine
Mref/Morpho	morphine
Nembies	pentobarbitone
Nitrous	nitrous oxide
Paki	cannabis
Paper acid	LSD
Paradise	cocaine
Peace	dimethoxymethyl amphetamine
Peace pill/PCP/weed	phencyclidine
Pep pills	amphetamine
Perote/buttons	mescaline
Puppers	amyl nitrate
Pot	cannabis
Purple haze	LSD
Quaas	methaqualone
Ruck	heroin
Rocks	amphetamines
Rocket fuel	phencyclidine
Rock 'n' roll	heroin
Rush	butyl nitrate
Shit	cannabis
Shrooms	psilocybin
Smack	cocaine/heroin
Smoke	cannabis
Snappers	amyl nitrate
Snort/Snow	cocaine
Sodies	sodium amylobarbitone
Soma	phencyclidine
Speed	amphetamine
Speedball	cocaine with heroin
STP	dimethoxymethyl amphetamine
Sulph/Sulphate	amphetamine
Supergrass/joint/weed/TAC	phencyclidine
Tea/Thai sticks	cannabis
Trips	hallucinogens
Uppers/up	amphetamine, caffeine, ephedrine, etc
Wake ups	amphetamine
Weed	cannabis
XTC	MDMA
Zoom	phencyclidine/gamma hydroxybutric acid

Foreign bodies

The variety of objects consumed by children is astonishing. Not all presentations are acute, e.g. chronic cough post-choking episode, and most do not require immediate intervention.

The typical CXR finding of a bronchial foreign body is hyperlucency of the obstructed segment, with opacification of the remaining segments because of their relative hyperperfusion (V/Q mismatch).

Management

- CXR ± AXR to determine position.
    - If inhaled foreign body suspected, expiratory CXR to confirm air trapping. If difficult to obtain, request lateral CXR with child lying on affected side, showing that the lung segment cannot deflate.
- Foreign bodies in the respiratory tract require bronchoscopic extraction.
- Oesophageal foreign bodies require endoscopy for removal or else displacement into the stomach.
- Gastrointestinal objects do not require surgical removal unless:
    - they are batteries (will be corroded by acid);
    - they could perforate the gut, e.g. nails, tacks.

Parents should be advised to check the child's stools to confirm the object has passed. In addition, they should return to hospital if the child develops abdominal pain.

Chapter 10

Cardiovascular

Assessment

Many congenital heart anomalies are identified antenatally. However, the clinician should be aware of cardiac conditions presenting via ED, e.g. the collapsed neonate whose duct has just closed (📖 p.32), the evolving cyanosis of Fallot's tetralogy, or the discovery of a murmur not previously heard.

History

Symptoms may be non-descript, e.g. feeding difficulties, recurrent chest infections, or else resemble other conditions, e.g. myocarditis having features of bronchiolitis or asthma.

If a child is known to have a cardiac condition, remember that medication can influence a child's clinical status, e.g. β blockers mask hypoglycaemia; digoxin, and amiodarone interact with other commonly used drugs.

Examination

The key features to determine are whether the child is:
- acyanotic or cyanotic (pink or blue);
- in cardiac failure;
- adequately perfused.

Other clinical signs such as growth failure, murmurs, or organomegaly not only are suggestive of cardiac disease, but also should alert the clinician to potential complications, e.g. susceptibility to fluid overload, risk of endocarditis.

The following should always be recorded.
- Skin colour: pale or pink or blue—oxygen saturations 85–95% are acceptable for cyanotic heart disease; ask the parents what are the usual saturations for their child.
- Pulse rate: too fast or slow, regular versus irregular.
- Respiratory rate: tachypnoea.
- Weight gain: too little; or too rapid = fluid retention due to congestive cardiac failure (📖 p.182).
- Perfusion: distal and central.
- Pulse presence especially femoral; character, e.g. bounding, weak.
- Blood pressure: cuff must cover 2/3 of the upper arm. Blood pressure is age-dependent and a lower BP than expected for age should be re-evaluated as hypotension is an alarming sign.
- Any precordial scars, thrills, murmurs (📖 p.184).
- The position of the apex beat, edge of the liver.

N.B. Temperature ± rash: consider acute rheumatic fever (📖 p.187), endocarditis (📖 p.188), Kawasaki's (📖 p.190).

Investigations

Perform CXR and ECG if cardiac failure, an arrhythmia, or a new murmur has been diagnosed. CXR and ECG can also be helpful in assessing children with known cardiovascular conditions whose clinical status has changed recently.

Cyanosis

Cyanosis of cardiac origin is due to a right to left shunt, and is usually detected during the neonatal period. Growth and development are adequate with saturations between 85 and 95% and interventions, such as Blalock–Taussig shunts, may be necessary to improve oxygenation to these levels. Cyanosis may be difficult to detect clinically if oxygen saturations are over 85% or if the child is anaemic.

Causes

Children with no known cardiac history presenting with cyanosis should be assessed for other causes:

- respiratory—hypoventilation versus pneumonic process;
- haematological—profound anaemia, methaemoglobinaemia;
- hypoperfusion causing cool peripheries and erroneous oximetry recordings.

Cardiac causes presenting outside of the neonatal period are due to the gradual increase in obstruction to pulmonary flow. These include:

- tetralogy of Fallot;
- total anomalous pulmonary venous drainage;
- truncus arteriosus;
- blocked Blalock–Taussig shunt;
- congenital cyanotic heart disease with respiratory illness or dehydration.

Examination

- The usual saturations for the child—from parents or the medical notes.
- BP and peripheral perfusion.
- Presence of pulses and precordial scars.
- Presence of murmurs. N.B. Obstructed flow means murmurs disappear!
- Presence of cardiac failure—common in AVSD, truncus.
- Neurological status—altered consciousness occurs with Fallot spells, and CVA secondary to polycythaemia.

Management

- Oxygen to keep saturations between 85 and 95% or 'usual' levels. Beware of hyper-oxygenation, which may decrease pulmonary vascular resistance and induce cardiac failure by increasing left to right shunting.
- CXR, ECG.
- Fluids—if cardiac failure, fluid restrict and diuretics (p.182); if dehydrated, careful use of fluid boluses to improve right-sided filling.
- Consult cardiologist for further advice.

Fallot spell

- Oxygen.
- Flex knees to chest to increase venous return.
- IV morphine 0.05mg/kg to minimize infundibular spasm.
- IV β blocker ± phenylephrine as advised by cardiologist.

ⓘ Chest pain

Usually benign in origin.[1] The majority have musculoskeletal causes and, in approximately one-third of patients, no reason will be found. However, acute chest pain causes great anxiety, especially if there has been a cardiac event in the family.

The differential diagnoses include the following.

- Musculoskeletal: unusual exercise, costochondritis, precordial catch.[2]
- Pulmonary: pneumothorax, pleuritic—viral illness, pneumonia, PE, exercise-induced asthma.
- Gastrointestinal: reflux, peptic ulcer, foreign body.
- Cardiac: arrhythmias, e.g. SVT, ventricular ectopics (📖 pp.78, 180); myocardial disease, e.g. cardiomyopathy, myocarditis (📖 p.191); valvular disease, e.g. MVP, AS, PS; ischaemia, e.g. anomalous origin of the left coronary artery, post- Kawasaki's, vasoconstrictor drugs such as cocaine.
- Psychosomatic: stressors such as school, illness in family.

History

- Note the distribution, radiation, intensity, and frequency of the pain.
- Any effect of changing position?
- Any provoking factors? For example, exercise, recent meals, intercurrent illness.
- Symptoms such as palpitations, cough, and shortness of breath are significant.
- Ask specifically if the child has ever had symptoms suggestive of Kawasaki disease (📖 p.190).

Examination

- Full examination of the chest, abdomen, and spine.
- Palpation of the ribs, especially at the costochondral junction, will be tender if there is a musculoskeletal cause.
- Carefully assess pulse rate, pulse volume, and apex position.
- Auscultate for a friction rub, a new murmur, muffling of heart sounds, and any respiratory signs.

Management

☠ If shock:

- ABC with oxygen;
- careful use of IV fluids until cardiac failure is excluded.

Consider rare conditions such as tension pneumothorax, massive pulmonary embolism, pancreatitis, aortic dissection—(Marfan's or traumatic).

1 Kocis, K.C. (1999). Chest pain in paediatrics. *Ped. Clin. N. Am.* **46**(2),189–203.

2 *Precordial catch.* A sudden stabbing pain lasting 30s to up to 3 minutes. It is usually left sternal or anterior on right and can be easily localized by the child, using one or two fingers. The patient usually breathes shallowly, but no colour change is noted.

In all cases, CXR and ECG are helpful as they can exclude pulmonary causes, along with ischaemia, which may be difficult to diagnose clinically.

:O: If ischaemia is found:

- insert cannula;
- bloods for cardiac enzymes and troponins;
- urgent cardiac consultation.

Musculoskeletal causes can be treated with NSAIDS. If no cause is found, parents often find a normal ECG reassuring and follow-up should be arranged with their general practitioner.

Arrhythmias

Sinus tachycardia Definition of tachycardia is age-dependent (p.523). If higher than expected for age, exclude SVT (p.78). Other causes are fever, pain, and shock. Determine cause and treat.

Atrial flutter and atrial fibrillation

Both rare in children. Usually secondary to atrial enlargement. Requires:

- 12 lead ECG;
- cannula—check UEC, thyroid function tests;
- digoxin—discuss doses with cardiologist;
- if unstable, treat as SVT ***but*** start with synchronized DC cardioversion starting at 0.5J/kg (p.78).

Bradycardia

Age-dependent rates (p.523). May be physiological, e.g. athletic children. Can arise with other conditions.

- Shock. Pre-terminal sign—resuscitate with oxygen and fluids.

> If pulse rate under 60, start CPR and treat as asystole (p.70)

- Raised intracranial pressure—stop any IV fluids, give mannitol 0.5g/kg IV. Notify ICU and neurosurgeon. Prepare to intubate.
- Myocardial infection, e.g. acute rheumatic fever, myocarditis. Check for pericardial effusion, perform ECG and CXR. Bloods as indicated (p.191).
- Vagal stimulation, e.g. intubation, suctioning. Usually transient. Give oxygen.
- Electrolyte anomalies, e.g. hypokalaemia, hypothyroidism. Check bloods.
- Poisonings—remember **PACED**.
  - **P** Propranolol (β blockers).
  - **A** Anticholinesterase drugs.
  - **C** Clonidine, calcium channel blockers.
  - **E** Ethanol/alcohols.
  - **D** Digoxin, druggies (opiates).

Continue cardiac monitoring until normal rate maintained.

Ventricular ectopics

Rare but normal in adolescence. Can cause chest pain. Usually resolve with exercise as normal sinus discharges prior to ectopic focus. However, treatment may be necessary in heart disease, e.g. myocarditis, cardiomyopathy, or post-cardiac surgery.

- Exclude catecholamine and digoxin toxicity.
- Perform ECG and discuss with cardiologist.

Long QT syndrome

Potentially life-threatening as Q on T phenomenon causes ventricular arrhythmias. There may be a family history of sudden death, e.g. Romano–Ward or deafness, e.g. Jervell–Lange–Nielsen.

Triggers include:

- a fright, e.g. alarm clock, sudden bang;
- exercise;
- raised intracranial pressure;
- hypocalcaemia;
- medications, e.g. antihistamines, anticholinergic antidepressants, amiodarone.

An ECG should be performed on every child presenting with collapse or first afebrile seizure

Duration over 440ms is pathological and will necessitate life-long β blockade (📖 p.192 for calculation of QTc).

Heart failure

☠ **Acute heart failure** is extremely rare and is a medical emergency.

- Notify ICU.
- Immediate intubation and ventilation (📖 p.474).
- IV access—UEC, cardiac enzymes, troponins.
- Titrated IV fluid boluses to assist pre-load.
- IV frusemide 0.5mg/kg.
- Inotropes as directed by cardiologist.
- CXR and ECG.

ⓘ **Congestive cardiac failure** is encountered more frequently. The infant may have poor feeding yet gains weight readily, or may experience episodes of clamminess when feeding. The older child may have poor exercise tolerance or frequent chest infections.

Causes include:

- <10 days of age:
  - left outflow tract obstruction, e.g. coarctation; hypoplastic left heart; critical aortic stenosis.
- Over 2 weeks:
  - left to right shunts;
  - rarely, cyanotic conditions, e.g. TAPVD, truncus arteriosus, single ventricle, TGA, and VSD.
- Older children:
  - arrhythmias (📖 p.180);
  - myocardial disease, e.g. myocarditis (📖 p.191); cardiomyopathy; ischaemia, e.g. post Kawasaki;
  - high output states, e.g. AV malformation, anaemia.

Examination

- Plot the child's growth parameters.
- Record pulse and respiratory rate.
- Document apex position, murmurs, and any rubs. Listen for 'gallop' rhythm.
- Check for signs of fluid overload—basal creps, hepatomegaly, peripheral oedema.
- Remember to auscultate the head—eyes, above ears—for intracranial bruits of AV malformation.

Management

- Oxygen if saturations under 85%. Do not exceed saturations of 95%.
- Correct any cause, i.e. stop arrhythmia, transfuse with diuretic cover.
- Take blood for UEC, calcium, magnesium; perform CXR, ECG.
- Start frusemide 1mg/kg/dose PO ± spironolactone 1mg/kg/dose PO. Dosing can be increased to bd and tds respectively, to a maximum of frusemide 4mg/kg/day and spironolactone 3mg/kg/day.
- If failure to thrive, arrange dietician review to increase caloric intake. NG feeds and admission may be necessary.
- Discuss with cardiologist and arrange follow-up.

Murmur

Over 50% of infants and children have 'innocent' murmurs that are usually heard during an intercurrent illness. Innocent murmurs tend to be:

- mid-systolic; no associated heave or thrill;
- soft—a 'musical' character;
- localized—radiation is unusual;
- affected by change in posture.

Further investigation may be needed if:

- the child is under 12 months;
- the child is dysmorphic;
- there are additional heart sounds;
- the murmur is loud;
- the murmur is diastolic.

Identifying a murmur requires a stepwise approach.

- Note the pulse volume, BP, and any thrills, e.g. water-hammer pulse with suprasternal thrill = aortic regurgitation.
- Distinguish the heart sounds and then the murmur.
- Try to relate the position where the murmur is loudest to the heart anatomy, e.g. interventricular flow of VSD heard at LLSE (see box).
- A continuous murmur indicates biphasic flow, e.g. AS with AR, PDA, shunt.

Correlation between position where murmur is loudest and cardiac malfunction

URSE (upper right sternal edge)
- Aortic stenosis(AS)
- Aortic regurgitation(AR)

ULSE (upper left sternal edge)
- Venous hum
- Innocent pulmonary flow murmur
- Pulmonary stenosis; valve or artery
- Coarctation, aortic stenosis
- Patent ductus arteriosus (PDA)
- ASD

LLSE (lower left sternal edge)
- Innocent murmur
- VSD
- Tricuspid regurgitation
- Fallot's

Back
- Pulmonary valve lesion
- PDA
- Coarctation

Apex
- Mitral regurgitation
- Mitral valve prolapse(MVP)
- Aortic stenosis

Management

- CXR.
- ECG.
- Arrange follow-up with cardiologist.
- If high-flow lesion suspected, e.g. PDA, VSD, or valvular disease, discuss endocarditis prophylaxis (📖 p.189).

Systolic

(a) Ejection systolic, e.g. AS, PS, innocent

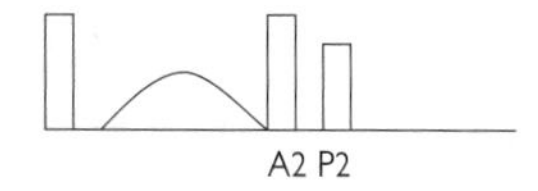

(b) Pansystolic, e.g. VSD, MR, TR

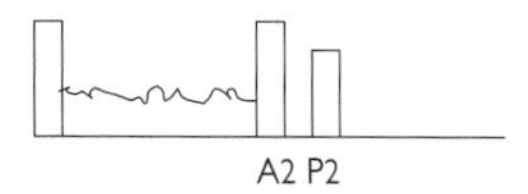

(c) Decrescendo, e.g. muscular VSD (maladie de Roger)

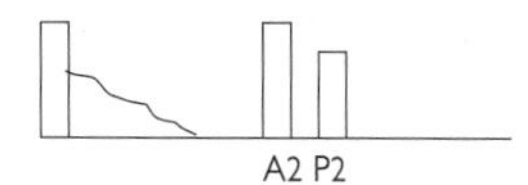

(d) Late systolic ± midsystolic click, e.g. MVP, HOCM especially on standing

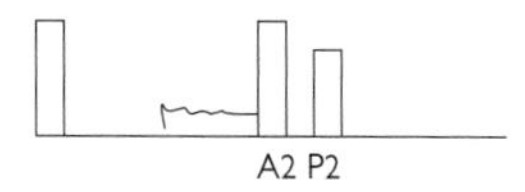

Diastolic

(a) Early diastolic (high pitched decrescendo), e.g. AR, PR, PR with MS

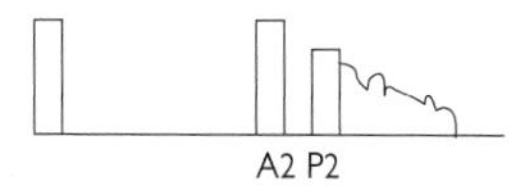

(b) Early diastolic (low pitched) e.g. PR

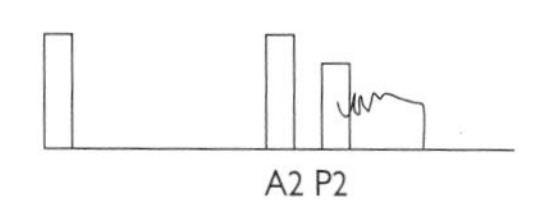

(c) Mid-diastolic (rumbling), e.g. MS

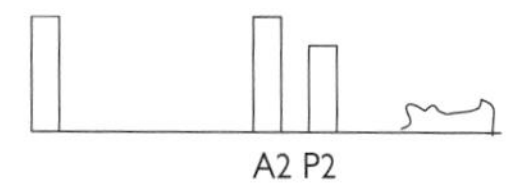

Fig. 10.1 Diagrammatic representations of murmurs.

ⓘ Hypertension

Blood pressure is age-dependent and hypertension is defined as being above the 95th centile for age. Blood pressure must be measured using a cuff that covers at least two-thirds of the child's arm—smaller cuffs will lead to elevated readings. Try to make it a game so that the child is not distressed.

The commonest cause of hypertension in children is renal disease. The other causes are in the acronym ERECT.

- **E** Essential—overweight.
- **R** Renal disease, especially glomerulonephritis, renal artery stenosis.
- **E** Endocrine, e.g. phaeochromocytoma, Cushings, thyrotoxicosis.
- **C** Co-arctation, intracranial pressure.
- **T** Toxins, e.g. cocaine, ecstasy, lead (📖 p.166).

A hypertensive emergency presents with headache, altered level of consciousness, or seizures. See renal chapter for management (📖 p.264). Otherwise symptoms are non-specific, e.g. poor feeding, vomiting, irritability in infants, whereas older children report headache, nausea, visual changes.

Blood pressure should always be documented in children presenting with a headache, a seizure, or cardiac failure

Examination

- Growth parameters.
- Phenotype—Turner's, neurofibromatosis, Cushing's.
- BP on at least two occasions and in different limbs.
- Peripheral pulses—radio-femoral delay can be detected in teenagers.
- Abdomen for masses.
- Renal and intracranial bruits.
- Fundi.
- Urine for dipstick analysis.

Management

- If renal disease is confirmed, see 📖 p.262.
- If coarctation is diagnosed, perform CXR and ECG and request cardiac consultation.
- Otherwise perform:
  - full blood count, UEC, plasma renin;
  - urine culture;
  - arrange renal ultrasound—Doppler of renal arteries;
  - suggest lifestyle changes such as more exercise, limiting sodium in diet, e.g. fewer pre-packaged foods;
  - arrange follow-up with paediatrician.

Rheumatic fever

Secondary to untreated group A streptococcus. Diagnosis depends on having 2 major criteria and 1 minor; or 1 major and 2 minor with supporting evidence of streptococcal infection. The symptoms may not arise concurrently.

Amended Duckett Jones criteria[3]

Major

- Carditis—a new murmur; pericarditis—an effusion or a rub; cardiac failure.
- Migratory polyarthritis.
- Sydenham's chorea—involuntary movements ± emotional lability; ataxia.
- Erythema marginatum—macular rash with distinct border, never on face.
- Subcutaneous nodules—non-tender, movable, palpated on scalp, spine, joints.

Minor

- Polyarthralgia—joints are tender without heat or swelling.
- Fever.
- Raised ESR and CRP.
- Prolonged PR interval (📖 p.192).
- Positive throat swab culture, or elevated ASOT/DNase B.
- History of acute rheumatic fever or rheumatic heart disease.

Investigations

- ECG, CXR.
- FBC, blood culture, ESR, CRP, ASOT, DNase B.
- Throat swab.
- Request cardiology assessment with echo, even if carditis cannot be detected clinically.

Treatment

- IV penicillin 30mg/kg/dose qds until afebrile. Then start oral penicillin 250mg bd until day 10 of treatment.
- Aspirin 7.5 to 15mg/kg/dose qds PO for arthritis and arthralgia.
- If carditis, prednisolone 2mg/kg PO daily.
- Bed rest.

Parents should be reminded that the disease can recur whenever the child has exposure to group A streptococcus, and the likelihood of developing rheumatic heart disease increases. Lifelong IM penicillin prophylaxis may be necessary.

3 Dajanii, A.S., Ayoub, E., Bierman, F.Z., *et al.* (1992). Guidelines for the diagnosis of rheumatic fever: Jones criteria, updated 1992. *J. Am. Med. Assoc.* **268,** 2069–73.

Infective endocarditis

Increasing incidence as more children survive with congenital heart disease or have central venous catheters *in situ*. Infection is usually with *Staphylococcus aureus*, coagulase negative staphylococci, *Streptococcus viridans* group, or even fungi, such as *Candida*[4].

Cardinal symptoms include:

- unexplained fever ± night sweats;
- weakness;
- myalgia, arthralgia;
- weight loss.

Septic emboli can cause cerebrovascular accidents or peripheral infarction.

Examination

Look for:

- petechiae;
- new murmurs (<50%);
- splenomegaly (70%).

Signs such as clubbing, Janeway lesions (flat, painless macules on thenar or hypothenar eminences), or Osler's nodes are unusual in children.

Investigations

- Full blood count, ESR, CRP.
- UEC—to check renal function.
- Blood cultures from at least two different sites.
- Urine analysis.
- ECG.
- CXR.

ECG is helpful for vegetations near the aortic valve that can disrupt conduction pathways. CXR is useful for monitoring right-sided lesions, which may send off pulmonary showers.

Treatment

- Request cardiac consultation with echo.
- Most centres have an established antibiotic regimen, e.g. IV penicillin 60mg/kg/dose qds and IV gentamicin 2.5mg/kg/dose (maximum 80mg) tds.
- IV vancomycin (15mg/kg loading dose) can be added on clinical suspicion.

Thereafter antibiotics are tailored to blood culture results[5].

4 Mylonakis, E. and Calderwood, S. (2001). *N. Engl. J. Med.* **345**(18), 1318–30.

5 Working Party of the British Society for Antimicrobial Chemotherapy (1998). Antibiotic treatment of streptococcal, enterococcal, and staphylococcal endocarditis. *Heart* **79**, 207–10.

Endocarditis prophylaxis[6]

High risk

- High flow congenital heart lesions, i.e. not ASD
- Complex cyanotic heart disease
- Previous endocarditis, even if structurally normal heart
- All prosthetic valves
- Presence of surgically created shunts and conduits

Moderate risk

- Acquired valvular dysfunction, including after surgery
- Hypertrophic cardiomyopathy
- Mitral valve prolapse with valvular regurgitation

Procedures not meriting prophylaxis Intubation, flexible bronchoscopy, grommets, endoscopy and biopsy, trans-oesphaegeal echo.
If there is no genitourinary infection: catheterization, micturating cystourethrogram, circumcision.

Dental, oral, oesophageal, respiratory procedures

Amoxycillin 50mg/kg PO 1 hour before procedure; repeat 6 hours afterwards

- If penicillin-allergic, use clindamycin 20mg/kg po or cephalexin 50mg/kg PO
- If unable to take oral medications, IV ampicillin 50mg/kg or IV clindamycin 20mg/kg infusion completed within 30 minutes before procedure.

GI/GU procedures

High risk

- IV ampicillin 50mg/kg (maximum 2g) + IV gentamicin 1.5mg/kg (maximum 120mg) within 30 minutes of procedure; 6 hours later IV ampicillin 25mg/kg or amoxycillin 25mg/kg PO
- If penicillin-allergic, IV vancomycin 20mg/kg (maximum 1g) over 1 to 2 hours + IV gentamicin 1.5mg/kg infusion completed within 30 minutes of procedure

Moderate risk

- IV ampicillin 50mg/kg (maximum 2g) within 30 minutes of procedure or oral amoxycillin 50mg/kg 1 hour before
- If penicillin-allergic, IV vancomycin 20mg/kg over 1 to 2 hours; infusion completed within 30 minutes of procedure.

6 Dajani, A.S., Taubert, K.A., Wilson, W., *et al.* (1997). Prevention of bacterial endocarditis: recommendations by the American Heart Association. *Circulation* **96**, 358–66.

Kawasaki's disease

Unknown aetiology but thought to be super-antigen phenomenon, which may be why clinical features resemble those of Group A streptococcus and measles. A vasculitic illness, which in the second week causes the formation of aneurysms, particularly of the coronary arteries. Prompt recognition and treatment minimize the chance of myocardial compromise.

There are six features.

- **Unremitting fever** over 5 days.
- **Eyes:** non-exudative conjunctivitis with limbic sparing.
- **Mucosa:** red lips ('lipstick' sign) with cracking and fissuring ± strawberry tongue ± pharyngitis.
- **Cervical lymphadenopathy:** nodes over 1.5cm width bilaterally or unilateral mass
- **Rash:** may be erythema, urticaria, follicular, or transient. Peeling in the nappy area of the groin is a significant finding.
- **Peripheral:** oedema of hands and feet ± red palms and soles.

Diagnosis requires the presence of fever along with four other clinical features.

Incidental findings include irritability, diarrhoea, cough, arthralgia. In the second week, desquamation of the finger tips develops, along with a progressive thrombocytosis.

Treatment

- IV immunoglobulin 2g/kg given over 8–12 hours. Repeat dose if fever does not settle in 48 hours.
- Oral aspirin to prevent thrombosis of any aneurysms. The benefit of high dose aspirin (20mg/kg/dose qds) over low dose (2–5mg/kg daily) is not known. Some prefer the low dose regime as it is better tolerated.
- Cardiology consult ± echo to monitor coronary arteries.

Myocarditis

Rare but has a mortality of 35%. Usually caused by viruses, e.g. adenovirus, coxsackie, echo; but also by bacteria such as *Haemophilus influenzae*. Initial symptoms of cough, wheeze, and tachypnoea may be misdiagnosed, and should be re-evaluated should the child appear disproportionately unwell for 'bronchiolitis' or if bronchodilator therapy is ineffective.

Cardiac manifestations include:

- weak pulses;
- hyperactive precordium;
- murmur ± quiet heart sounds;
- signs of congestive cardiac failure.

Investigations

- CXR—cardiomegaly with pulmonary congestion.
- ECG—ST changes, arrhythmias such as AV block, ventricular ectopics.
- Blood for UEC; viral serology and blood cultures.

Treatment

- Treat cardiac failure (📖 p.182).
- Continuous cardiac monitoring for arrhythmias. Ectopics are a poor prognostic indicator.
- Discuss urgently with cardiologist.

Arrange admission to high dependency unit or ICU.

ECG guide

Normal paediatric ECGs differ from adult ECGs, e.g. right axis deviation (>110°) until 3 months, inverted T waves until 10 years, and certain parameters have age-dependent values. However the approach is the same.

- Calculate rate—is there sinus rhythm?
- Calculate axis.
- Measure PR interval—start of P to start of QRS (Table 10.1).
- Calculate QTc—start of QRS until the end of T, divided by the square root of the R–R1 interval, i.e. time between successive R waves.
- Look for biphasic or raised P waves, abnormal Q waves, δ waves.
- Prolonged PR interval.
  - Endocardial cushion defect.
  - Ebstein's anomaly—congenital tricuspid regurgitation.
  - Acute rheumatic fever, myocarditis.
  - Congenital block secondary to maternal lupus.
- Short PR interval.
  - Wolff–Parkinson–White.
  - Glycogen storage disease.
  - Low atrial pacemaker.
- Prolonged QRS.
  - Myocardial disease, ventricular hypertrophy.
  - Bundle branch block (BBB) e.g. post-operative.
  - Digoxin toxicity, hyperkalaemia, hypothyroidism.
- Atrial enlargement.
  - P wave >2.5mm at 6 months = RAH, e.g. Ebstein's, tricuspid atresia, Fallot's tetralogy.
  - P wave >0.1s in lead II = LAH, e.g. cardiomyopathy, mitral valve disease, large PDA.
- Partial right BBB.
  - With left axis deviation: ostium primum ASD.
  - With right axis deviation: ostium secundum ASD.
  - With RAH, δ waves: Ebstein's.
- Complete right BBB: post-ventriculotomy.
- Right ventricular hypertrophy.
  - R>S in V1 after 1 year; upright T waves in right chest leads after 1 week of age; S in V6 >15mm at 1 week, >10mm at 6 months, >5mm at 1 year.
- Left ventricular hypertrophy.
  - Under 1 year, S in V1 and R in V6 > 30mm.
  - Over 1 year, S in V1 and R in V6 > 40mm.
- **Q waves are normal in II, III, AVF, V5, V6.** If elsewhere, think of HOCM, anomalous left coronary artery, congenitally corrected transposition, infarction.

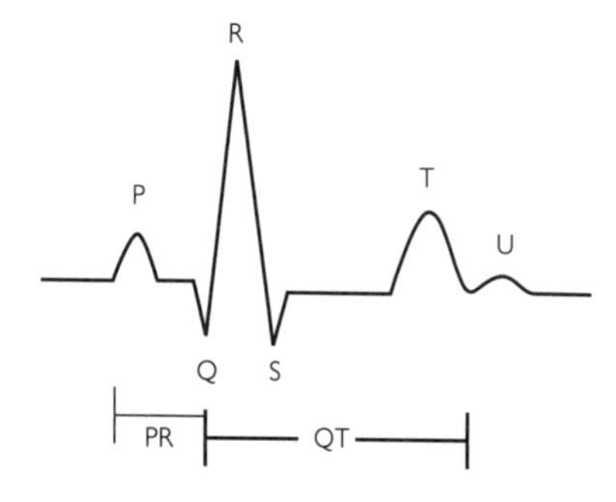

Fig. 10.2 Depiction of ECG intervals.

Table 10.1 Duration of ECG components

	Duration (seconds) at age		
ECG component	**Under 1 year**	**1–5 years**	**5–15 years**
PR interval	0.08–0.13	0.1–0.15	0.12–17
QRS	0.04–0.08	0.05–0.09	0.05–0.09
QTc	0.3–0.5	0.34–0.43	0.35–0.4

Chapter 11

Respiratory

Assessment

Respiratory illnesses make up the bulk of paediatric admissions to hospital. Most are mild and self-limiting, requiring little if any intervention. However, the differential is wide and includes serious diseases that may rapidly deteriorate if not managed expertly. Taking an appropriately detailed history, whilst performing a rapid initial assessment to pick out those who are worryingly unwell, requires a systematic but flexible approach.

Children with respiratory problems present with one or more of the following symptoms/signs:

- Stridor (📖 p.202).
- Wheeze (📖 p.210).
- Tachypnoea (📖 p.220).
- Cough (📖 p.226).
- Haemoptysis (📖 p.230).

These are discussed individually in subsequent pages but the key features of the history and examination remain the same.

History

Elicit details of the present complaint(s), as well any previous symptoms and also look for risk factors for respiratory illness.

- Tachypnoea—is there persistent or intermittent breathlessness? Does it reduce activity or feeding?
- Cough —is it productive, paroxysmal, or does the child change colour? Is it a barking cough (upper airway) or a chesty cough (lower airway)?
- Other noises.
  - Stridor—an inspiratory noise, ± hoarse voice/cry.
  - Wheeze—an expiratory noise.
  - Snoring—intermittent or persistent.
- Precipitants—does anything make the problem worse?
  - Colds, pollen, exercise, cold air, feeding, lying flat.
  - Cigarette smoke (child or parent). Outside is better than indoors, but it is rare to see parents standing in the rain outside the back door, having a smoke in the UK!
- Was the onset acute? E.g. epiglottitis, foreign body (N.B. missing small toys), juggling peanuts?
- Family history—are the family well? Are there illnesses that run in the family?
  - Asthma, hay fever, eczema.
  - CF, immunodeficiency, chronic cough (TB).
- Are there pets? N.B. birds and farm animals (psitticosis and brucellosis).
- Immunity—is the child fully immunized; are there chronic infections suggestive of immuno-incompetence (📖 p.148)?
- Interim symptoms—is there cough, wheeze, or breathlessness, when the child is well or exercising?

Examination

Much is learned by observation. Once a child is approached, auscultation, amid the cries, can become challenging

Look and listen

Posture Beware the child sitting upright or forwards, supporting their weight on their arms ('tripod position'). They are fixing their pectoral muscles in an attempt to optimize a failing respiratory system.

Level of consciousness Restless, agitated, drowsy.
- Secondary to hypoxia, hypercapnia, or just tired?

Colour Pink, blue, pale.

Respiratory rate age-dependent (Table 11.1).

Beware a normal respiratory rate in an ill and tiring child!

Work of breathing Signs of respiratory distress (Table 11.2).
- Nasal flaring, head bobbing.
- Use of accessory muscles.
- Intercostal recession.
- Sternal tug.
- Grunting—attempting to provide extra PEEP as small airways collapse.
- Prolonged expiratory phase—precedes or coincident with wheeze.

Expansion
- Symmetry. N.B. Chest deformities, e.g. scoliosis, gibbus.
- Hyperinflation.

Table 11.1 Respiratory rate at different ages

	Neonate	**<1 year**	**1–5 years**	**>5 years**
Breaths/minute	30–50	25–45	20–30	15–25

Physiological factors increasing respiratory rate

Factors increasing respiratory rate
- Fever
- Agitation
- Fear
- Hyperventilation
- Pain

Factors decreasing respiratory rate
- Impending respiratory collapse
- Raised intracranial pressure

Table 11.2 Assessment of work of breathing

	Mild	Moderate	Severe
Feeding/drinking	Normal	Reduced	Unable
Ability to talk	Sentences	Phrases	Words
Respiratory rate	May be increased slightly	Much faster than expected	Very fast, or worryingly normal
Heart rate			
<5 years old	<100	100–120	>120
>5 years old	<80	80–110	>110
Altered level of consciousness	No	No	Yes
Exhaustion	No	No	Yes
Central cyanosis	Absent	Absent	Present
Accessory muscle use	None/minimal	Moderate	Severe
Hyperinflation	None	Lots	Marked
Recession	Absent	Moderate	Marked
Wheeze	Moderate	Loud	Often quiet

Added sounds

Beware the silent chest or one that is less wheezy than expected

- Hoarse cry/voice.
- Inspiratory.
  - Stertor—pharyngeal obstruction, e.g. tonsils.
  - Stridor—reflects supraglottic narrowing. Biphasic stridor = tracheal pathology.
- Expiratory.
  - Wheeze—polyphonic. Bronchiolar pathology.
  - Crepitations—crackles. Alveolar pathology.
- Cough—distinguish between pharyngeal (harsh or barking), and bronchial ('chesty').

Other

- Harrison sulci.
  - Grooves parallel and above costal margin, caused by excessive diaphragmatic activity in chronic respiratory insufficiency.
- Clubbing.
- Palpable pulsus paradoxus (increase in the normal drop in systolic pressure on inspiration; causes reduction in pulse volume from beat to beat) seen with extreme respiratory effort.

Feel

- Tracheal position—be gentle, it's an unpleasant sensation.
  - Deviated away by tension pneumothorax, large effusion (fluid or blood).
  - Pulled towards significant collapse.
- Apex beat—5th intercostal space, mid-axillary line (4th in >5 years). More lateral with right ventricular hypertrophy.
- Expansion—>1cm in >5 years.

Percuss

Compare sides.

- Hyperresonance—air-trapping or pneumothorax (📖 p.103).
- Dull—consolidation and/or collapse.
- Stony dull—fluid—pleural effusion, haemothorax, empyema.

Ausculate

Compare sides.

- Stridor—upper airway obstruction (📖 p.202).
- Bronchial breathing—infection, or above fluid collection.
- Wheeze (or prolonged expiratory phase)—small airway obstruction (📖 p.210).
- Crackles—atelectasis, infection, fluid.

Common investigations

FBC, CRP, ESR

- Non-specific increase in WCC in inflammation and infection. Raised neutrophils do not confirm bacterial infection.
- Raised eosinophils in allergy, asthma, and parasitic infection.
- Role of pro-calcitonin yet to be confirmed in clinical practice.

Oxygen saturation Non-invasive measure of difference in light absorption between oxygenated and de-oxygenated blood.

- Allow pulse oximeter to 'settle' before reading.
- Compare reading with the colour/clinical state of child.
- If poor signal, do not believe result.
  - Try warmer, better perfused digit or ear lobe.
- Inaccurate at extremes of range.

Chest x-ray (CXR)

Only order a CXR when you suspect it will provide information that will change your management, e.g. where diagnosis unclear or child very ill.

Stridor CXR or lateral neck x-ray not required routinely and ***never*** if suspect epiglottitis.

Asthma Only when:

- unilateral signs that persist after initial treatment. Areas of atelectasis are very common and are mechanical, rather than infective;
- acute severe asthma, to exclude pneumothorax.

If tension pneumothorax diagnosed clinically, ***must*** treat with insertion of intercostal drain (📖 p.478) before ordering CXR

Bronchiolitis Rarely need CXR. Necessary if sudden deterioration—exclude pneumothorax or lobar collapse.

Pneumonia If the diagnosis is clinically apparent, children ***do not*** routinely need CXR. Only required if unsure and child tachypnoeic and/or febrile.

Foreign body Mandatory. Ideally inspiratory and expiratory films. Otherwise, lying on affected side to demonstrate that lobe does not deflate.

Cough Rarely helpful, but usually done to exclude foreign body.

Haemoptysis If significant amount of blood.

Blood gas

Blood gas analysis rarely alters management. The decision to instigate respiratory support is always a clinical one made by an experienced paediatrician.

Venous blood gas results will usually suffice in the first instance. They may overestimate acidosis and give little indication of oxygen level. Venous samples are a reasonable alternative to arterial stabs, especially if watching a trend, e.g. DKA. If the result does not fit the clinical picture, then an arterial sample is needed. However, arterial samples are painful, even with EMLA.

Capillary sample from a well-perfused heel provides reliable acid–base data only.

Lung function tests

Rarely useful in acute setting and difficult for children under 7 to do.

- PEFR—effort-dependent and unlikely to be reliable in sick children. Hospitalization is usually required if the post-bronchodilator PEFR is <60% of recent best.
- FEV_1—as for PEFR.
- FVC—Useful in respiratory assessment of neuromuscular conditions e.g. worsening ascending paralysis in Guillain–Barré syndrome.

Stridor

Stridor is a high-pitched, harsh noise, secondary to turbulent flow through a partially obstructed upper airway. Stertor is a coarse inspiratory noise through a narrowed nose/pharynx ('Darth-Vader like'). Ask parent to demonstrate noise to be sure they are describing inspiratory noise.

Usually inspiratory, but may be biphasic and variable.

- Inspiratory. Usually extra-thoracic lesion, at or above glottis. During inspiration, extra-thoracic intraluminal airway pressure is negative, relative to atmospheric pressure, leading to collapse of supraglottal structures.
- Biphasic—glottic, subglottic, tracheal. A fixed obstruction resulting in a fixed calibre airway.

Typically arises in children aged 6 months to 5 years. Stridor in children under 6 months is suggestive of congenital defects, e.g. laryngomalacia, vascular ring, and warrants investigation. Older children suffering stridor tend to have airway sensitivity, e.g. hay fever, asthma, and have recurrent episodes. Stridor may be more severe in ex-premature infants and those with low muscle tone, e.g. Down's syndrome, myotonias.

Table 11.3 covers possible differential diagnoses of stridor, but the commonest causes are:

- croup;
- epiglottitis;
- foreign body;
- anaphylaxis;
- laryngomalacia.

Of these, epiglottitis, anaphylaxis, and foreign body inhalation are potentially life-threatening. Make certain that you have excluded them all before treating as 'croup'.

Table 11.3 Differential diagnosis of stridor

Common	Uncommon	Rare	Very rare
Supralaryngeal			
Hypertrophic adenoids	Macroglossia, e.g. Down's, Beckwith–Wiedeman	Choanal atresia	Vallecular cyst
		Thyroglossal cyst	Tongue dermoid
			Tongue teratoma
Laryngeal			
Viral croup	Spasmodic croup	Epiglottitis	Laryngeal cleft
Laryngomalacia	Foreign body	Retropharyngeal abscess	Bilateral vocal cord palsy
Hypertrophic tonsils	Anaphylaxis—angioneurotic oedema	Subglottic stenosis	Laryngeal web
		Peritonsillar abscess	Cyst/hygroma
		Hysterical	Haemangioma
		Hypocalcaemic laryngospasm	Papillomata
Tracheal			
	Foreign body	Double aortic arch	Deep strawberry naevus
Tracheomalacia	Bacterial tracheitis	Aberrant innominate artery	Bronchogenic cyst
	Tracheal stenosis	Aberrant subclavian vein	
		Pulmonary artery sling (sling–ring complex)	

Viral croup (laryngotracheobronchitis)

Commonest cause of stridor in children, aged 6 months to 3 years. May recur in older children.

History Usually coryzal for preceding days, with acute onset barking cough, often in middle of night. Often well during day. Can deteriorate rapidly.

Examination Characteristic seal-like, barking cough, when upset, or when supine. Low grade fever, but usually not systemically ill. Respiratory distress is usually mild. If severe, consider possibility of epiglottitis and enlist senior help urgently (Table 11.4 and 11.5).

Investigation Pulse oximetry, if tolerated.

Treatment

See algorithm in Fig. 11.1 for management of croup.

- Oxygen, if saturation <92%.
- Oral steroids:
  - dexamethasone 0.15mg/kg PO, one or two doses;
  - budesonide nebulized is an expensive, and no more effective alternative.

Epiglottitis

Increasing prevalence because of decreasing immunization rates.

History Typically arises in children aged 2–5 years old. High fever with child rapidly becoming unwell. Complains of sore throat, dysphagia. May not have been immunized to *Haemophilus influenzae B*.

Examination Flushed, drooling, toxic-looking child. Sitting upright, in tripod position, with soft stridor. ***Only touch child if respiratory arrest.***

Investigation

Only performed when airway controlled by intubation.

- FBC, blood cultures, and throat swab.
- Immunoglobulins, anti-tetanus, and Hib antibody levels—markers of ability to mount immune response post-immunization.

Treatment

- Summon most senior anaesthetist and ENT surgeon available.
- Arrange for careful transfer to area where gaseous induction of anaesthesia possible, and where emergency tracheostomy can be performed (p.476), if intubation impossible.
- Start IV cefotaxime 50mg/kg/dose tds before transfer to PICU.

Table 11.4 Distinguishing croup and epiglottitis

	Croup	Epiglottitis
Onset	Acute/sub-acute	Hours
Cough	Barking	Weak
Fever	None or mild	>38°
General appearance	Well	Ill, with drooling
Timing	Worse at night	No diurnal variation
Cyanosis	Rare	Common
Treatment	Supportive, steroids	Intubation and antibiotics

Table 11.5 Assessment of severity of croup

	Mild	Moderate	Severe
Stridor	±	+	++
Sternal tug	–	+	++
Recession	–	+	++
Accessory muscles	–	+	++
Nasal flare	–	+	++
Cyanosis	–	–	+
Drooling	–	–	+
Air entry	Normal	Reduced	Poor
Hydration	Normal	Normal/reduced	Reduced
If the child does not object:			
Saturation	Normal	Normal/reduced	Reduced
Heart rate	Normal	Raised	Raised (bradycardia is a pre-terminal event)

Foreign body aspiration

If child presents acutely, treat as for choking (p.58)

- If maintaining own airway, but unwell, do not move. Inform senior colleague and ENT team.
- O_2 as tolerated, without upsetting child.
- ***Do not blindly finger sweep mouth*** as this may force FB more distal.

History
- Commonest between 6 months and 3 years.
- Symptoms may be transient but ask whether there is:
  - persistent cough;
  - purulent sputum or bad breath.

Examination
Signs depend on level of obstruction.
- Laryngeal/tracheal.
  - Croupy cough, stridor, tachypnoea ± hypoxaemia/cyanosis.
  - Chest often clear, or transmitted noises.
- Lower trachea/bronchial. Initial cough, choking, or wheeze may settle, followed by minimal symptoms over the following days or weeks. Atelectasis will develop with a bronchial cough ± wheeze and signs resembling a lower respiratory tract infection, e.g. temperature, crackles, bronchial breathing, decreased air entry on affected side, and/or hyperresonance of affected side.

Investigation
- Expiratory CXR—unilateral hyperexpansion of affected lobes ± atelectasis distal to the obstruction.
- Alternatively, lateral CXR with child lying on affected side to confirm lack of deflation.
- In 20% of cases, foreign body visible. If doubt about position, a lateral CXR will confirm if it is bronchial or oesophageal.
- Pulse oximetry—may be normal.

Treatment Very rarely, urgent tracheostomy required. Bronchoscopy—usually rigid, under general anaesthetic—to remove foreign body.

Anaphylaxis

Rapid onset of wheeze, which may be accompanied by urticaria and swelling of lips, mouth, and face. Stridor develops when airway compromised. At risk of circulatory collapse. Enquire about potential precipitants and remove any still present, e.g. bee stings. IM adrenaline necessary (p.62).

Upper airway constriction

This can be either congenital or acquired. Laryngomalacia is the commonest congenital airway malformation. Infectious causes include retropharyngeal and peritonsillar abscesses.

ⓘ *Laryngomalacia*

History

- Often chronic stridor, with acute exacerbations secondary to respiratory infection.
- May be present from birth or appear in first few days.
- Exacerbated by feeding, crying, or lying supine.
- If present at all times, or biphasic consider fixed anatomical obstruction, e.g. ring–sling complex, with aberrant left pulmonary artery.

Examination Often mild respiratory distress; worse when upset. Positional stridor, i.e. improves when sat upright. Plot growth on percentile chart.

Investigation None, unless to exclude other causes of airway malformation.

Treatment Nil but admission necessary if significant respiratory signs or failure to thrive.

ⓘ *Other airway malformations*

All these are rare, but may cause persistent non-positional stridor in children under 6 months. If lower airway compressed, can also cause chronic wheeze.

- Extrinsic compression of airway:
    - mediastinal tumour;
    - T-cell lymphoma;
    - neuroblastoma.
- Aberrant blood vessels:
    - pulmonary artery;
    - double aortic arch.
- Intrinsic abnormality:
    - congenital cystic adenomatous malformation;
    - congenital lobar emphysema.

Investigation CXR. If abnormal, refer to respiratory team. May need barium swallow ± chest CT.

Retropharyngeal abscess (📖 p.314)

ⓘ *Peritonsillar abscess* (📖 p.312)

Immediate management of stridor

Make certain that you are dealing with croup. Assess severity, from the end of the cot, without disturbing child (Table 11.5).

- ☠ If severe, emergency treatment with O_2 and adrenaline (Fig. 11.1).
- Otherwise, take history and examine
- Do not disturb child—leave on carer's lap, in position of comfort.

History

- Is it definitely stridor, not wheeze? Has the child's cry/voice changed?
- When was the onset? Has the severity changed?
- Any precipitants, e.g. URTI, contact with peanuts, playing with small toy?
- Any effect on activity, talking?
- Any cough, vomiting, or diarrhoea? Any rash noticed?
- Any drooling?
- Any possibility of foreign body? N.B. Choking episode in past months.
- Any previous episodes of stridor?
- Ask about neonatal events, particularly if ventilation was required and its duration. N.B. Ventilation may be ongoing but non-invasive.
- Is the child fully immunized?
- Any congenital abnormalities?
- Is the child thriving?

Examination

General

- Level of consciousness—less responsive, if hypoxic.
- Drooling.
- Fever.
- Dysmorphic features (Down syndrome, cranio-facial), cutaneous naevi (capillary haemangioma may be deep and involve underlying structures).

Specific

- Any respiratory distress; tachypnoea, tracheal tug, recession, poor air entry.
- Barking cough, hoarse cry.
- Tachycardia, murmur.

Stridor

- At rest or intermittent; worse with crying or anxiety?
- Timing.
- Loudness ***not*** indicative of severity.

Investigation

- If *in extremis*, none necessary before treatment.
- Otherwise only saturations, if probe tolerated.
- Neck x-rays never indicated.
- Other tests may be indicated for rarer causes (see individual disease).

Treatment See Fig. 11.1 for treatment of stridor. See individual diseases for specific treatment.

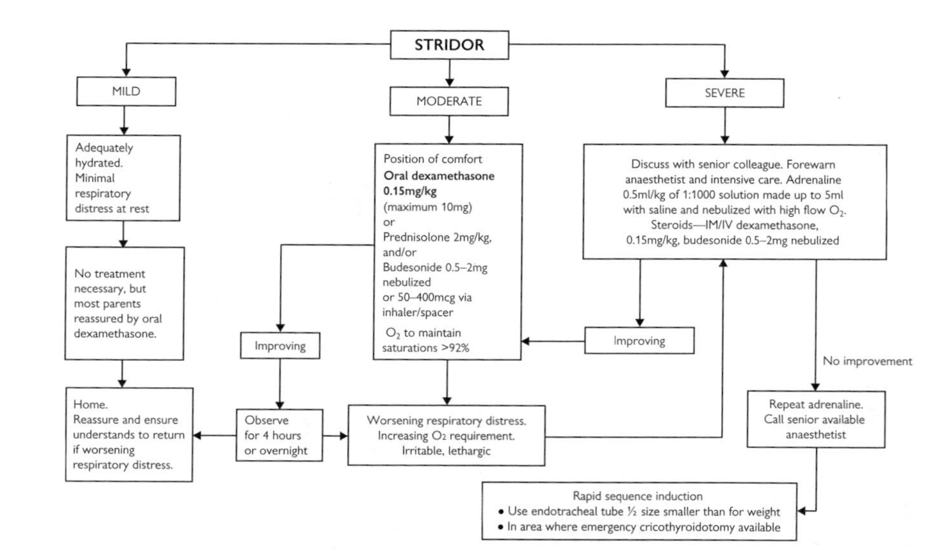

Fig. 11.1 Algorithm for treatment of stridor.

Wheeze

Ask carer to demonstrate the noise they call wheeze—they sometimes mean upper airways noise or stridor.

Predominantly expiratory, but may be biphasic.

> Do not presume that all that wheezes is asthma!

Causes may be acute:

- viral-induced wheeze;
- bronchiolitis (📖 p.218);
- foreign body (📖 p.219);
- aspiration (📖 p.219);
- anaphylaxis (📖 p.62);
- air pollutants—sulphur dioxide.

However, causes may also be acute exacerbations of a chronic problem:

- asthma;
- airway malformation—intrinsic or extrinsic (📖 p.207);
- chronic lung disease (bronchopulmonary dysplasia) (📖 p.219);
- cystic fibrosis;
- post-viral airway sensitivity (📖 p.219).

These may be distinguished by the history and examination, as discussed in the following pages.

However, the life-threatening forms of wheeze are:

- ☠ anaphylaxis. Rapid onset of wheeze, which may be accompanied by urticaria and swelling of lips, mouth, and face. At risk of airway compromise and circulatory collapse. Enquire about potential precipitants and remove any still present, e.g. bee stings. IM adrenaline necessary (📖 p.62).
- ☠ acute severe asthma.

Foreign body Requires a high index of suspicion, as initial incident may have occurred many days prior to onset of symptoms and may have been forgotten. See p.206.

Aspiration pneumonitis

Typically seen in children with impaired swallowing.

History

Key factors

- Temporal relation between feeds and respiratory distress.
- Cough, choke, splutter with feeds.
- Recurrent regurgitation of feeds or vomiting.
- Proven gastro-oesophageal regurgitation:
  - barium swallow or pH study.

Examination

- Signs of pre-existing neurological abnormality.
- Often febrile.
- Wide spectrum—minimal signs to severe respiratory distress.
- Crackles ± wheeze.

Investigations

- Pulse oximetry normal or reduced.
  - Check what is the patient's usual saturation.
- CXR—focal (often right upper) or diffuse changes.

Treatment If ill, IV cefuroxime and metronidazole. Respiratory support, such as CPAP or invasive ventilation, if child still suitable for full life-support measures.

Airway malformation See p.207.

Chronic lung disease Chronic lung disease or bronchopulmonary dysplasia develops in preterm neonates treated with oxygen and positive pressure ventilation. It is loosely defined as an oxygen requirement at 28 days of life. They are more prone to wheeze as infants and, importantly, they are more likely to need respiratory support if they catch a respiratory virus, such as RSV. Some may benefit from prophylactic passive immunization with RSV-specific immunoglobulin and/or early treatment with drugs active against influenza (palivizumab).

Post-viral Wheeze may persist after a viral upper or lower respiratory infection has resolved. Equally, subsequent infections may be associated with worse wheeze. Maternal smoking during pregnancy reduces airway diameter, predisposing to viral-induced wheeze. Bronchiolitis also increases the risk of subsequent wheeze.

Tachypnoea

From the safety of the end of the cot, assess the respiratory system. Important to assess the work of breathing, as well as rate and oxygen saturation by pulse oximetry (see Tables 11.1 and 11.2).

If tachypnoeic, consider non-respiratory causes (see box).

The commonest respiratory cause is pneumonia but remember to exclude a foreign body (📖 p.206) and asthma (📖 p.212)

Causes of tachypnoea

Respiratory
- Upper respiratory tract infection
- Lower respiratory tract infection
- Foreign body
- Asthma

Non-respiratory
- Cardiac failure
- Metabolic acidosis, e.g. DKA
- Intracranial pathology ± raised ICP—rate may increase, decrease, or become irregular
- Raised temperature
- Anxiety/fear
- Hyperventilation

☼ Pneumonia

- Common; incidence 40 per 1000 in pre-school children.
- Mainly viral, various bacteria, atypicals (*Mycoplasma* spp.). See Table 11.8.
- Depends on seasons, age, immune susceptibility.

History

Often recent viral URTI, which allows commensal organisms access to the lower respiratory tract. Increased risk of pneumonia if:
- ex-premature babies;
- the very young, with poor socio-economic background;
- lots of siblings;
- parents who smoke.

Further risk factors are:
- impaired local defences—recent URTI;
- immunocompromised;
- neurological deficits—poor cough reflex, muscle weakness;
- mucociliary abnormality.

Ask about:

- pyrexia—not always present in viral illness or *Chlamydia*. Rigors suggest either lower lobe pneumonia or bacteraemia;
- cough—intermittent or paroxysmal;
- coryza;
- increased work of breathing, e.g. is there exercise limitation?
- impaired feeding—any vomiting? Are they feeding less than usual? Were they thriving before this illness?
- any associated symptoms, e.g. abdominal pain is indicative of lower lobe pneumonia or else *Staph. aureus* infection; diarrhoea occurs with pneumococcal sepsis, as well as viral illness or after oral antibiotics.

Examination

- Document work of breathing, respiratory rate, presence of crackles, or bronchial breathing.
- Assess level of hydration and nutrition.
- ***No signs are sensitive or specific for bacterial rather than viral infection.***

Investigation

- Pulse oximetry—less than 92% requires supplemental O_2.
- FBC—neutrophilia is suggestive, but not diagnostic, of bacterial infection.
- CRP—does not differentiate viral from bacterial.
- Blood cultures—positive in 10–30% bacterial pneumonia.
- ± serology for viruses, *Mycoplasma, Chlamydia*.
- CXR—no pathognomonic features.
  - Lobar changes suggest Pneumococcus or *Haemophilus influenzae*.
  - Pneumatoceles common with *Staphylococcus aureus*.
  - Large pleural effusions are usually bacterial (*Pneumococcus*).
  - Patchy, perihilar changes suggestive of *Mycoplasma* or virus.
- ± NPA—immunofluorescence or PCR, for RSV, human metapneumovirus (HMPV), 'flu and paraflu', adenovirus.

Treatment

- **Oxygen** saves lives—give generously to all those with saturations <92%.
- Assess hydration. If dehydrated, ideally, rehydrate by mouth or orogastric tube. If IV fluids given, reduce to 80% maintenance and check UEC daily as at risk of SIADH.

Table 11.7 Common causes of LRTI

Pathogen	Distinguishing clinical features	Risk factors	Key investigations	Treatment	Complications
Viral 'bronchiolitis' if <2 years 'Viral pneumonitis' if >2 years	• Under 4 years • Apnoea in children under 3 months • Only 50% will be febrile • Wheeze progressing to crackles	• Ex-premature • Overcrowding, e.g. daycare, deprived domestic circumstances	• NPA • CXR if necessary—hyperinflated with bilateral infiltrates	If required • Oxygen if SpO_2 <92% • Orogastric feeds • IV fluids—80% maintenance • Antivirals (seldom indicated)	• Post-viral wheeze • SIADH • Bronchiolitis obliterans, especially post-adenovirus
Pneumococcus	Diarrhoea	• Immunocompromised, e.g. asplenic, nephrotic syndrome • Post-varicella	• CXR—lobar consolidation	• Oral amoxycillin **or** erythromycin if penicillin allergy • IV penicillin **or** cefuroxime if local resistance	• Pleural effusion (25%) • Disseminated disease in immunocompromised
Haemophilus influenzae (Hib)		• Overcrowding, e.g. daycare, deprived domestic circumstances • Recent viral illness	• CXR—lobar consolidation	• Amoxycillin/clavulanic acid • Ceftriaxone	• Invasive Hib disease—all household contacts and children <4 to receive Hib booster

Staph. aureus	• Rapid progression to very sick child • Abdominal pain		• CXR—pneumatoceles	• IV flucloxacillin ± rifampicin ± vancomycin if resistance	• Pleural effusion (55%) • Lung abscess • Empyema • Disseminated disease
Mycoplasma	• Viral URTI-like symptoms but *no* runny nose • Headache • Myalgia • Diffuse crackles	• Summer epidemics	• CXR—perihilar interstitial shadowing; may be unilateral • Mycoplasma serology • IgM cold agglutinins if child over 5 years	• Azithromycin 5 days **or** • Clarithromycin 7 days	• Arthralgia • Pericarditis • Aseptic meningitis • Chronic reversible small airways disease
Chlamydia	• Dry, staccato cough • Tachypnoea with minimal signs on auscultation • Muco-purulent conjunctivitis in neonates	• Neonatal presentation means congenital exposure. Treat both parents (📖 p.362).	• CXR—interstitial shadowing • Chlamydia serology • If conjunctivitis, use specific swabs and culture medium	• Erythromycin 5 days • Tetracycline ointment qds for conjunctivitis	

Bronchiolitis/viral pneumonia (📖 p.218)

Discharge home if clinical diagnosis is clear and:

- >3 months.
- No O_2 requirement.
- Adequately hydrated.
- No underlying medical condition, e.g. cardiac, chronic lung disease.
- Safe social circumstances, with parent who understands to return, if worsens.

Bacterial pneumonia

There may be textbook clinical features to help you to determine the nature of the illness (Table 11.7 and 11.8). Often, you will have to resort to 'best-guess' antibiotics, according to local resistance. A suggested regimen is:

- mild pneumonia—oral amoxycillin or erythromycin;
- moderate—admit. IV penicillin;
- severe—admit. IV cefotaxime ± flucloxacillin.

Complications: pleural effusions/empyema

Clinical diagnosis with reduced air entry and stony dullness on percussion. Confirm on US and ask radiographer to mark spot for drain. Aspiration with large cannula may be diagnostic and therapeutic, but intercostal drain (📖 p.478) is optimal. Intrapleural urokinase may expedite drainage.

Table 11.8 Best guess antibiotics

Age	Signs and symptoms	CXR appearance	Likely organism	Therapy
Neonate	Respiratory distress Lethargy Fever	Reticular pattern or lobar	Group B streptococcus *Listeria*	Ampicillin + gentamicin
Infant	Cough Tachypnoea Minimal fever Wheeze	Hyperinflated, with bilateral infiltrates	Viral or *Chlamydia*	Supportive Consider erythromycin
Infant	High fever Cough Tachypnoea	Lobar or segmental ± effusion	*Pneumococcus, Haemophilus influenzae, Staphylococcus aureus*	Cefuroxime
Child	Abrupt onset High fever Cough Tachypnoea	Lobar	*Pneumococcus*	Amoxicillin if well, or IV benzyl penicillin or ampicillin
Child	Post-viral Fever Tachypnoea Bilateral signs	Patchy consolidation	*Pneumococcus, Haemophilus influenzae, Staphylococcus aureus* Viral	Cefuroxime
Child	Post viral Fever Tachypnoea Unilateral or bilateral signs Hypoxic	Lobar/ segmental ± effusion	*Pneumococcus, Haemophilus influenzae, Staphylococcus aureus*	Third generation cephalosporin + flucloxacillin
Child	Malaise, cough, wheeze, mild fever, myalgia	Segmental or patchy consolidation, reticular shadowing	Mycoplasma, viral	Macrolide

Reproduced with permission from Dr A Thomson, Consultant Respiratory Paediatrician, Oxford Children's Hospital, Oxford, UK.

ⓘ Cough

Rarely presents as primary problem to emergency department, but may be associated with respiratory distress or apnoea/cyanosis.

History

Quality

- Barking—croup, or in those with repaired tracheo-oesophageal fistula ('TOF-cough').
- Paroxysms ± vomiting/'whoop'/cyanosis/apnoea—whooping cough (📖 p.228)
- Short, sharp 'staccato'—*Mycoplasma*, *Chlamydia*.
- Loud, 'honking' – psychogenic.

Timing

- Associated with feeds ± vomits ± choking:
  - gastro-oesophageal reflux (GOR);
  - H-type tracheo-oesophageal fistula;
  - neurological impairment resulting in discoordinate swallow and chronic micro-aspiration.
- Night-time:
  - post-nasal drip;
  - asthma;
  - sinusitis;
  - GOR;
  - croup;
  - cardiac failure.
- Early morning:
  - LRTI;
  - cystic fibrosis;
  - bronchiectasis.
- Exercise/cold-induced:
  - asthma
  - cardiac failure.
- Only when awake ± school days, when observed:
  - psychogenic.

Examination

- Listen to cough.
- Associated symptoms such as pharyngitis, laryngitis, tender sinuses, snoring, stridor all suggest upper airway. Wheeze, crackles, reduced air entry, suggest LRTI.
- Big liver, gallop rhythm suggest cardiac failure.
- Upper quadrant abdominal tenderness is indicative of diaphragmatic irritation.

Investigations

- Pulse oximetry in all.
- Consider CXR (📖 p.200).

Treatment

If predominant symptom/sign is stridor/wheeze or LRTI, see also 📖 p.202, p.210.

Treatment of chronic cough is frequently ineffective. Codeine-based medication may help, particularly at night. Nasal steroids or anti-histamines may reduce postnasal drip.

Table 11.9 Differential diagnosis of cough based on age and anatomy

	Location		
Age	**Upper airway**	**Lower airway**	**Non-respiratory**
Infancy	URTI	Bronchiolitis	Impaired gag/cough
	GOR	LRTI	
	Croup		
	Foreign body		
	Whooping cough	TOF	
	Laryngeal oedema	Tracheal compression	
	Aspiration	Pulmonary oedema	
Pre-school	URTI	Asthma	
	Croup	LRTI	
	Foreign body	CF	
	Laryngeal oedema	Acute bronchitis	Heart failure
		Aspiration	Phrenic or vagal nerve irritation
		Noxious fume inhalation	
School age	URTI	Asthma	
	Sinusitis	LRTI	
	Post-nasal drip	Noxious fume inhalation	
	Smoking		
			Psychogenic

Whooping cough

Caused by *Bordetella pertussis* or *B. parapertussis*, which are Gram-negative bacilli. *B. parapertussis* produces a similar, but milder clinical picture. Vaccination provides >90% protection from disease and reduces the morbidity if the child contracts *B. pertussis*. Unimmunized infants or those with underlying cardiorespiratory disease are most likely to die or suffer significant morbidity, such as bronchiectasis. Whooping cough is highly infectious by droplets, but antibiotics reduce the risk of transmission.

There are three indistinct phases.

- **Catarrhal phase.**
  - Dry cough, with coryza.
  - Macrolide antibiotics at this stage may attenuate course.
- **Paroxysmal phase.**
  - Increasing cough with paroxysms of continuous cough, followed by inspiratory 'whoop' and/or vomiting.
  - Babies may have apnoea instead of whoop.
  - May go blue.
- **Recovery phase.**
  - Chronic cough that may last up to 3 months (was known as the 'hundred day cough').

Complications Subconjunctival haemorrhage, pneumothorax, surgical emphysema.
1 in 10 000 have fits or encephalitis.

History Check risk factors in perinatal and past medical history. Alarming symptoms include episodes of apnoea or cyanosis, along with impaired feeding.

Examination ABC and oximetry, particularly during coughing. Assess adequacy of feeding and check for chest signs of unilateral collapse or atelectasis.

Investigation

- CXR—if unilateral signs, or concerns over air leaks.
- FBC—relative lymphocytosis at 2 weeks, which may be very high (normal in *B. parapertussis*).
- IgA serology.
- Pernasal swab—many labs accept NPA, so check first. Culture only positive in 50% after 5 days incubation.
- PCR increasingly available and will supercede culture.

Management

- Always admit babies under 6 months. Observation necessary for apnoea, bradycardia or severe desaturation when coughing.
- Give oxygen if saturations persistently <92%.
- Orogastric feeds if dehydrated or FTT. If frequently coughs up tube, or working hard, then IV fluids at 75% maintenance as at risk of SIADH.

- If frequent bradycardia, hypoxia, or tiring, request PICU review as may require assisted ventilation.
- Macrolide antibiotic to reduce infectivity.
- Prophylactic treatment with erythromycin for 10 days:
  - household contacts under 5 years;
  - immunocompromised contacts;
  - contacts with underlying chronic illness.

Adults lose their immunity with time, but suffer a milder illness of chronic cough. They are a source of infection.

Haemoptysis

Causes

Infectious

- Bacterial LRTI.
- Viral, e.g. measles.
- Tuberculosis.
- Suppuration, e.g. cystic fibrosis, bronchiectasis.

Non-infectious

- Inhaled foreign body.
- Pulmonary embolus.
- Pulmonary contusion, e.g. trauma, fractured rib.
- Airway compression, e.g. cystic adenomatous malformation, large left atrium, anomalous vessels.
- Arteriovenous malformation.
- Bleeding diathesis.
- Wegener's granulomatosis.
- Pulmonary haemosiderosis (very rare).

History Determine whether this is haemoptysis or coughing up swallowed blood from nasal trauma. With haematemesis, the blood will be altered by stomach acid. Variceal bleeds in children with chronic liver disease do occur but are rare.

Check if any antecedent illness, abdominal pain, cough, choking, calf pain, chronic medical problems (cough, diarrhoea, FTT), fever, medications such as OCP.

Examination

- Evaluate ABCs—if in shock, manage as p.94.
- Usually not hypovolaemic, but may be hypoxic with respiratory distress.
- Signs depend on cause, e.g. tenderness and/or erythema over fractured rib; swollen, tender calf if DVT.

Investigation None necessary, if small amount. Otherwise, consider:

- FBC, cross-match, clotting;
- CXR.

Management

- Resuscitate, as needed.
- In emergency, replace lost blood with saline and with blood as soon as available.
- Inform anaesthetist and ENT ± general/paediatric surgeons, if significant haemorrhage.

Chapter 12

Gastroenterology

Many thanks to South Wales Network in Paediatric Gastroenterology and Dr Ike Lagunju for reviewing this chapter.

Assessment

There are three key areas:
- current nutritional status;
- growth;
- hydration status.

Current nutritional status
- Plot weight, length, and OFC (<2 years); weight and standing height (≥2 years) on growth chart. Correct for prematurity to 2 years.
  - Weight centile lower than centiles for length and OFC suggests recent weight loss.
  - Low height for age suggests long-term growth failure.
- Look for signs of protein–energy malnutrition.
  - Misery, apathy, and anorexia.
  - Pallor
  - Reduced muscle and subcutaneous fat, e.g. wasting of buttocks.

Children 1–5 years should have mid-upper arm circumference >13.5cm.
  - Depigmented, thin, sparse hair.
  - Nutritional oedema.
  - Hepatomegaly.
  - Signs of specific vitamin deficiencies, e.g. tibial bowing (D); corneal clouding (A); ataxia (E).

Growth Compare current indices with as many previous measurements as possible to assess trend of growth and growth velocity.

Hydration status Assess dehydration from difference between present and recent weight together with clinical signs (📖 p.239, Table 12.2).

Basic investigations
- FBC, UEC, creatinine.
- LFT including plasma albumin ± coagulation screen.
- Stool microscopy and culture.
- Urinalysis and urine culture.

Further assessment if undernourished
- Haematinics (ferritin, red cell folate, vitamin B_{12}).
- CRP and ESR.
- Bone profile (Ca^{2+}, PO_4^-, alkaline phosphatase).
- Anti-tissue transglutaminase (TTG) IgA antibodies plus total IgA—to exclude IgA deficiency. (IgA deficiency is more common in coeliac disease).
- Inspect stool, e.g. fat, blood; send for pH, reducing substances, fat.
- Consider sweat test, CXR for CF screening; karyotype.
- Measurement of selenium, zinc, and vitamins A, D, E requires consultation with laboratory.

Vomiting and GOR

Vomiting may result from diseases in many of the body systems. It may occur as one of a typical constellation of symptoms and signs, e.g. early morning vomiting ± headache suggests raised ICP. However, identifying the cause can be difficult and requires a thorough clinical assessment.

Try to differentiate the effortless regurgitation of gastro-oesophageal reflux (GOR) from the nausea, retching, and forceful vomiting that occur in the emetic reflex.

Assess carefully for dehydration and electrolyte imbalance. Consider finger prick glucose to exclude hypo- or hyperglycaemia (📖 p.404, p.413). Thereafter, management depends on the underlying cause. Anti-emetics are reserved for specific indications, e.g. cytotoxic therapy, central causes.

Common causes

- Infection—especially UTI, URTI, and meningitis. Low threshold for full septic screen including LP, if no contraindications (📖 p.470).
- Raised ICP—neurological assessment, BP, and consider CT scan brain.
- Drugs, e.g. cytotoxics, theophylline, digoxin, iron.
- Metabolic—uraemia; inherited metabolic disease such as urea cycle defects, organic acidaemias.
- Hormonal—diabetes mellitus (📖 p.404), adrenal insufficiency (📖 p.410).
- Psychogenic—especially if spitting saliva or retching.

Important gastroenterological causes include:

- acute gastroenteritis (📖 p.238);
- food intolerance—cow's milk protein, soya, egg;
- pyloric stenosis;
- gastro-oesophageal reflux—uncomplicated and complicated;
- cyclical vomiting;
- bulimia;
- peptic ulcer disease;
- rumination;
- pancreatitis (📖 p.250);
- intestinal obstruction (📖 p.274).

ⓘ Food allergy

Food-allergic enteropathy describes inflammation of the intestinal mucosa that resolves when the offending protein is withdrawn from the diet. The child develops chronic diarrhoea ± vomiting with poor weight gain. Other features may include colic, abdominal distension, gastro-oesophageal reflux, blood in the stools, eczema, perianal erythema, and nappy rash. Food-allergic enteropathy can occur without any immediate allergic manifestations, e.g. rash, urticaria, angio-oedema, anaphylaxis. Moreover, skin prick tests, and specific IgE may be negative.

The commonest clinical scenario is cow's milk protein-intolerance after a bout of gastroenteritis in a formula-fed infant. Other food proteins that commonly cause food-allergic enteropathy in young children are nuts, soya, eggs, and fish. Diagnosis depends on a detailed history and may require referral for blinded food challenges.

Management is by exclusion of the offending food and, in cow's milk-sensitive enteropathy, there is usually a marked clinical response when the infant is changed to an extensively hydrolysed milk formula. Dietetic advice is required to ensure that the diet remains adequate. Usually, the food is tolerated when introduced at age 2–3 years but intolerance persists in some children.

ⓘ Lactose intolerance

May be a congenital or acquired reduction in lactase levels, due to absence of enzyme, or damage to the small intestine mucosa. Bacteria in gut utilize the lactose forming glucose, galactose, and hydrogen; symptoms include bloating, flatulence, diarrhoea, and faltering growth.

Commonest presentation is with persistent or recurrent diarrhoea, following gastroenteritis. Diagnosis is on basis of history and presence of reducing sugars in (liquid portion of) faeces. It resolves with time, with or without a temporary lactose-free diet.

Other causes include the following.

- Primary or congenital alactasia; rare and presents with watery diarrhoea from birth.
- Acquired causes:
  - coeliac disease, IBD, allergic or auto-immune enteropathy, eosinophilic gastroenteritis;
  - reduced bowel surface area—short bowel syndrome;
  - rapid gut transit—thyrotoxicosis, dumping syndrome (gastrostomy fed child).
- Late onset—race-specific reduction in lactase activity with age.

ⓘ **Pyloric stenosis** Vomiting is post-prandial, non-bilious, and forceful. Usually presents between ages 2 and 8 weeks, and is more common in boys, especially the firstborn. The baby remains eager to feed. For further clinical features and management see 📖 p.276.

ⓘ Gastro-oesophageal reflux (GOR)—uncomplicated

'Posseting', even if frequent, does not require any investigation if the infant is well and gaining weight.

- Reassure parents.
- Exclude overfeeding—bottle-fed infants take up to 150ml/kg/day.
- Frequent small feeds and place prone or left-lateral after feeds.

If symptoms persist, use thickened feeds.

- Add thickener (e.g. Carobel®) to infant formula and use enlarged teat-hole. Breast-fed babies require thickener administered by spoon prior to breastfeeds.

- Change to pre-thickened feeds, e.g. Enfamil AR, SMA Staydown.
- Infant Gaviscon works as a thickener; beware sodium overload if cardiac/renal disease.

ⓘ Gastro-oesophageal reflux (GOR)—complicated

More common in preterm infants with chronic lung disease, cerebral palsy, or after GI surgery, e.g. oesophageal atresia, diaphragmatic hernia. Symptoms include: oesophagitis—retrosternal pain, irritability, blood in the vomit, anaemia; aspiration pneumonia; or weight loss. 'Reflux' with colic, diarrhoea, or eczema raises the possibility of food intolerance.

- Perform CXR for suspected pulmonary aspiration.
- Treat as for uncomplicated GOR.
- Add ranitidine
  - 1–6 months 1mg/kg 3 times daily;
  - 6 months–12 years 2–4mg/kg twice daily (maximum 150mg);
  - 12–18 years 150mg twice daily
- or proton-pump inhibitor e.g. Omeprazole
  - 1 month–2 years 700 mcg/kg once daily, increased if necessary to 3mg/kg, (maximum 20mg) once daily;
  - 10–20kg child 10mg once daily, increased to 20mg once daily if necessary;
  - >20kg 20mg once daily, increased to 40mg once daily if necessary. (Losec 10, 20, or 40mg can be dissolved in 10ml water; then take appropriate dose from that solution.)
- Refer for specialist investigation—24 hour oesophageal pH study, endoscopy, barium swallow or video fluoroscopy, speech therapy assessment.

ⓘ Cyclical vomiting

Recurrent episodes of nausea, vomiting, and abdominal pain lasting for hours or days with no identifiable organic cause and completely symptom-free intervals.

- Usual onset between ages 3 and 7 years.
- A personal or family history of migraine.
- May be an obvious trigger, e.g. infection, emotional stress, excitement.
- May be a prodrome, e.g. abdominal pain.
- Pallor, lethargy can arise ± fever and diarrhoea.

Exclude other causes of recurrent vomiting—especially gastrointestinal, renal, and metabolic.

If persistent vomiting and/or dehydration:

- check UEC;
- IV fluids: rehydrate with 0.45% saline/2.5% dextrose;
- nasogastric suction often helps;
- IV anti-emetics after correction of fluid balance.

After recovery, discuss how to avoid triggers, prophylaxis with migraine medicines (e.g. pizotifen), and early administration of anti-emetics during prodrome.

ⓘ Bulimia

Binge eating followed by vomiting, diarrhoea, dieting, and exercise. Most commonly found in adolescent girls with anxiety about body size and shape.

- Vomiting may be induced by gagging, saline, or other emetics.
- Vague gastrointestinal symptoms common.
- Often dysfunctional family, substance abuse, sexual abuse.
- Note loss of enamel on back of teeth and hypophosphataemia.
- Refer for expert child psychiatry assessment—psychotherapy and antidepressants.

? **Peptic ulcer disease** Rare in children. Epigastric pain prominent; may radiate to the back and wake from sleep. There may be blood in vomitus and epigastric tenderness. Refer for specialist assessment: C^{13} urea breath test for presence of *H. pylori*, endoscopy, barium studies. N.B. *H. pylori* serology does not reliably differentiate between current and past infection.

? **Rumination** The frequent regurgitation of previously ingested food into the mouth. Food may be spat out but without nausea or forceful vomiting. Occurs in GOR, mental retardation, bulimia, neglect—including prolonged hospitalization.

- Assess and manage underlying and associated causes.
- If neglect, increase attention especially during feeding.
- Supportive measures, e.g. community nurses, social workers.

Diarrhoea

The passage of 3 or more liquid stools in 24 hour period. For breastfed babies, the stools are more liquid than normal. Infection is the commonest cause of diarrhoea (Table 12.1), but may be outside the GI tract, e.g. UTI. Also consider other GI pathology, e.g. malabsorption, IBD in older children.

- Differentiate between acute (<14 days) and persistent (≥14 days) diarrhoea. The latter will require careful feeding after rehydration.
- Assess hydration status (Table 12.2). Two or more clinical signs are required for determination of severity.
- Record baseline weight.
- Check blood glucose and manage accordingly (📖 p.413).

Management

Young infants and children debilitated by chronic illness are at greater risk of a complicated course and should be reviewed frequently. Enteral rehydration is the safest treatment, whether oral or nasogastric. Breast feeding should be continued.

Severe dehydration (>10%) is rare in First World countries. However, shock, secondary to dehydration with sepsis, may be encountered. IV rehydration is undertaken with great care—if too rapid, it can result in hyponatraemia with devastating neurological sequelae. Babies under 3 months may require additional glucose supplementation.

Anti-emetics and anti-diarrhoeal drugs are not safe for use in children. Antibiotics are seldom used except in sepsis; dysentery; giardiasis; or *Clostridium difficile* infection (📖 p.490).

Severe dehydration (>10%)

- The child requires 100ml/kg, which is given over 3 to 6 hours depending on their age.
- Offer oral rehydration formula (ORF) whilst preparing IV.
- Give IV N/saline 30ml/kg over 1 hour in children <12 months or over 30 mins if ≥12 months.
- After infusion, reassess pulse, RR, perfusion and repeat if no response.
- Then, give 70ml/kg over 5 hours in children <12 months or over 2.5 hours in children ≥12 months.
- Give ORF 5ml/kg/hour as soon as child can drink.
- Check UEC and glucose 4 hourly—consider sampling cannula.
- Reassess frequently and adjust treatment accordingly.
- If unable to tolerate adequate oral intake, continue to rehydrate over 48 hours assuming 10% dry, using 0.45% saline + 2.5% dextrose (📖. p.507). Add potassium once UEC known.
- Consult with PICU if no improvement.

Table 12.1 Clinical features of common infectious diarrhoeal agents

Characteristics	Likely organisms
Watery stools	Viruses: rotavirus, enterovirus, adenovirus, norovirus Protozoa: *Cryptosporidium* spp
Bloody stools ± high fever, abdominal pain ± tenderness, guarding	Bacteria: *Shigella*, entero-invasive *Escherichia coli*, *Salmonella*, *Campylobacter* spp, *Staphylococcus aureus* Parasites: *Entamoeba histolytica*
Persistent diarrhoea	*Giardia lamblia*, rotavirus
After antibiotics	*Clostridium difficile*

Table 12.2 Clinical features of dehydration[1]. Assessment of hydration status requires 2 or more clinical features—WHO advocates the clinical features marked by an asterisk.

	Mild	Moderate	Severe
Behaviour*	Normal	Thirsty, restless, irritable	Lethargic, drowsy, cold
Willingness to drink*	Drinks	Thirsty—drinks eagerly	Unable to drink
Eyes*	Normal	Sunken	Very sunken
Tears	Normal	Reduced	Absent
Skin turgor after pinch*	<1s	1 to 2s	>2s
Mucosae	Normal	Dry	Very dry
Fontanelle	Normal	Sunken	Very sunken
Weight loss	<5%	5–10 %	>10%
Pulse	Normal	Rapid, normal volume	Rapid, weak, thready
Blood pressure	Normal	Normal or low	Low or unrecordable
Central capillary refill	<2s	2–4s	>4s
Urine output	Normal	Reduced	Very reduced, anuria

1 World Health Organization Division of Child Health and Development (1990). *A manual for the treatment of diarrhoea*, WHO/CDD/SER 80.2 Rev 2. WHO, Geneva.

Mild and moderate dehydration

- Start with a trial of enteral rehydration using oral rehydration formula, e.g. ReSoMal; Gastrolyte.
- Aim for child to drink 20ml/kg/h of ORF.
  - Children often dislike ORF as it is salty, so ask parents to offer ORF 'little and often'.
- Continue breastfeeding ± full strength bottle feeds.
- Place local anaesthetic (e.g. EMLA) patch and review after 1 hour.
- If oral intake inadequate, offer NGT rehydration with ORF; IV rehydration with 0.45% saline + 2.5% dextrose should be a last resort.
  - Check UEC and glucose.
  - Calculate fluids as maintenance plus deficit (maximum 5%).
  - Consider further trial of ORF after 4 hours.
- If child tolerates ORF trial, discharge home with written advice:
  - continue ORF and breast/bottle feeds;
  - offer simple foods, e.g. toast, crackers when vomiting settles;
  - warn that diarrhoea may continue for several days;
  - child should be reviewed if parents are concerned.

Complications

Hyponatraemic dehydration (serum Na^+ <130mmol/l)
- Stop IV fluids and review degree of dehydration.
- Check glucose and BP—exclude adrenal failure (p.410).
- Change to 0.9% saline and rehydrate over 48 hours (p.507).
- Check UEC 4 hourly.

Hypernatraemic dehydration (serum Na^+ >150mmol/l)
Clinical signs of dehydration are less reliable and mortality is higher. Aim to reduce serum sodium gradually, i.e. by less than 10mmol/l in 24 h.
- Seek senior advice early.
- Correct estimated fluid deficit over 48 hours (p.507)
  - If severe: contact consultant; use IV 0.45% saline + 2.5% dextrose with added K^+.
  - If mild/moderate dehydration: use ORF.
- Measure serum sodium every 4 hours.

Haemolytic uraemic syndrome
Bloody diarrhoea followed a week later by haemolytic anaemia, acute renal failure, thrombocytopenia. Usually secondary to toxin-producing *Escherichia coli*, but has also been described with *Campybolacter, Shigella,* and *Streptococcus pneumoniae*. (p.261).

Further information

Murphy, M.S. (1998). Guidelines for managing acute gastroenteritis based on a systematic review of published research. *Arch. Dis. Child.* **79**, 279–84.

? Faltering growth

Gain in weight and height less than expected in a young child.

Growth faltering should be assessed promptly because:

- it may be the presenting feature of numerous underlying pathologies;
- neglect or abuse should be considered;
- complex interactions between several interrelated factors often contribute to poor growth in an individual child, e.g. domestic violence in an economically deprived family;
- poor growth and micronutrient deficiency may require intervention.

Assess current nutritional status and trend of growth since birth (📖 p.232).

- Account for effects of prematurity and intra-uterine growth retardation
- Beware 'catch-down' growth occurring up to age 2 years.
  - Anthropometric indices fall from birth centiles (determined by intra-uterine environment) to those determined by genetic potential (estimated from mid-parental height).

Useful to think of 3 areas.

- ***Calories in***: feeding—from birth to present. Observe feeding, detailed assessment of adequacy of diet by a dietician.
- ***Calories out***: GI losses—vomiting, gastro-oesophageal reflux, malabsorption.
- ***Organ systems and other factors***.
  - Increased energy expenditure, e.g. chronic conditions (congenital heart disease, thyrotoxicosis).
  - CNS: developmental delay with feeding difficulties.
  - Chromosome/genetic abnormalities, e.g. Turner's syndrome.
  - Metabolic, e.g. renal tubular acidosis, diabetes insipidus.
  - Congenital, e.g. heart disease, obstructive uropathy.
  - Psychosocial, behaviour and interaction between child and mother or other carers.

Multidisciplinary assessment and management—paediatrician, dietician, speech and language therapists, social workers—is required in most children and can usually be performed on an out-patient basis.

Admission is indicated:

- for detailed investigation of underlying causes, e.g. imaging;
- if intensive nutritional repletion is required;
- if there are child protection issues. Child/parent interaction can be observed in a place of safety for the child.

? Hepatosplenomegaly

Numerous causes, many rare (Table 12.3).

- Ascertain if acute or chronic.
- Exclude apparent hepatomegaly where pulmonary hyperinflation pushes liver down ('ptosis' of the liver).
- Management according to cause.

Table 12.3 Causes of hepatosplenomegaly

	Hepatomegaly	Hepatosplenomegaly	Splenomegaly
Infection	Congenital—TORCH Abscess Hepatitis Parasites	EBV Abdominal TB	EBV Malaria SBE
Haematological	Neonatal haemolysis	Thalassaemia Sickle cell disease—especially <5 years	Spherocytosis Leukaemia Sickle cell disease
Malignancy	Hepatoblastoma Neuroblastoma	Leukaemia Lymphoma	Histiocytosis Lymphoma Neuroblastoma (stage IV)
Congestion	CCF Biliary atresia	Budd–Chiari Pericarditis	Causes of portal hypertension Kassabach–Merrit syndrome
Inflammation	JIA Early cirrhosis		
Metabolic	α1-antitrypsin deficiency Galactosaemia Glycogen storage disorders Reye's Wilson's	Mucopolysaccharidoses	Lipid storage disorders

Jaundice

Jaundice is clinically detectable when serum bilirubin >50 μmol/l. The causes of jaundice can be divided according to age at presentation (Table 12.4), and anatomical aetiology. (Table 12.5) Investigations and management of neonatal jaundice are covered on 📖 p.42.

Table 12.4 Jaundice according to age

Typical age	Cause and distinguishing features
Day 1	***Jaundice always abnormal at this age*** Haemolysis (e.g. RhD, ABO): well infant with anaemia Infection: signs may be subtle but may include fever and acute phase response Crigler–Najjar disease type 1 causes unrelenting unconjugated hyperbilirubinaemia in the absence of haemolytic or liver disease. Type 2 results in milder jaundice that responds to enzyme induction with phenobarbitone
Days 2–14	Physiological jaundice: ***diagnosis of exclusion***, unconjugated hyperbilirubinaemia in an otherwise well infant. Usually resolves by d10 in term and d14 in preterm infants
>Day 14	***'Prolonged jaundice' requires urgent investigation + early consultation with specialist unit if appropriate*** Causes of conjugated hyperbilirubinaemia include: • syndromic bile duct paucity—Alagille's syndrome • non-syndromic bile duct paucity, e.g. biliary atresia • α_1-antitrypsin deficiency, metabolic disease • choledochal cyst • sepsis (inc. UTI), congenital infections, and idiopathic neonatal hepatitis (diagnosis of exclusion) Causes of unconjugated hyperbilirubinaemia include haemolysis, hypothyroidism, prolonged physiological jaundice (esp. if breastfed), and upper GI obstruction (e.g. pyloric stenosis)
Neonate/infancy	Galactosaemia: measure serum galactose-1-phosphate uridyl transferase in any sick infant (feeding difficulty, signs of liver disease, sepsis, hypoglycaemia, haemolysis)
Puberty	Gilbert's syndrome: recurrent, mild, unconjugated hyperbilirubinaemia with otherwise normal LFT. Jaundice may be precipitated by viral infection or fasting and there may be a positive family history

Table 12.5 Jaundice classified according to major cause

	Pre-hepatic	Hepatic	Post-hepatic
Causes	Haemolysis	See next section	Biliary tract obstruction e.g. choledochal cyst, biliary atresia
Clinical signs	Pale yellow	Tender hepatomegaly ± dark urine, pale stools	Abdominal pain, hepatomegaly, dark urine, pale stools
Investigations	Unconjugated bilirubin ↑, indices of haemolysis (reticulocytosis, AST ↑, Coombs' test positive)	Conjugated bilirubin ↑, AST ↑, ALT ↑, urine positive for bilirubin	ALP ↑ ***plus*** GGT ↑, urine positive for bilirubin

Hepatic causes of jaundice

- Infection—hepatitis A, B, C, E; EBV, CMV, HHV6; malaria.
- Drugs—paracetamol, valproate, halothane.
- Toxins—solvents, iron, arsenic.
- Chronic disease with acute decompensation:
  - α_1-antitrypsin deficiency;
  - Wilson's disease;
  - metabolic—galactosaemia, fatty acid oxidation defects, urea cycle disorders, organic acidaemias, mitochondrial disease.
- Auto-immune.

Sick child with jaundice Consider:
- infection: bacterial/viral sepsis;
- haematological disorders, e.g. sickle cell disease;
- metabolic disorders, e.g. galactosaemia, amino/organic acidaemias;
- drug poisoning;
- cholangitis especially if previous Kasai procedure for biliary atresia.

Ask about changes in urine and stool; any recent infections; any travel abroad; family history including consanguinity; drug exposure including illicit; note any developmental delay.

Look for stigmata of chronic disease, e.g. spider naevi, caput medusae; dysmorphism, e.g. Alagille's. Document any bruising or ascites.

Investigations
- FBC and film, UEC, LFT, glucose ± blood cultures.
- Clotting screen.
- Ammonia—consult with laboratory.
- Viral serology—hepatitis viruses, CMV, EBV—monospot if over 4 years.
- Urine—dipstick, send for urinary metabolic and toxicology screen.
- Arrange USS of liver and spleen.

Specific tests usually require prior notification of laboratory.

Hepatitis C

Ask about maternal HCV infection, IV drug abuse, and therapy with blood products. Measure anti-HCV antibodies. PCR for HCV is required if:
- presents early after exposure—antibody response may not have started;
- in immunocompromised children—antibody response may be impaired;
- in the presence of maternal antibodies.

Hepatitis E (HEV) Faecal–oral transmission—ask about foreign travel to India, central and Southeast Asia, China, and Africa. Measure anti-HEV antibodies.

Alpha-1-anti-trypsin deficiency Liver disease ± lung disease.
- Serum α1AT: classify variant by electrophoresis.

Wilson's Liver disease with later onset of CNS/psychiatric signs. Usually seen in children over the age of 5. Wing beat tremor if arms held out to the sides, Kayser–Fleischer rings on slit-lamp examination.

- Serum copper and ceruloplasmin.
- Urinary copper excretion.

Autoimmune hepatitis Rare, often in conjunction with other auto-immune diseases, e.g. JIA, diabetes type I.

- Immunoglobulins—raised IgG.
- Auto-antibodies—ANA, SMA, LKM (liver kidney microsomal antibodies).
- Complement (C3, C4).
- Urine—dipstick for glomerulonephritis screen.

Alagille's syndrome Intrahepatic cholestasis with congenital heart disease, typically peripheral pulmonary stenosis. Facial features include prominent forehead, long nose, and deep set eyes. Skeletal abnormalities include butterfly vertebrae. Intraocular anomalies such as posterior embryotoxon are best identified by ophthalmologists. Diagnosis is confirmed by analysis of JAG1 gene.

Liver failure[1]

Rare; typically arises when chronic liver disease decompensates. Prompt recognition vital for prevention of complications, e.g. gastrointestinal bleeding, renal failure, cerebral oedema; and early referral for liver transplantation.

Clinical features

- Coagulopathy—constant feature.
- Jaundice—variable.
- Encephalopathy—onset may be acute or gradual. Difficult to assess:
  - infants: early signs—poor feeding, vomiting; later signs—irritability, reversal of day/night sleep pattern;
  - older children: abnormal behaviour, e.g. aggression; convulsions.

Investigations Perform jaundice screen if cause unknown (p.246).

Laboratory features

- Conjugated hyperbilirubinaemia.
- ALT, AST >10 000IU/l.
- Hypoalbuminaemia.
- Plasma ammonia >100μmol/l.
- Prothrombin time (PT) >40 seconds.

Management

Discuss with specialist centre early for advice on management and assessment for liver transplant. Consider possibility of paracetamol poisoning (p.160). Review medications for hepatotoxicity or causing GI irritation. Admit ICU.

- Ventilate if GCS < 8.
- Prevent cerebral oedema: fluid restriction to 75% of maintenance.
- Prevent hypoglycaemia: IV 10–20% glucose—keep glucose >4mmol/l.
- Prevent gastrointestinal bleeding: IV Ranitidine 3mg/kg.
- Prevent sepsis:
  - broad spectrum antibiotics until bacterial cultures are available:
  - IV cefuroxime 20mg/kg/dose tds ***plus*** Amoxil 25mg/kg/dose tds ***plus*** metronidazole 8mg/kg/dose tds;
  - Consider antifungal agents: fluconazole.
- Control coagulopathy.
  - PT >40s: IV vitamin K. Neonate, 1mg; 1 month to 11 years, 250–300mcg/kg; 12–18 years, 10mg.
  - Repeat IV vitamin K if PT still prolonged at 3 hours.
  - PT >60s or active bleeding: add fresh frozen plasma and cryoprecipitate.
- Reduce production of amines in bowel: oral lactulose (5–20ml/day) if child conscious.
- Urgent dietitian referral to arrange nutritional support.

1 Kelly, D.A. (2002). Managing liver failure. *Postgrad. Med. J* **78,** 660–7.

ⓘ Constipation

Pain or difficulty in the passage of stools. Prolonged faecal retention results in a megarectum, with loss of sensation that further impairs the urge to defecate. Beware spurious diarrhoea—the overflow of liquid stools as a result of faecal retention. Enemas and suppositories may exacerbate any fears of defecation, so their use should be avoided.

Confirm diagnosis.

- History of large hard stools or 'rabbit pellets'; stool withholding; red blood on surface of stools or toilet paper from anal fissure.
- The abdomen may be distended and faeces palpable. N.B. Abdominal examination often normal, especially if already on faecal softener.
- Inspect anus for fissures, skin tags, infection, and anal ectopia.
- If diagnosis unclear, consider:
  - gentle rectal examination to detect retained stools;
  - AXR to show faecal loading and megarectum.

The great majority of children have functional constipation. However, the following danger signs should prompt specialist referral to exclude anorectal malformation, Hirschsprung's disease, neurological problem, coeliac disease:

- meconium not passed within 48 hours of birth in term infants;
- constipation starting in the neonatal period;
- previous anorectal surgery;
- pit/dimple, hairy patch, or pigmentation overlying the spine;
- neurological abnormalities in the lower limbs;
- underweight or short stature.

Functional constipation

Maintenance therapy with regular follow-up is likely to be needed for several months.

- Explain pathophysiology. Exclude opiate and anticholinergic drugs
- High fibre diet: refer to dietician if necessary.
- Adequate water intake: ≤5 years, 5 cups/day; 6 years and over, 7 cups/day.
- Regular toileting: sit on toilet 5–10 minutes after breakfast and evening meal; ensure that child's feet are supported when on the toilet.
- Use stool softeners to overcome child's fear of pain. If no improvement after 1 week, consider adding stimulant laxatives to regime.
- Ensure follow-up arranged, e.g. GP, paediatrician.

Faecal impaction Retained faeces may cause the child to walk on tiptoes to minimize discomfort and may impair appetite and mood. Evacuation is an essential first step. Can usually be achieved by oral osmotic laxatives, e.g. polyethylene glycol. Attempt at home and repeat in hospital if required. Enemas are only required in extreme cases and should be administered under sedation.

Pancreatitis

Uncommon—diagnosis requires a high index of suspicion. Complications include pancreatic haemorrhage, pleural effusion, and multiorgan failure.

Acute pancreatitis

Clinical presentation

- Severe epigastric or periumbilical pain:
  - may radiate to back, chest, or lower abdomen;
  - worse on eating;
  - relieved by drawing up knees.
- Persistent nausea and vomiting.
- Fever.
- Abdomen may be distended with tenderness/guarding especially in the epigastrium.
- Bowel sounds either decreased or increased.

Causes Blunt abdominal trauma; viral infection (mumps, chickenpox); congenital abnormalities of the pancreato-biliary ducts; drugs, e.g. asparaginase; idiopathic (25%).

Investigation

- Elevated pancreatic enzymes. N.B. Levels may not be grossly elevated.
  - Serum amylase—levels peak within 24–48 hours and may remain elevated for up to 4 days.
  - Serum lipase—more specific than amylase and remain elevated for longer.
- Hyperglycaemia, hypocalcaemia, hyperbilirubinaemia, coagulopathy, raised γ GT.
- Enlarged, oedematous pancreas on USS or CT scan.

Management

- Consult with gastroenterology ± surgeons.
- Analgesia.
- NBM; NGT suction if persistent vomiting or ileus; IV ranitidine to reduce gastric acid production and prevent gastritis.
- IV fluids—correct electrolyte abnormalities and consider parenteral nutrition; strict fluid balance.
- Consider IV antibiotics.

Chronic pancreatitis Very rare—may occur in cystic fibrosis or hereditary pancreatitis.

Management

- Adequate analgesia.
- Low fat diet.
- Pancreatic enzyme supplements.
- Surgical assessment.

Chapter 13
Renal

Renal colic

Classically, in adults, renal colic starts as loin pain that radiates around the flank to the anterior abdomen. Children seldom describe this progression of pain, so the diagnosis of renal pathology must be considered in any child who presents with abdominal pain, even central.

In children, renal colic is most commonly secondary to infection, rather than stones. Other causes of right upper quadrant pain include the following.

- Renal pathology.
  - Infection—UTI (p.254) or pyelonephritis.
  - Stones—acute, severe colic.
  - Papillary necrosis—analgesia abuse, recurrent pyelonephritis, sickle cell disease, obstruction.
  - Renal vein thrombosis—pain with gross haematuria, flank mass. Arises in newborn with shock/dehydration or asphyxia. In older child with nephrotic syndrome (p.260); cyanotic heart disease (polycythaemia secondary to hypoxia); recent IV contrast administration. Platelets are low and diagnosis can be confirmed by USS.
- Musculoskeletal—from vomiting, coughing or trauma (fracture or muscle tear on ribs 10–12).
- Shingles—painful vesicles in a band along one or two dermatomes.
- Referred pleuritic pain—lower lobe pneumonia, pulmonary embolus
- GIT—appendicitis, Crohn's, cholecystitis.
- Idiopathic loin pain haematuria syndrome—diagnosis of exclusion.

Investigations

- Blood: FBC, UEC, CRP, Ca^{2+}, PO_4, urate, ± cultures.
- Urine.
  - Urinalysis, M, C, & S, looking for casts, cells, organisms, and crystals N.B. pH: <6 with urate stones; > 8 urea-splitting organisms, e.g. *Proteus, Pseudomonas, Klebsiella.*
  - Urinary calcium, phosphate, oxalate, and urate.
  - Start 24 hour collection for creatinine clearance. Consider sieving urine for stones.
- X-ray: KUB—70% stones radio-opaque. N.B. phleboliths look similar.
- Ultrasound: hydronephrosis, stones.
- Consider abdominal CT, IVP, retrograde pyelogram to locate stone, if required, but significant radiation.

Treatment

Analgesia is the patient's prime concern and should be generous. NSAIDs are as efficacious as opiates in most cases.

Treatment depends on diagnosis.

- UTI (p.254).
- Stones—adequate hydration and discuss with surgeon ± renal team and gastroenterologist.

ⓘ Urinary tract infection

- UTI is more common in males in the first 3 months, but thereafter females predominate
- 65 to 85% of UTIs are caused by *E. coli*. Other common pathogens include *Proteus, Klebsiella, Pseudomonas*
- The possibility of sexual abuse should always be borne in mind
- Up to 2% of pre-school children may have asymptomatic bacteriuria, so this may not be the cause of their symptoms

History The typical history of frequency, dysuria, temperature ± nocturia may not always be present. Neonates may present with septicaemia, diarrhoea and vomiting, prolonged jaundice, or failure to thrive. Older children may present with abdominal pain, enuresis, or vomiting. Systemic features such as rigors, loin pain, with fever and vomiting are suggestive of pyelonephritis. The reported colour or smell of urine is a poor discriminator.

Examination

- ABC including BP. Gram-negative shock is rare, but may be life-threatening.
- Assess hydration status.
- Palpate abdomen—loin or upper quadrant tenderness ± mass; note any faecal masses.
- Inspect and palpate spine; then assess lower limb neurology to exclude neuropathic bladder.
- Inspect genitalia.
  - Fused labia—treat with topical oestrogen cream for a fortnight; then paediatric review.
  - Exclude phimosis—circumcised boys have 90% fewer UTIs.

Investigations

Collecting an uncontaminated sample of urine is crucial

Methods of collection in order of precision.

- Suprapubic aspirate (SPA) (📖 p.472)—up to 18 months of age. Higher success rate with USS guidance.
- Catheter sample (in and out)—invasive and unpleasant, but gives immediate definitive answer.
- Mid-stream urine—in children with good bladder control.
- Clean catch urine—sit child on parent's knee on a towel and parents attempt to catch in a sterile container. 80% of babies will pass urine within 10 minutes of a feed.
- Pad—sterile cotton wool ball in nappy.
- Bag urine—if clear on dip or microscopy, then excludes UTI. However, high risk of false positive, so ***never base diagnosis on bag sample***.

Inspect the urine, noting any cloudiness; then dipstick.

Urinalysis—testing negative to leucocytes ***and*** nitrites makes UTI highly unlikely. However, any febrile child may have leucocytes on dipstick or microscopy and this is not diagnostic of UTI. Moreover, certain bacteria, e.g. *Enterococci, Proteus* cannot reduce nitrates, so will be nitrite negative.

Microscopy seldom detects organisms. Leucocytes will be present in most febrile children.

Culture. Any growth on a SPA or clean catch urine is significant. Otherwise, pure growth of $>10^8$ colony-forming units is diagnostic.

FBC, UEC, blood cultures should be taken if possibility of bacteraemia, i.e. child is under 6 months of age; or has temperature over 38°C; or looks unwell, e.g. vomiting profusely.

- USS only required acutely if:
  - any suggestion of obstruction;
  - under 3 months, looking for hydronephrosis, ureteric dilatation, or anatomical anomalies, e.g. duplex system. If hydronephrosis, arrange urgent MCUG looking for posterior urethral valves.

Management

- Resuscitate if necessary.
  - Apply oxygen, give 20ml/kg 0.9% saline IV.
- Try to obtain blood and urine cultures before giving IV antibiotics. Do not delay treatment, so obtain urine sample from SPA or catheter.

In those under 6 months, or unable to tolerate oral fluids, or systemic symptoms suggestive of pyelonephritis

- IV gentamicin 7mg/kg once daily + IV ampicillin 50mg/kg/dose tds or a cephalosporin.
- Once afebrile and feeding, change to oral antibiotic (see below).

If febrile but tolerating fluids

- Consider a single dose of IM gentamicin before sending home with a course of oral antibiotics.
- Oral antibiotics should be guided by local practice, but trimethoprim 4mg/kg/dose bd or cephalosporins often suffice.
- Treatment is for 7–10 days, guided by bacterial sensitivities.
- When child discharged home, arrange follow-up with GP to ensure urine culture result is reviewed in next few days.

Ongoing management

Prophylactic antibiotics, MCUG after 6 weeks, and DMSA after 4 months, ***used*** to be standard in all those under 5 with first UTI. This is no longer the case, as our ability to prevent renal scarring has been called into question. Investigation and on-going prophylactic antibiotics is therefore at the discretion of the paediatric consultant.

Under 3 years

In those under 3, it is reasonable to start prophylactic trimethoprim 2mg/kg at night, having completed the treatment course, and continue until reviewed by local paediatrician.

- Arrange renal USS if not done acutely; then local paediatrician follow-up
- Repeat urine culture after treatment course, to ensure bugs have gone.

Over 3 years

- Arrange renal USS if not done acutely; then GP follow-up.
- Repeat urine culture after treatment course, to ensure bugs have gone.
- May be prudent to suggest an annual check of blood pressure once adult, to pick up the few who subsequently develop hypertension.

ⓘ Dysuria and urinary frequency

Dysuria often arises in conjunction with urinary frequency. These symptoms are indicative of lower renal tract pathology, and causes other than UTI must be considered.

Urinary frequency is defined as passing urine on more than eight occasions per day. Usually the child with urinary frequency passes small volumes of urine repeatedly during an hour.

Dysuria

- Bladder irritation—UTI, fizzy drinks, bladder stones.
- Skin irritation: vulvovaginitis (learning toileting, secondary to bubble baths); perianal (threadworms, nappy rash; sexual abuse).

Frequency

- Impaired bladder emptying.
  - Intrinsic—neuropathic, dysfunctional bladder; congenital anomalies e.g. vaginal insertion of ureter.
  - Extrinsic—compression from external mass, e.g. constipation, tumour.
- Urinary.
  - Causes of dysuria.
  - Osmotic—hyperglycaemia, hypercalcaemia.

History

Older children may be able to state when during the urinary stream they notice their urine 'stinging'—the earlier, the more proximal the pathology. With urinary frequency, it is important to determine whether the child has daytime urinary continence—usually attained by 4 years. If the child has never been continent ('primary incontinence') and is developmentally appropriate, bladder functional anomalies should be considered.

Examination

- Abdomen—palpate for masses, e.g. bladder, faecal.
- Spine.
  - Inspect—sacral tuft of hair = spina bifida occulta; café au lait spots.
  - Palpate—vertebral anomalies.
- Check lower limb reflexes and sensation.
- Inspect genitalia and perineum; check perineal sensation.

Investigation Urinalysis and urine culture.

Management Most causes will be evident on examination. Bladder functional anomalies require referral to either renal team or urology for urodynamic studies ± renal tract imaging.

Haematuria

Less than 1ml of blood is required to change the colour of urine. As a general rule, the more obvious the blood, the lower the renal tract pathology, e.g. tea-coloured urine of glomerulonephritis versus bloody urine of haemorrhagic cystitis.

Other causes of a red appearance of the urine include:

- gross haematuria:
  - from renal tract, e.g. tumour, trauma;
  - from vagina or rectum—exclude NAI/abuse.
- haemoglobinuria—haemolysis;
- myoglobinuria—post-muscular trauma or prolonged exercise;
- drugs—rifampicin;
- food—beetroot;
- urate crystals—'brick dust' in a baby's nappy.

These can be distinguished by urinary dipstick followed by microscopy.

N.B. Urine dipsticks are exquisitely sensitive: blood positive with fewer than 5 red blood cells per high power field (up to 10 RBC/hpf is normal). If positive for blood on dipstick, request urinary microscopy to confirm the presence of multiple red blood cells, e.g. myoglobinuria positive for blood on dipstick, but negative on microscopy.

Once certain that this is haematuria, proceed with history.

History

- Ask about recent health, specifically about any URTI, sore throat, diarrhoeal illness, skin infection.
- Ask about any weight loss or lethargy.
- Any symptoms of a UTI (📖 p.254).
- Any renal trauma, e.g. rugby tackle.
- Is there bleeding elsewhere, e.g. mouth, nose, skin—bleeding disorder, vasculitis, Henoch–Schönlein purpura (HSP).
- Is this a recurrent problem, e.g. IgA nephritis (📖 p.259).
- Any history of joint pain/swelling—HSP; arthritides such as lupus, JIA.
- Any recent medications—cyclophosphamide.

Examination

- Vital signs including BP. Hypertension is glomerulonephritis until proven otherwise; unwell, pale child—think HUS (📖 p.240).
- Skin for rash or bruising.
  - HSP—on extensor surfaces of lower limb/buttocks, with joint and abdominal pain.
  - ITP—widespread petechiae, purpura, ecchymoses in well child.
  - Bleeding disorder—nose bleeds, swollen joints.
  - Vasculitis—joint pain.
  - Nappy rash—common cause of microscopic haematuria.
- Assess peripheries for oedema.
- Palpate abdomen.
  - Loin pain—UTI/pyelonephritis; stones.
  - Loin mass—renal vein thrombosis; Wilms' tumour; hydronephrosis; polycystic kidney disease.

History

- Any history of renal damage, e.g. UTIs, trauma, or radiotherapy.
- Any history of aortic trauma, e.g. umbilical artery catheter, or coarctation repair.
- Are there symptoms of palpitations or sweating?
- Does the child suffer headaches? If so, are there additional symptoms of raised ICP?
- Does the child have frequent nosebleeds?
- Is the child on any medication, e.g. steroids or stimulants for ADHD.
- Is the teenager a smoker?
- Is there a family history of hypertension or renal disease?

Examination

- Exclude Turner's, neurofibromatosis type I—both associated with coarctation; any features of Cushing's—hirsute, acne, buffalo hump.
- Check BP in right arm.
- Check limb pulses normal or, if child over 10 years, exclude radio-femoral delay.
  - If previous coarctation repair, left radial pulse usually absent with no recordable BP in that arm.
- Palpate abdomen for masses or tenderness.
- Check for renal bruit of renal artery stenosis.
- Full neurological examination to exclude focal pathology causing raised ICP and to exclude hemiplegia secondary to hypertensive intracranial bleed.
- Perform fundoscopy for papilloedema and to exclude retinal haemorrhages.
- Check growth parameters, e.g. short—Turner's, chronic renal failure, Cushing's; tall—neurofibromatosis; overweight—essential hypertension, Cushing's.

Investigations

- UEC—K^+ raised with renal insufficiency and low in hyperaldosteronism.
- Aldosterone and renin are difficult to measure, so discuss with endocrinologist and/or biochemist first.
- ECG—often normal, but may show left ventricular hypertrophy. Symptomatic COA may see RVH or RBBB.
- Urine—dipstick and microscopy to exclude glomerulonephritis (📖 p.259)
- Abdominal USS ± Doppler studies of renal vessels—tumours, renal vascular disease.
- Head CT—if signs of raised ICP or intracranial bleed.

Non-emergency investigations

- Urine—steroids (17-β hydroxyl-steroids) and catecholamines.
- Echocardiogram: exclude COA and quantify ventricular mass.

Treatment

Hypertensive crisis; see next section. If symptomatic, consult with renal team. Otherwise, refer to paediatrician for follow-up. If no cause evident, i.e. essential hypertension, suggest dietary modification, e.g. low salt, low fat, and increased exercise to lower BP without medication.

☠ Hypertensive crisis

BP > 180/110 and symptoms.

- Severe headache.
- Vomiting.
- Irritability.
- Lethargy.
- Seizures.
- Papilloedema.
- Retinal haemorrhages.
- Cardiac failure.

Swift intervention is necessary but rapid reduction in BP may lead to reduced organ perfusion.

Management

- Discuss with cardiology/renal.
- Obtain IV access. Treatment options include:
  - nitroprusside, 0.5–1mcg/kg/min infusion, 3mg/kg made up to 50ml with 5% dextrose. 1ml/h = 1mcg/kg/min; maximum 10ml/h;
  - hydralazine, 0.15mg/kg 4–6 hourly;
  - ± frusemide 1mg/kg.
  - Older children may also manage oral treatment, e.g. nifedipine 'crunch', 250–500mcg/kg PO.
- Restrict fluid intake and monitor balance.
- Control fits with conventional drugs (📖 p.286).
- Move to PICU for invasive blood pressure monitoring.

Chapter 14

Urology

Trauma of urinary tract

The urinary tract is vulnerable to injury from the kidney to the urethral meatus. Trauma can be caused by blunt or penetrating injuries. When dealing with the following mechanisms of injury, careful history and thorough investigation are paramount to avoid missing urinary tract trauma.

- Direct blow to loin (renal).
- Lap-belt injury (bladder).
- Fracture of pelvis (bladder and urethra).
- Falling astride object on to perineum (urethra).
- Penetrating injury (renal, bladder, urethra).

Types of injury

- Renal haematoma.
- Renal avulsion.
- Transection of ureter.
- Bladder haematoma.
- Bladder perforation.
- Urethral transection.

Presentation

- Haemodynamic instability—resuscitate before investigation!
- Haematuria.
- Acute abdomen.
- Abdominal mass.
- Blood at urethral meatus.

Investigations

- CT scan with double contrast.
- Intravenous urogram (IVU).
- Cystoscopy.

Management

- Resuscitate as required.
- Careful systematic examination to exclude other injuries (often multi-trauma).
- Most renal trauma is initially treated non-operatively. Urgent surgical intervention required for renal avulsion with major bleeding and major renal parenchymal injuries resulting in significant urinary leak.
- Bladder perforations require drainage or surgical repair.
- Primary realignment or delayed repair are both options for treating urethral injury.

ⓘ Painful (acute) scrotum

Acute scrotum is the commonest urological emergency in children requiring surgery. Whilst testicular torsion is the most urgent to treat, it is rare in the pre-pubertal age group. However, acute scrotum is considered to be torsion until proved otherwise and urgent exploration of the scrotum is often indicated.

Causes

- Testicular torsion.
- Torted hydatid of Morgagni (testicular appendage).
- Epididymo-orchitis.
- Irreducible inguinal hernia.
- Idiopathic scrotal oedema.
- Varicocele.
- Trauma.
- Henoch–Schönlein purpura (HSP).
- Tumour (primary or secondary).
- Referred pain (e.g. from renal calculus).

History

- Did the pain start suddenly?
- Is it confined to the scrotum or does it radiate into the abdomen?
  - Adolescent torsion can be associated with loin or abdominal pain.
- Is it associated with urinary symptoms or pyrexia?
- Is it associated with nausea?
- Is it associated with a groin swelling?
- Does pain increase with movement?
- Is there a history of trauma?
- Is there a history of malignancy (leukaemic deposits, etc.)?

Examination

- Hemi-scrotum may be enlarged and erythematous. HSP may present as a vasculitic rash.
- Testicular torsion is usually associated with swollen testis sitting high within the scrotum.
- With torted testicular appendage, testicular tenderness is often confined to the upper pole of the testis. A 'blue pea' sign is confirmatory.
- Idiopathic scrotal oedema is associated with florid scrotal erythema and oedema radiating into perineum and groin, but surprisingly minimal testicular tenderness.
- Irreducible inguinal hernia presents with swelling of groin/scrotum. It is not possible to get above the swelling when examined from the scrotum.

Investigations

- Urinalysis to exclude infection, HSP.
- No other routine investigations required. Note that ultrasound for torsion can be misleading and may give false negative result.
- If acute episode is confirmed to be epididymo-orchitis, elective renal tract investigations necessary.

Treatment

- If torsion present or if torsion cannot be excluded, immediate surgical exploration of scrotum required. Surgery needs to be within 8 hours of torsion to salvage testis.
- Torted testicular appendage usually treated surgically but does not have to be done as emergency.
- Oral or intravenous Augmentin required for epididymo-orchitis.
- Irreducible inguinal hernia needs reduction after administration of analgesia or sedation. If reduction successful, herniotomy performed after 24–48 hours to enable oedema to settle. Failed reduction requires emergency herniotomy.
- Systemic causes of acute scrotum treated accordingly.

ⓘ Urinary retention

Retention of urine can occur for a number of reasons. These include mechanical and functional causes.

Causes

- Pathological phimosis including balanitis xerotica obliterans (BXO).
- Balanoprosthitis.
- Urethral meatal stenosis.
- Urethral stricture.
- Haematuria causing 'clot retention'.
- Pelvic tumour.
- Neurological disorders.
- Postoperative—epidural, post-operative pain.

Management

- Examination includes full neurological assessment including sensation up to S1 to S5. Examine spine looking for scoliosis, local tenderness.
- If short history, give analgesia and attempt conservative approach, e.g. warm bath, running water.
- If conservative approach fails or longer history, catheterization required—urethral if possible, otherwise suprapubic.
- Treat underlying cause.

Balanitis xerotica obliterans

- This is recognized by the appearance of dense, white scar tissue occluding the end of the foreskin.
- Of unknown aetiology but thought to be equivalent to lichen sclerosis in females.
- Potentially pre-malignant and can extend along the whole urethra.
- Absolute indication for circumcision.

Priapism

This rare condition is defined as a 'persistent and painful erection'. It occurs as a result of venous thrombosis or venous obstruction.

Causes

- Sickle-cell disease.
- Leukaemia.
- Post-splenectomy thrombocytosis.
- Tumours of urethra or perineal structures.

Management

- Needle aspiration of blood from corpora cavernosa sometimes required in acute phase.
- Recurrent or persistent priapism treated with surgical venous bypass.
- Treat underlying cause.

ⓘ Paraphimosis and balanoprosthitis

Paraphimosis

Occurs when tight foreskin retracts but then fails to protract. The foreskin rapidly becomes oedematous and painful. The oedema may restrict blood flow and therefore urgent management is required.

Treatment

- Attempt to reduce swelling, e.g. with icepacks. If fail, attempt reduction under sedation/analgesia.
- Failure to reduce paraphimosis requires surgical intervention with either a dorsal-slit or acute circumcision under general anaesthesia.
- If reduction achieved, elective circumcision often required, especially if scar tissue developed.

Balanoprosthitis

Mild inflammation of the foreskin is common and is often due to ammoniacal dermatitis. This is to be distinguished from an infection of the foreskin (prosthitis) or glans (balanitis), which is usually associated with a non-retractile foreskin. Although the infection is usually localized, it can sometimes be more severe and associated with systemic signs. Recurrent balanoprosthitis *per se* is not an indication for circumcision.

Causes

- Usually associated with non-retractile foreskin.
- Sometimes due to poor hygiene in older child.
- Balanitis xerotica obliterans (BXO) may be present.

Presentation

- Swollen, erythematous foreskin ± glans .
- Pus present in severe forms.
- Can present with urinary retention.
- Pyrexia in severe cases.

Investigation

- Microbiology swab.
- Urinalysis—if UTI confirmed, renal tract investigations required.

Treatment

- Topical or oral antibiotics for mild cases—IV antibiotics sometimes required for severe cases.
- Regular bathing during acute episode for symptom relief.
- Once acute episode has resolved, encourage regular retraction of foreskin ± a course of 0.1% Betnovate ointment to increase foreskin retractility and prevent further episodes of infection.
- Elective circumcision indicated if episode results in scarring of foreskin or if associated with recurrent UTIs.

Chapter 15

General surgery

Intestinal obstruction

Intestinal obstruction in infants and children can be caused by a number of different conditions that are either congenital or acquired. Many of these can result in bowel ischaemia and must be managed urgently, e.g. malrotation volvulus requires laparotomy within 4 hours to restore blood supply to the midgut.

The age of the child influences the possible cause of the obstruction.

Neonatal

- Pyloric stenosis.
- Obstructed inguinal hernia.
- Malrotation volvulus.
- Intestinal atresias—duodenal, jejuno-ileal, colonic.
- Meconium ileus—associated with cystic fibrosis.
- Necrotizing enterocolitis (NEC) (📖 p.41).
- Hirschsprung's disease (📖 p.41).
- Meconium plug syndrome.
- Anorectal malformation/imperforate anus.

Older child

- Intussusception.
- Adhesional obstruction.
- Obstructed inguinal hernia.
- Small bowel volvulus.
- Appendix mass.
- Meckel's diverticulitis.

Examination

- ABCD—babies with malrotation volvulus and NEC are often profoundly shocked.
  - Occasionally, bowel obstruction can also cause an acute confusional state or altered level of consciousness.
- Note any dysmorphic features, e.g. Down's syndrome associated with duodenal atresia, Hirschsprung's.
- Remember: the more distal the obstruction, the greater the degree of abdominal distension but the later the onset of vomiting.
- Determine if true bile-stained vomiting is present, i.e. green rather than yellow—distinguishes obstruction from gastroenteritis.
- Erythema or 'shininess' of abdominal wall suggests acute abdomen.

Investigations

- AXR AP—lateral views if perforation suspected.
- FBC, UEC, glucose, CRP, cross-match.
- Blood cultures if febrile or in all newborns, even if afebrile.
- Urinanalysis.

Further investigations as indicated, e.g. contrast studies, rectal biopsy for Hirschsprung's.

Treatment

- Resuscitation often required, particularly in babies.
  - Give 20ml/kg bolus of 0.9% saline.
- Nil by mouth, IV fluids—0.45% saline + 2.5% dextrose.
- Insertion of wide-bore nasogastric tube, kept on free drainage and aspirated hourly.
- Refer immediately to a paediatric surgeon.

Noenates may also require glucose supplementation up to 10% dextrose (📖 p.506) and prophylactic IV antibiotics e.g. 3rd generation cephalosporin plus gentamicin plus metronidazole.

Pyloric stenosis and intussusception

ⓘ Pyloric stenosis

Usually presents between ages 2 and 8 weeks, and is more common in boys, especially the firstborn. There is often a family history. The vomiting is non-bilious but is postprandial and forceful (projectile). If presentation is delayed, there is poor weight gain and possibly a history of constipation. On examination, the baby is hungry with an anxious expression. Observe for visible peristalsis, do a test feed, and palpate deeply for a pyloric 'olive'.

Management

- If mass impalpable, confirm diagnosis by USS. If USS equivocal, arrange upper GI contrast study.
- Check UEC and blood gas: classically hypochloraemic, hypokalaemic metabolic alkalosis.
- Correct dehydration and acid–base balance.
  - If shocked, 20ml/kg 0.9% saline bolus.
  - IV 0.45% saline + 5% dextrose, and add KCl 10mmol/500ml bag once passing urine (📖 p.506).
  - Insert NG tube, place on free drainage, and replace NG losses ml for ml with IV 0.9% saline.
  - Monitor UEC, bicarbonate, and pH every 4–6h and adjust IV fluids accordingly.
- Early discussion with surgeons *re* pyloromyotomy. Surgery only performed when dehydration fully corrected.

Intussusception

Typically presents during first year of life (peak age is 9 months) but can arise at any age. Often preceded by upper respiratory tract infection and 'idiopathic' in cause. If a child has had a previous episode, there is a 5% chance of recurrence. If recurrent intussusception, consider presence of 'lead point', e.g. Meckel's diverticulum, etc.

History The pain is colicky and bile-stained vomiting is frequently present. The child usually draws up legs during painful episodes.

Examination

The child can appear very pale and shocked.

> The diagnosis of intussusception must be considered when dealing with any vomiting child, who looks 'too unwell'

The classic 'sausage-shaped' mass may be palpable, but commonly a tender fullness is found. Red currant jelly stool may be present in the nappy.

Management

- ABC.
- Insert IV cannula—fluid resuscitation as necessary ***plus*** IV access obligatory before attempted reduction.
- Take blood for FBC, UEC, glucose, cross-match.
- Urgent surgical opinion.
- AXR and USS to confirm diagnosis and to exclude perforation.
- Reduction by air enema with surgeons present in case procedure unsuccessful. If perforation occurs, an IV cannula is inserted immediately into the peritoneum and aspirated.
    - Post-reduction, child will require additional fluids because of third-spacing, so review frequently. The chance of recurrence is greatest in the first 24 hours post-reduction.

Acute abdomen

There is a wide number of different conditions that present with an acute abdomen during childhood (see box). In young children, the presentation is often different from that in older children or adults and can lead to delayed diagnosis, e.g. appendicitis. Always remember that 'common things occur commonly', but rare things do occur!

Some causes of acute abdomen

Gastrointestinal
- Appendicitis
- Mesenteric Adenitis
- Malrotation volvulus
- Intussusception
- Adhesive obstruction
- Meckel's Diverticulitis
- Inflammatory Bowel Disease
- Acute pancreatitis
- Cholecystitis
- Trauma

Pulmonary
- Lower lobe pneumonia

Renal
- Urinary tract infection (UTI)
- Pyelonephritis
- Renal colic

Ovarian
- Ovarian torsion

Systemic illness
- Sickle cell crisis
- Henoch-Schönlein Purpura
- Metabolic disorders, e.g. diabetic ketoacidosis, porphyria

History

The cause of an acute abdomen is influenced by the age of the child, e.g. appendicitis is rare in children <5 years, and can often be determined from the history. The following questions are useful.
- Did the pain start suddenly or gradually?
  - Pain associated with intussusception, volvulus, and perforation starts suddenly.
- Where is the pain located and has this position changed?
  - Visceral pain is referred to central abdomen, whereas inflammation of peritoneum is localized to site of condition.
- Is the pain colicky or constant in nature?
  - Colicky pain suggests luminal pain rather than peritonitis.
- Is the pain increased with movement?
  - Increased pain with movement suggests localized or generalized peritonitis.
- Is the pain accompanied by other symptoms, e.g. nausea, dysuria?
- Has there been a preceding viral illness?
  - Mesenteric adenitis and intussusception are frequently preceded by an upper respiratory tract infection.
- Is there a history of trauma?
- Has there been previous abdominal surgery?
  - Possibility of adhesional obstruction.

Examination

- Inspect for general well-being, anaemia, and jaundice.
- Temperature.
  - A temperature of >39°C suggests either a viral infection, e.g. mesenteric adenitis, or severe bacterial infection, e.g. perforated appendicitis or pyelonephritis.
  - Uncomplicated appendicitis usually causes a low grade pyrexia, but adolescents may be afebrile.
- Careful respiratory examination.
  - Lower lobe pneumonia can present with abdominal signs in the young child.
  - Tachypnoea may be due to anxiety, sepsis, acidosis, e.g. DKA.
- Locate site of maximal abdominal tenderness.
  - Distraction techniques are useful when examining young children.
- Examine for peritonitis by getting child to cough or jump on the spot
  - This way of testing for peritonism is much kinder than suddenly releasing the examining hand and elicits signs as effectively.
- Palpate for abdominal mass.
  - If mass identified, define its position, size, and consistency.
- Rectal examination is rarely indicated in children with abdominal pain and should only ever be performed by an experienced doctor.

Investigation

Investigations are undertaken if the diagnosis is uncertain, to determine exact anatomy, e.g. defining a mass, or as part of the anaesthetic assessment. All children with acute abdomen should have urinalysis performed to check particularly for white cells, nitrites, blood, and glucose.

If the diagnosis has been made clinically, no further investigations may be required, e.g. appendicitis or mesenteric adenitis. Otherwise, consider performing:

- FBC, CRP ± amylase, glucose to exclude pancreatitis (📖 p.250), DKA (📖 p.404);
- AXR ± CXR if lower lobe signs;
- abdominal ultrasound;
- CT scan if mass identified.

Treatment

- Adequate resuscitation is vital for all children with an acute abdomen.
- Analgesia to be given once abdominal examination has been performed by surgeon. Analgesia can mask clinical signs, but withholding it unnecessarily is cruel.
- Definitive treatment depends on underlying cause but most will need a laparotomy.
- Consider antibiotics (📖 p.490).

ⓘ Gastrointestinal bleeding

GI bleeding can present in a number of different ways during childhood according to the site within the GI tract of the underlying condition and the age of the child. Do not forget that 'vomited blood' may have originally been swallowed e.g. by breastfed baby from cracked nipple, post-tonsillectomy.

Causes include the following.

Vomiting blood

- Ingested blood.
- Oesophagitis.
- Mallory–Weiss tear.
- Gastritis and peptic ulceration.
- Oesophageal varices secondary to portal hypertension.
- Haemangiomas.

Rectal bleeding

- Anal fissure:
  - fresh blood following defecation 'in pan and on paper'.
- Haemorrhoids—as for fissure.
- Intestinal polyps (single or multiple):
  - often associated with passage of mucus.
- Meckel's diverticulum:
  - usually significant amount of altered blood passed.
- Intussusception:
  - 'red currant jelly' stool passed.
- Gastrointestinal duplication cyst.

History

- Enquire how much blood has been lost and whether vomited or passed per rectum.
- Confirm whether bleeding is fresh blood (bright red) or altered blood (maroon, coffee grounds), or black tarry stool of melaena. N.B. The appearance is influenced by rate of bleeding as well as how close lesion is to mouth or rectum.
- Take careful past medical history.
  - Note family history of IBD, bowel malignancies.
  - Medications including iron, NSAIDs.

Examination

- ABC—assess haemodynamic state of child.
- Skin—look for petechiae, jaundice. Perioral hyperpigmentation may be Peutz–Jeghers, associated with intestinal polyps.
- Look in mouth and nose:
  - any bleeding points—blood may be ingested rather than from GIT;
  - mouth ulcers may be indicative of inflammatory bowel disease.
- Abdominal examination including inspection of anus.
  - Note size and consistency of liver.

Investigations

The investigations performed depend on the suspected underlying cause.

- FBC, cross-match ± coagulation studies.
- Specific investigations include Meckel's technetium scan, endoscopy (upper or lower GI), angiography.

Treatment

- Resuscitation as required.
- Bleeding from oesophageal varices can be torrential and may require insertion of Sengstaken–Blakemore tube.
- Major bleeding may require laparotomy before definitive diagnosis confirmed.
- Definitive treatment based on underlying cause.

? Abscess

An abscess is 'a localized collection of pus anywhere in the body, surrounded by damaged and inflamed tissues'.

Presentation

- Painful swelling.
- Swinging, spiking pyrexia.
- Superficial abscesses present as warm, erythematous, fluctuant swellings. The exception to this is the 'cold abscess' of tuberculosis.

Treatment

- Broad-spectrum antibiotics are indicated in the early stages of infection.
    - **Face**: IV penicillin and flucloxacillin.
    - **Elsewhere**: IV augmentin + metronidazole, if perianal.
- Despite the introduction of newer, more powerful, antibiotics, once a formal abscess has developed, the surgical axiom 'if there is pus about, let it out', i.e. incision and drainage still applies in most cases.
- Microbiology of pus will determine causative organism, and which antibiotics required.

Assessment

When taking a history, gain information from the parents and child. If questions are phrased appropriately, children can describe events, e.g. unusual sensations before a seizure, tingling ('shooting') pain of neuralgia.

The antenatal and developmental history are key elements. If parents cannot remember milestones, ask them to compare the child's development with that of his/her siblings. Other significant factors include family history of neurological events, e.g. seizures, migraines, and if there is any parental consanguinity.

The examination cannot always be conducted as with an adult patient, as a child may not cooperate. However, information can be gained from watching the child play, e.g. hand preference, ataxic movements. Devise games to help your assessment, e.g. finger puppets for ocular movements, putting the lid on a biro to assess ataxia.

Leave scary procedures such as fundoscopy until the end.

Examination

Observe:

- mental state—alert, confused, unconscious (AVPU);
- posture—frog's legs of hypotonia, truncal ataxia;
- gait—proximal weakness, neuropathic, spasticity;
- dysmorphic features;
- Neurocutaneous stigmata—café-au-lait spots, hypopigmented macules, angiomas.

Particular features of the physical examination should be noted.

- Head—size, shape, palpation of fontanelles, auscultation of bruits.
- Chest—cardiac murmur, e.g. mucopolysaccharidoses (MPS), acute rheumatic fever.
- Abdomen—organomegaly, e.g. congenital infection, MPS, urea cycle defects; abnormal genitalia, e.g. fragile X, (macro-orchidism) hypothalamic disorders.
- Limbs—asymmetry (growth arrest of hypertonic limb); muscle tenderness; nerve thickening.
- Spine—scoliosis, kyphosis, spina bifida occulta, gibbus.
- Growth parameters, especially head circumference.

Cranial nerves (CN I–CN XII). Sit level with the child and ask t
to assist, e.g. holding the head still, covering eye. CN I is seldo
in an emergency; CN II requires visual acuity charts or d
whether a child can grab a small toy. Light perception can be a
asking whether an ophthalmoscope light is on or off. The ren
the examination is similar to that in adults, with most child
happy to show their tongue!

Peripheral nervous system

Assessment is easily made into a game—'make your legs go fl
spaghetti and let me wobble them'; 'let's see how strong you are
and tone in babies can be assessed by the 180° examination:

- pull to sit;
- maintenance of sitting position;
- attempted weight bearing (hold under arms);
- ventral suspension;
- position when prone.

Eliciting reflexes should be demonstrated on the parents before th
Sensation can only be checked in the older child and if there is
tracting injury. Most children enjoy finger–nose and heel–shin testi
children over the age of 5 can participate in joint position assessme

Specific manoeuvres

Fog test To elicit UMN signs in upper limbs.

Ask the child to walk on the outer sides of their feet. The affecte
will assume a position of spasticity.

Gowers manoeuvre To assess strength of muscles in lower limbs.

Ask the child to lie down and then get up ***without*** pushing their h
on the floor. If there is proximal weakness, the child will crouch and
push on their thighs and 'climb' upwards. If there is generalized weak
the child may be unable to sit up but will roll on to hands and k
before 'climbing' up their thighs.

Romberg's sign To determine if proprioception is normal.

Ask child to stand with feet together and then close their e
Romberg's sign is positive if the child sways, i.e. can only stand stea
with eyes open.

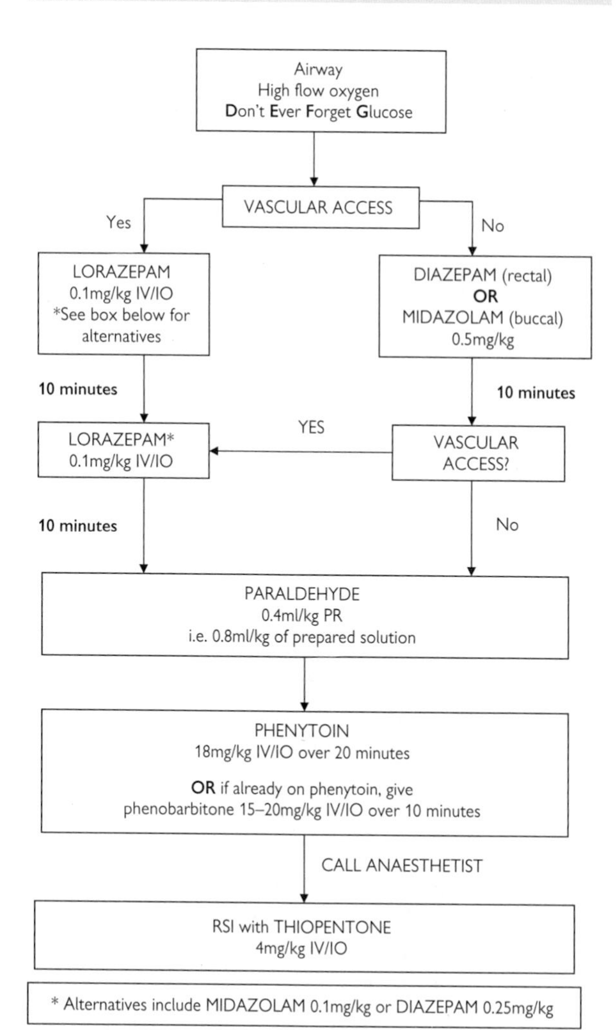

Fig. 16.1 Algorithm for management of status epilepticus. (reproduced with permission from Wieteska, S., Mackway-Jones, K., and Phillips, B. (eds.) (2005). *Advanced paediatric life support*, 4th edn. BMJ Books and Blackwell Publishing, Oxford.

Investigations

Blood tests

- Any electrolyte imbalance can precipitate a seizure. Hypoglycaemia must be urgently corrected (📖 p.413).
- Liver function tests are helpful as a base line in case anticonvulsants are subsequently required.
- Anticonvulsant levels are a means of assessing medication compliance. Only phenytoin has a reliable therapeutic range.
- Most febrile convulsions are caused by viruses. But if the child appears septic, give IV cefotaxime 50mg/kg/dose after blood cultures have been taken.

ECG ECG should be performed if this is the first afebrile seizure, in order to exclude arrhythmia (📖 p.181).

Cranial CT ± lumbar puncture An urgent head CT is indicated if there are signs of raised ICP or neck stiffness. The latter may be secondary to meningitis or an intracranial bleed. Having excluded a bleed by cranial CT, check fundi to exclude raised ICP and, if GCS is >13, do an LP.

Management

Admit if:

- medication required to stop seizure;
- increasing frequency of seizures;
- child appears toxic;
- parental anxiety.

Focal seizure A focal seizure is suggestive of localized intracranial pathology, which necessitates investigation with EEG and cranial imaging. A consultant should decide whether admission is necessary.
N.B. Not all focal seizures are bad news, e.g. mouthing and grimacing of Rolandic epilepsy in adolescents.
N.B. A generalized seizure may have a focal onset, which is either witnessed or else revealed by localizing neurological signs. Paralysis of a limb, persisting after a generalized seizure is over ('Todd's paresis'), is indicative of a focal onset. These necessitate investigation.

Afebrile seizure If the seizure is self-limiting, the child can be discharged home with follow-up by their GP. Paediatric follow-up is recommended if this is the second afebrile seizure or if there are risk factors, e.g. history of prolonged febrile convulsions, developmental delay, significant family history. Discuss with a consultant whether to make an EEG referral and whether medication is required.

Febrile seizure These seldom recur in the same illness. Thus, if the seizure is self-limiting, the child can be discharged home, with GP review in the following days. However, paediatric follow-up is indicated if there are risk factors (see 'Afebrile seizure', above). Discuss with a consultant whether an EEG is necessary.

Advice to parents

In all cases, parents should be educated about what to do if a further seizure occurs, e.g. 60% of children who have a febrile convulsion will have at least one more before they are 6 years old.

- Place child in the recovery position, where they cannot harm themselves, e.g. on floor rather than on bed.
- Clear area around child.
- Call for help. Assistant should summon ambulance.
- Do not attempt to assist breathing by placing items in child's mouth.
- Stay with the child until the ambulance arrives.

Altered level of consciousness

An altered level of consciousness in children is usually caused by a diffuse insult to the brain, e.g. infection, poisoning. Structural intracranial anomalies, e.g. AVM or tumour, have a focal onset and then progress globally. Evidence of confusion and impaired cognition, particularly if they fluctuate, is suggestive of delirium—an acute confusional state (📖 p.424).

Any child with a decreased conscious level should be repeatedly assessed using ABC, with disability being evaluated by either the Glasgow coma scale (modified for children under the age of 4), or by the AVPU scale (📖 p.520).

- A child with a GCS < 8 or only responding to pain is at risk of losing their airway and should be intubated electively
- An LP should not be undertaken if the GCS is <13

History

Perform any resuscitative manoeuvres necessary, whilst asking about:

- any recent trauma;
- any pre-existing neurological condition, e.g. epilepsy, developmental delay;
- any medical conditions, e.g. diabetes, renal disease;
- any medications being taken or accessible at home, e.g. opiates, β blockers;
- when the child last ate—metabolic conditions can be unmasked with starvation;
- any recent exotic travel, e.g. malaria.

Examination

Assess in particular:

- skin—neurocutaneous stigmata, rash, e.g. herpes, petechiae;
- odour—metabolic disorder, poisonings;
- skull—deficits, intracranial bruits;
- neck—rigidity is suggestive of either meningitis or intracerebral bleed;
- abdomen—hepatomegaly (possible metabolic illness); bowel obstruction, e.g. intussusception (📖 p.274);
- neurology—pupillary responses, fundoscopy, tone, posture, and tendon reflexes.

Usually a cause can be found and management directed accordingly. If no cause can be found, investigate as encephalitis (📖 p.142).

ⓘ Headache

A headache can be caused by any pain-sensitive structure in the skull, i.e. scalp, eyes, sinuses, teeth, nose, throat; as well as by infections, dehydration, or poisonings. Recurrent headaches can also have a psychological component.

The key features in the history include:

- chronicity of the headache;
- whether the headache is changing in nature;
- whether the headache wakes the child from sleep;
- whether the headache can be exacerbated, e.g. straining, lying down;
- any associated behavioural changes;
- a family history of migraine.

Examination

Full neurological examination, along with a thorough examination of the head.

- Check BP (📖 p.523).
- Measure head circumference.
- Inspect scalp and skin for infections, rashes.
- Palpate skull and sinuses for muscle tension and tenderness.
- Auscultate for intracranial bruits.
- Check dentition, ENT.
- Check for neck stiffness.
- Neurological examination—visual acuity, fundoscopy, tendon reflexes.

Management

CT head should be performed if the history and examination are suggestive of:

- intracranial bleed;
- raised ICP;
- evolving neurological signs.

Many centres prefer CT for sinus imaging rather than x-ray. N.B. Sinusitis is rare under the age of 7 and may not be a febrile illness (📖 p.318).

An LP should be performed if the child:

- is febrile with neck stiffness;
- is confused—to exclude encephalitis (📖 pp.142, 424).

Contraindications to LP are covered on 📖 p.470. N.B. Pseudotumour cerebri (benign intracranial hypertension) will resemble raised ICP, yet have a normal scan. LP will be diagnostic (pressure over 20mmHg) and therapeutic.

If the child has a BP over the 95th percentile for age, assess for potential causes (📖 p.262) and treat any hypertensive emergency ☠. If no cause is found, treat with NSAIDs and arrange follow-up with GP to see if other factors emerge, e.g. stressors, depression.

Tension headache Usually chronic, bandlike, or generalized. They are non-progressive.

Migraine Over 75% have a family history. Usually unilateral, throbbing, and eased by sleep. Auras may not be present. Children may vomit repeatedly. Rarely, children can present with acute confusional states or focal neurology, e.g. hemiplegia. Such complex migraines should be considered a diagnosis of exclusion.

Raised intracranial pressure (ICP) Progressive, worse on lying down. May be accompanied by vomiting, especially in the morning. Papilloedema is a late sign.

Acute intracranial bleed Headache of sudden onset, 'worst ever'.

ⓘ Weakness

Weakness can be generalized or, more usually, confined to an extremity.

History

With a child with generalized weakness, enquire whether there has been progression from a focal onset. If not, consider neurodegenerative diseases and metabolic illnesses such as Addison's, periodic paralysis.

With weakness that began focally, the history should determine:

- the progression of the weakness, e.g. distal onset moving proximally (Guillain–Barré (GBS));
  - proximal weakness rather than distal (myositis, Duchenne's muscular dystrophy);
  - eye muscles then generalized (myasthenia).

Ask in particular if there have been increased drooling, choking episodes, episodes of incontinence, and:

- whether it is painful—pain is associated with tumours, GBS, myositis but not with myasthenia or toxins, e.g. botulism[1];
- any recent illness or fever, e.g. spinal abscess, GBS;
- any recent head or spinal trauma;
- any medical history of note, e.g. sickle cell disease;
- any family history of weakness, e.g. muscular dystrophy, myotonias;
- any medications, e.g. heavy metals such as lead;
- any exotic travel, e.g. tick bite[2] (US and Australia), polio[3].

Examination

Key features include the following.

- Vital signs especially respiratory rate and BP.
- Face: expressionless, ptosis, squint, drooling.
- Chest: respiratory distress, bell-shape—myopathy.
- Spine: scoliosis, lordosis.
- Muscles. Observe for fasciculations, wasting. Palpate for tenderness, e.g. myositis, polio, and nerve thickening, e.g. Charcot–Marie–Tooth.
- Power: use 1 to 5 grading for older children. For babies, perform 180° examination (📖 p.285). Note tone and any anti-gravity movements. Ask older children to perform Gowers manoeuvre (📖 p.285).
- Reflexes: increased = CNS pathology; decreased—neuropathies, e.g. spinal muscular atrophy, GBS, or late myopathies; normal—muscular.

Use reflexes ± sensation to determine the level of the lesion. A rectal examination may be necessary to determine sphincter tone.

1 Botulism: spore in undercooked food or honey. Starts with diarrhoea, then has ocular signs progressing to generalized weakness. Will then be constipated. Check stool for toxin. Anti-toxin not effective.

2 Tick bite: progressive weakness from bite outwards. Look on scalp, in ears, and rectum for tick. Remove head of tick. Anti-toxin seldom beneficial.

3 Polio: vomiting and diarrhoea, then asymmetric ascending paralysis with muscle pain and fasciculations.

Management

If generalized or progressive weakness, place on continuous oximetry monitoring. If oxygen saturations <95%, obtain a blood gas; perform spirometry if child is over 7 years. Notify ICU and arrange high-dependency care.

If a spinal level is determined, perform x-rays and request MRI. CT may be helpful. Arrange admission with neurology ± neurosurgical consultation.

Proximal weakness is associated with myopathies—perform a CK. Distal weakness is common with neuropathies. Both require discussion with a neurologist for further management such as EMG, nerve conduction tests.

ⓘ Ataxia

Unsteadiness may be due to weakness (📖 p.294), loss of proprioception, or, most commonly, cerebellar dysfunction. These can be distinguished from the history and also by observing the child, e.g. inability to rise from floor (weakness); wide-based gait (proprioceptive or cerebellar dysfunction). A child unable to steadily move from lying to sitting has truncal ataxia, which is indicative of a midline cerebellar lesion.

History

- Duration—acute versus chronic.
- Any head or spinal injuries.
- Any recent infections, e.g. VZV,[4] EBV, or Guillain-Barré.
- Any headaches, e.g. intracerebral bleed, basilar artery migraine.
- Any medications at home, e.g. phenytoin, antihistamines, alcohol.

Examination

- Odour: alcohol, inborn error of metabolism, e.g. MSUD.
- Skin: e.g. angiomas (ataxia telangiectasia); viral lesions (VZV, herpes).
- BP: may be raised with intracerebral lesion, neuroblastoma.
- Abdomen: hepatomegaly (Wilson's); mass (neuroblastoma).
- Visual acuity and fields: intracerebral lesion.
- Fundoscopy: papilloedema; optic atrophy (Friedreich's).
- Eye movements: opsoclonus (📖 p.298), nystagmus—horizontal or vertical.
  - No nystagmus = chronic ataxia.
  - Horizontal nystagmus = cerebellar lesion.
  - Vertical nystagmus = brainstem lesion.
- Reflexes: brisk (intracerebral lesion); absent (neuropathy, e.g. GBS, late myopathy).
- Peripheral sensation especially joint position sense, vibration. Lost in vitamin B_{12} deficiency, Friedreich's. Note wide-based, slapping gait.
- Loss of perception of pain and temperature indicative of neuropathy, e.g. diabetes mellitus, abetalipoproteinaemia.

Assess speech by getting the child to talk about books and toys; check dysmetria by getting them to reach for objects. Younger children can be asked to put the lid on the pen held by the examiner; older children can perform finger–nose, heel–shin, and dysdiadokinesis.

Management

All cases should be discussed with a neurologist. Children with acute or progressive ataxia and no evident cause, will require an urgent CT or MRI. Obtain blood to exclude hypoglycaemia or electrolyte disturbances. A urinary drug screen may also be necessary.

Admission will be necessary if there is associated vomiting requiring rehydration, or if the children cannot be safely cared for at home. If fit for discharge, follow-up should be arranged after discussion with a neurologist.

4 VZV can cause ataxia before, during, and up to 2 weeks after the appearance of the skin lesions. Classically, a truncal ataxia that becomes generalized.

ⓘ Dizziness

The term 'dizziness' needs to be clarified whether it is the perception of:
- feeling faint—cardiovascular;
- being unbalanced—cerebellar and proprioceptive disorders;
- light headedness—hypoglycaemia, possible psychiatric cause;
- vertigo—the sensation of spinning, either of the child ('central vertigo') or the world around them ('peripheral vertigo').

Central vertigo is less common and has a more gradual onset. It is due to lesions of the cortex, cerebellum, or brainstem and there will be associated symptoms, such as diplopia, facial numbness, dysphagia. Peripheral vertigo has an acute onset and is secondary to vestibular disease, usually post-viral.

Also note if the child is on any ototoxic medication, e.g. frusemide.

Examination

On examination, check:
- BP: postural drop;
- cardiovascular: pulses, murmurs for aortic stenosis;
- neurological: ocular movements, fundoscopy, fields, cerebellar and proprioceptive function. Romberg's is useful—with vertigo, the child will sway to the affected side;
- Ears: hearing acuity, otitis media.

With vertigo, the child will also have nystagmus and ataxia on standing. On lying down, the ataxia associated with vertigo will improve.

With central vertigo, the child will have multidirectional nystagmus. Peripheral vertigo will have nystagmus most pronounced on looking to the side that is affected. If there is difficulty discerning the two, turn the child's head to one side—central vertigo will cause the nystagmus to start instantly and will not settle, whereas peripheral has a latency of a couple of seconds and will subside with gaze fixation.

Management

By the end of the examination, the cause should be evident and appropriate investigations instigated.

Children with peripheral vertigo and no hearing loss have vestibular neuronitis. Symptoms should settle over the next few days but many prefer to use promethazine 0.5mg/kg/dose maximum 12 hourly to alleviate the acute symptoms. Children should be encouraged not to sleep on the affected side.

Children with peripheral vertigo and hearing loss may have acute labyrinthitis. However, they should be reviewed by the GP to ensure that the hearing recovers. If not, the child should be investigated for an acoustic neuroma.

ⓘ Abnormal movements

Chorea

Unusual jerking movements that appear to flow, changing in speed and direction. May be accompanied by writhing movements of proximal limbs ('choreo-athetoid'). Associated with acute rheumatic fever (📖 p.187), Wilson's, and lupus.

Check the history for any recent sore throat or skin infection, and any family history such as Huntington's. Assess for:

- skin: rashes, jaundice, angiomas—ataxia telangiectasia;
- cardiovascular: murmurs;
- abdomen: chronic liver disease stigmata.

Specific manoeuvres to amplify chorea

- Child squeezes your fingers ('milkmaid's grip').
- Holds arms above head ('pronator sign').
- Sticks tongue out ('jack-in-the-box').

Investigations Take blood for ASOT, DNase B. Consider caeruloplasmin and copper levels. Discuss neuroimaging with neurologist and whether IV penicillin should be started (📖 p.187).

Dystonia

Abnormal posturing that usually comes on in spasms, e.g. arms extended, teeth bared, eyes rolling, yet patient is still conscious.

Acute presentations are invariably due to medication, e.g. prochlorperazine, antipsychotic medications.

- **Give procylidine 0.1mg/kg/dose IM or IV or benztropine 20mcg/kg/dose oral, IM, or IV.**

Myoclonus

Sudden, irregular contractions of muscles in disorganized manner. Usually seen in chronic conditions such as brain malformations, neurodegenerative disorders, or inborn errors of metabolism.

Acute presentations are rare.

- Under 4 years, consider neuroblastoma. Examine for hypertension, abdominal mass, 'dancing eyes' (opsoclonus myoclonus). Discuss with neurologist ± oncologist for further imaging and investigations
- Over 6 years, consider juvenile myoclonic epilepsy. Usually has jerks on awakening. Take blood for glucose, UEC, calcium, magnesium, phosphate, and liver function tests. Arrange EEG, ideally sleep-deprived, and follow-up with neurologist.

ⓘ Palsies

Facial nerve palsy (CN VII)

Although Bell's palsy is common, a central lesion of VII needs to be excluded. Check:

- BP;
- function of V sensory, VII, and VIII as all emerge from cerebellopontine angle. Partial sparing of the forehead muscles is indicative of a central lesion;
- ears—otitis media, herpetic lesions (Ramsay Hunt).

If lower motor lesion confirmed see 📖 p.322. If central lesion identified arrange CT or MRI brain and specify that cerebellum is to be included.

Radial, median, and ulnar nerve palsies

These nerves are most commonly damaged with supracondylar fractures of the humerus. Children will need the fracture immobilized and analgesia given, before assessment is attempted.

Ask the child to:

- Stop—extend hand dorsally at wrist (radial).
- Make an 'L'—abduct the thumb at 90° to index finger (median).
- Make a fist (median) and open it (radial). Stretch all fingers out (ulnar).
- Make an 'O'—touch thumb to index finger (ulnar). If this is too painful, try to encourage the child to hold a piece of paper between two fingers whilst you pull it out (Froment's sign). Sensation is difficult to assess satisfactorily if the child is in pain.

Check two point discrimination in:

- thumb web space (radial);
- volar surface of index finger (median);
- volar surface of little finger (ulnar).

Any neurovascular compromise necessitates urgent orthopaedic consultation and preparation for operative reduction.

ⓘ Big head

Macrocephaly is unlikely to be the primary reason for presentation but can be an unexpected finding at the end of an examination. The majority will have familial macrocephaly, but there is a known association with several conditions, e.g. NF1, achondroplasia.

Causes for concern include:

- rapidly increasing head circumference crossing percentiles;
- growth that is disproportionate to the rest of the body;
- signs of raised intracranial pressure, e.g. headache, lethargy, vomiting.

Examination

Repeat the measurement twice and check that it has been plotted correctly on percentile charts. Compare with other growth parameters.

On examination, look for:

- skin: neurocutaneous stigmata—NF1, tuberous sclerosis;
- skull: palpate for suture separation, bulging fontanelles. Anterior fontanelle should close at 18 months, posterior fontanelle at 4 months;
  - if any shunts are present, see 📖 p.302;
  - auscultate for bruits—AVM;
- spine: spina bifida occulta; gibbus—mucopolysaccharidosis;
- eyes: visual fields; fundoscopy (papilloedema); movements (cranial nerve palsies due to tumour or raised ICP). Inability to look upwards may be third nerve palsy or because frontal bossing of the skull obscures the visual target;
- reflexes: exclude hyperreflexia.

Also check and plot parents' head circumference to exclude familial macrocephaly.

Management

The examination findings dictate the urgency of further imaging. Any suggestion of a rapidly increasing OFC or an intracerebral lesion merits an urgent USS + CT and neurosurgical consultation.

Hydrocephalus with signs of raised ICP necessitates insertion of a shunt or reservoir. Cannulate and take blood for FBC, cross-match, and UEC.

All other conditions require follow-up, either with a neurologist or paediatrician.

Shunt malfunctions

Typically, CSF shunts run between the cerebral ventricle and the peritoneum. They are composed of three parts:

- proximal tubing—ventricle to scalp;
- valve chamber ± reservoir—usually palpable above right ear;
- distal tubing—tunnelled subcutaneously.

The valve chamber enables a pressure gradient to be established so that the CSF drains. It is also enables patency to be assessed, CSF to be sampled, and even medications to be administered.

Shunt malfunctions are:

- obstruction;
- infection.

Shunt obstruction

As a general rule, obstruction in the first 2 years after insertion will be due to problems with the proximal shunt—debris in tubing, catheter tip migration. After this period, distal obstruction—secondary to tube disconnection or pseudocyst formation around the distal tip—is more likely. Also remember that infection can cause shunt obstruction.

Obstructed shunts are difficult to diagnose, despite careful clinical evaluation and radiological investigation.

- *Always* consult with neurosurgery.

The presentation may be one of acutely raised ICP, but generally the symptoms are vague and insidious and may be mistaken for mundane illness such as gastroenteritis. So beware the child with a shunt *in situ* who presents with:

- vomiting;
- lethargy;
- headache;
- abdominal pain;
- ataxia;
- altered consciousness.

Slit ventricle syndrome

This needs to be considered when the child presents with symptoms that fluctuate. The drainage functions 'too well' and the surrounding cerebral tissue occludes the tip of the drain. The CSF accumulates until the CSF gains sufficient pressure to overcome the obstruction.

A further factor for confusion is that cerebral tissue loses compliance. So even with increased CSF volume, the ventricles may appear to have a normal appearance on CT.

Fortunately, newer shunt systems are less prone to this complication.

Examination

- GCS—if GCS < 8, summon help and intubate.
- Measure OFC.
- If child under 12 months, palpate anterior fontanelle.

- Inspect the shunt site for infection or tracking of CSF along the tubing.
- Full neurological examination, noting ocular movements and UMN signs in lower limbs.
  Third nerve compression—pupillary dilatation, and an inability to look upwards—is an early sign.
- With slit ventricle syndrome, the signs are accentuated by standing up and will improve on lying down.
- Locate the shunt reservoir, compress and see how quickly it refills. Typically, if it is hard to compress there is a distal obstruction and if it takes over 3s to fill, there is a proximal obstruction. N.B. Only 50% of obstructed shunts will be identified by this method.

Management

- If GCS fluctuating and signs of raised ICP, give iv mannitol 250mg/kg. Urgently consult with neurosurgery whether shunt tap should be performed.

Shunt tap

Sterile procedure that neurosurgeons prefer to perform themselves. But may be necessary if shunt obstruction causing life-threatening raised ICP.

You will need:

- gown, gloves, mask, drapes as fully sterile procedure
- 22G butterfly needle
- 5ml syringe
- CSF manometer

Technique

- Clean and drape skin overlying reservoir
- Shave hair
- Attach hub of butterfly needle to manometer
- Insert butterfly needle into reservoir
- Occlude reservoir outflow and read CSF pressure
  - <12mmHg—proximal obstruction
  - >20mmHg—distal obstruction
- If distal obstruction, attach syringe and aspirate CSF slowly until CSF pressure below 20mmHg
- If CSF cloudy, send for glucose, protein, M, C, & S.

- If child stable, arrange:
  - shunt series x-rays—AP and lateral skull, CXR, AXR—looking for catheter kinking, disconnection, abdominal pseudocyst;
  - head CT—to assess ventricular size. Previous studies will be necessary for comparison;
  - consult with neurosurgery.

Shunt infection

The majority of shunt infections are caused by skin pathogens (*S. epidermidis, S. aureus*) so the clinical features may be muted, e.g. absence of fever, vague localizing signs. Bacterial meningitis pathogens (*N. meningitidis*, Hib, *S. pneumoniae*) tend to cause more overt symptoms.

Shunt infections can manifest as:

- local infection around shunt insertion site;
- meningitis;
- abdominal pain or even peritonitis;
- shunt obstruction.

Examination

Look for:

- redness and swelling around reservoir;
- neck stiffness—not a consistent sign;
- abdominal tenderness, guarding;
- signs of raised ICP.

Management

The diagnosis can only be confirmed by shunt tap. Do not perform an LP—it may not be diagnostic and is contraindicated if there is raised ICP.

- Investigate as for shunt obstruction.
- If abdominal signs, arrange USS/CT to exclude intra-abdominal collection.
- Consult with neurosurgery—determine who will perform shunt tap (📖 p.303).
- When shunt tap performed, send CSF for glucose, protein, M, C, & S.
    - Infection = normal glucose, raised protein, raised leucocyte count.
- If infection confirmed, admit and start IV antibiotics as advised, e.g. cefotaxime and vancomycin.
- Intrathecal antibiotics via reservoir ± surgical shunt removal may be necessary.

Chapter 17

Otolaryngology

Assessment

To examine the ears, position the child on their parent's lap:

- side on;
- child's arm under parent's arm—parent's arm across child;
- child's head on parent's shoulder, held gently but firmly by parent's free hand. Fingers may need to be splayed so you can access the ear. This immobilizes the child in a cuddle position, which is then reversed for the other ear. You gain further brownie points for examining the least tender ear first! Remember you pull the ear back and down (gently) to examine a child's ear.

To examine the nose and throat, position the child sitting on parent's lap and facing you. Ask the parent to hold the child's arms with one arm and rest the child's head back on the parent's chest with the parent's hand on the child's forehead. Most children will clamp their mouths tightly shut at this point.

- Throat—insert tongue depressor in the corner of the child's mouth and advance towards the molars. As the mouth opens, move the depressor rapidly medially and depress the tongue. A gag reflex or crying gives you an excellent view! Don't forget to look at the gums, teeth, and palate en route to the throat.
- Nose—the easiest way to examine a nose is to use the auroscope! To assess patency of airway use a shiny surface, e.g. metal tongue depressor mists over when held under the child's nose with the child's mouth shut.

ⓘ Acute sore throat

Causes

- Acute tonsillitis—viral (especially <5 years, but rare <2 years), or bacterial.
- Quinsy—peritonsillar abscess, with deviation of uvula by enlarged tonsil with local bulging mass.
- Glandular fever.
- Diphtheria—very rare.

Symptoms

- Painful swallowing—young children may refuse to eat.
- Smelly breath.
- Fever.
- Otalgia.
- Difficulty in speaking or breathing.

Signs

- Fetor, fever, unwell.
- Enlarged red tonsils ± exudates.
    - Huge red tonsils with white/grey membrane and petechial haemorrhages on palate are characteristic of glandular fever.
- Enlarged tender nodes.
- Snoring (stertor) ± apnoeic episodes.

Management

- Admit if enlarged tonsils are causing respiratory compromise:
    - hot potato voice;
    - muffled voice with snoring and apnoeic episodes.
- You will need:
    - oxygen saturation monitoring, especially when asleep;
    - IV dexamethasone to reduce tonsil oedema;
    - ENT review.
    - if dips in oxygen saturations not self-correcting, or increasing pulse and respiratory rate, needs anaesthetic review as well. Options include nasopharyngeal prong, intubation in theatre, and 'hot' tonsillectomy or, rarely, tracheostomy.
- Also admit if:
    - child unwell;
    - not drinking;
    - significant palatal cellulitis or possible quinsy.
- For all admissions consider:
    - performing blood cultures, FBC, CRP ± UEC;
    - glandular fever (📖 p.151). If suspected, perform FBC, LFT, and EBV/CMV serology. Monospot is seldom positive in children under the age of 5 years;
    - IV antibiotics—penicillin or cefuroxime ± metronidazole if quinsy suspected. Erythromycin if penicillin allergy;
    - ENT review if suspect quinsy.

- Otherwise, illness usually self-limiting and child can go home with:
  - pain relief and antipyretics;
  - possibly antibiotics.

Dilemma of whether to give antibiotics

There is limited evidence in children for use of antibiotics; they probably reduce overall length of sore throat by 1 day but no evidence that they lessen severity. Complications, such as rheumatic fever, are very rare; therefore it is necessary to treat a very high number to prevent one case. Moreover, treating EBV with Augmentin gives the patient an annoying rash!

Suggest give antibiotics—penicillin or augmentin—if:

- symptoms >48 hours;
- history of febrile convulsions;
- borderline oral intake;
- already had a lot of time off school;
- immunocompromised;
- valvular heart disease.

Drooling

Causes

- Acute epiglottitis (p.204).
- Retropharyngeal abscess.
- Foreign body in pharynx (p.315).

Acute epiglottitis is a medical emergency. The child will be:
- deteriorating rapidly;
- looking toxic;
- drooling;
- stridulous;
- sitting in tripod position.

Do not approach unless respiratory arrest!

Acute retropharyngeal abscess

URTI causes adenitis, then suppuration in retropharyngeal nodes.

Symptoms
- URTI followed by increasing dysphagia and dribbling.
- The child may become increasingly unwilling to open their mouth (trismus).

Signs
- Child may look unwell with high temperature.
- Head may be held on one side.
- Bulging posterior pharyngeal wall on one side of midline.

Management
- Refer urgently to ENT and involve anaesthetist. Will need incision and drainage under GA.
- If child well enough, may request CT scan first.
- If pyrexial do blood cultures and start antibiotics—IV cefuroxime and metronidazole.

Foreign bodies

ⓘ Ear

- History of putting something in the ear.
- Occasionally pain, bleeding, discharge, or tinnitus.

Remove if possible or refer to ENT clinic. If live insect visible, drown in olive oil before attempting extraction.

ⓘ Nose

- Unilateral purulent discharge from nose or excoriation around nose.
- The object is usually visible.
- If long history of unilateral discharge and no visible object, consider unilateral choanal stenosis.

Apply otrivine nose drops to reduce surrounding oedema. Wrap child in blanket and ask experienced nurse to hold on couch. Ensure adequate light and use forceps or a hook to remove object. If in doubt refer to ENT and consider GA.

ⓘ Pharynx and oesophagus

- History of something stuck in throat.
- Didn't finish meal.
- Unable to swallow.
- Drooling.
- There may be tenderness on palpation.
- Look for evidence of perforation (fever); chest or back pain; neck swelling; or surgical emphysema.

Investigation Lateral soft tissue of neck ± CXR. Look for:

- foreign body if opaque—confirm with parent if foreign body resembles missing object;
- air in the pharynx or oesophagus;
- loss of curvature of cervical spine;
- widening of soft tissue anterior to the cervical spine—retropharyngeal abscess.

If foreign body present or high index of suspicion will need rigid endoscopy.

Larynx, trachea, and bronchi See 📖 p.206 and p.216.

ⓘ Epistaxis

History

- When did bleeding start?
- How much blood might have been lost (can be difficult to estimate)?
- Is bleeding from nostril or down the back of the throat?
- Right, left, or both nostrils?
- Any history of excessive bleeding or bruising, e.g. following immunizations?
- Any family history of bleeding disorders?

Management

- Look for signs of shock—resuscitate as needed. Call for help from senior colleagues and ENT.
  - Bleeding anteriorly from one nostril in an otherwise fit child is usually from Little's area (anterior nasal septum).
- Apply steady pressure by pinching the front of the nose for 10 minutes and apply ice pack to dorsum of nose. Keep child nil by mouth until bleeding stopped.
- When bleeding stops, wait at least half an hour and then send home; if history of recurrent episodes, refer to ENT clinic for interval cautery. Prescribe Naseptin cream once a day for 2 weeks (if no peanut allergy).
- If fails to stop, look for bleeding point on nasal septum. If visible, consider cautery using a silver nitrate stick under local anaesthetic. If not visible, consider packing the nose with expandable nasal tampon.
- If unsuccessful, summon ENT. Reassess vital signs, establish IV access, check FBC and clotting, group and save.

Trauma

ⓘ Ear

Sharp or blunt injury to pinna

- If superficial, clean laceration and steristrip or suture under local anaesthetic. If extensive involvement of cartilage or tissue loss, refer to ENT.
- Blunt injuries produce bruising but may also cause a haematoma—look for tender discoloured fluctuant swelling. Usually needs incision and drainage under GA; therefore refer to ENT.

Perforation of ear drum

- Either from sharp object or slapping injury, e.g. fall into water on to ear. Exclude physical abuse.
- Look for a perforation with ragged edges and signs of recent bleeding.
- Ask about hearing loss.
- Advise to keep ear dry and prescribe 10 day course of ciprofloxacin ear drops.
- Refer to ENT clinic for interval hearing test.

ⓘ Nose

- Stop bleeding (see opposite).
- Inspect nasal septum to exclude a septal haematoma—red swelling blocking airway of both nostrils. This will need incision and drainage to prevent cartilage necrosis; therefore refer to ENT.
- Check orbital margins and eye movements.
- Refer to ENT to be seen in 5 days when swelling settled.

Neck

Lacerations

- Assess vital signs.
- Assess position relative to airway and depth.
  - Superficial—steristrips or suture.
  - Deep—compromised airway and/or suspect vascular injury. Contact ENT/vascular surgeons/anaesthetists.

Blunt injury

This can occur after strangulation or from seatbelt injuries.

- Assess vital signs.
- **Airway**. Careful assessment and review—swelling not always immediate.
- Look for evidence of:
  - bruising;
  - local tenderness;
  - fractured thyroid cartilage;
  - surgical emphysema.
- Call anaesthetist/ENT early if any signs of trauma. Anaesthetist may decide to electively intubate if concerned airway may swell.

? Acute sinusitis

Often a secondary bacterial infection following an URTI. Complications arise due to the close proximity of the eye and intracranial cavity. Young children get maxillary or ethmoidal sinusitis; frontal sinusitis is rare before puberty.

Symptoms and signs of sinusitis

- Severe URTI with purulent nasal discharge.
- Sometimes report facial pain or headache.
- High temperature.
- Periorbital swelling (may fluctuate).
- Neurological exam to exclude complications.

Complications

! *Eye complications*

Usually due to ethmoiditis. See 📖 p.349 for further clinical details.

- Preseptal cellulitis—oedema of the eyelids, minimal tenderness, normal globe, normal eye movements.
- Orbital cellulitis—increasing oedema, erythema, and pain with proptosis. Pus collects between the sinus and the orbit initially stripping off the periosteum from the lamina papyracea—subperiosteal abscess. This causes further displacement of the globe and, together with the oedema, restriction of eye movements.
- Intra-orbital abscess—the pus breaches the periosteum causing further displacement of the globe, ophthalmoplegia, and a significant risk of visual loss.
- Cavernous sinus thrombosis—thrombophlebitis spreading posteriorly from the orbit to the cavernous sinus. Headache and Vth nerve signs followed by other cranial nerves (II–VI). Can cause bilateral blindness plus significant mortality.

Beware the sudden development of bilateral orbital signs

! *Intracranial complications*

Less common but may occur simultaneously with orbital complications.

- Subdural or frontal lobe abscess via septic thrombophlebitis. Initial symptoms not specific—fever, headache—followed by focal neurology, including fits and, ultimately, signs of raised intracranial pressure. Can present chronically some time after sinusitis has resolved.
- Meningitis.

Management

- Admit if unwell or suspect complications.
- Blood cultures, nasal swab, FBC, CRP.
- IV antibiotics—cefuroxime and metronidazole.
- Nasal decongestants, e.g. otrivine.
- ENT/ophthalmology review if suspect eye complications.
- Neurosugery/ENT review if suspect intracranial complications.

- Perform CT scan of sinuses and brain if:
  - proptosis;
  - restriction of eye movements (may complain of diplopia);
  - chemosis;
  - neurological signs.
- ***Urgent*** ophthalmology/ENT referral if:
  - loss of afferent pupillary reflex (📖 p.342);
  - loss of red reflex.
- Surgical drainage will be necessary to prevent permanent loss of vision.

Don't wait for the CT scan to be done before referring.

ⓘ Neck lumps

Causes

- Reactive lymph nodes secondary to common bacterial, e.g. acute tonsillitis, and viral infections, e.g. glandular fever. Lymph nodes may suppurate.

Don't forget TB or atypical TB

- If solitary can be congenital cysts—first presentation may follow URTI, when an abscess forms.
  - Thyroglossal cyst found anteriorly in neck; classically moves upwards when child protrudes tongue.
  - Branchial cyst found more laterally at anterior border upper third sternomastoid muscle.
- Malignant—not always obvious; features that are suspicious include increase in size over 4–6 week period, anorexia and weight loss, night sweats and fever, signs of local compression, e.g. nerve palsy, unilateral glue ear.

Symptoms and signs

- Systemic.
- Local—single or multiple lumps:
  - tenderness;
  - skin red and hot;
  - tense or fluctuant;
  - transilluminates.
- Look for primary source of infection—ENT, scalp, teeth.

Management

- If child toxic, or signs of infection admit for investigation—FBC, CRP, cultures ± UEC ± monospot and IV antibiotics.
- If suspect abscess, consider USS or CT scan and contact ENT.
- If not acutely unwell, management depends on presumptive diagnosis.
  - Glandular fever—rest and GP follow-up.
  - Tonsillitis.
  - Infected congenital cyst (no abscess)—Augmentin, ENT follow-up.
  - Malignant—assess for other masses (lymph nodes, hepatosplenomegaly); note any anaemia, petechiae, bony tenderness (📖 p.386).
  - Investigations will be directed by findings but CXR and FBC and film will be required as a minimum. Contact oncology and thereafter follow protocol.

Acute facial nerve palsy

Causes

- Bell's palsy.
- Herpes zoster oticus (Ramsay Hunt syndrome).
- Acute otitis media.
- Chronic otitis media (cholesteatoma).
- Lyme disease—acute facial palsy is the most common focal neurological manifestation.
- Trauma—temporal bone fractures. Facial injuries in parotid region.
- Melkersson–Rosenthal syndrome—relapsing, alternating facial paralysis with facial oedema and fissured tongue.

History

Establish when it started and any progression. Note any:

- associated earache or facial pain;
- alterations in taste;
- dry eyes;
- hearing loss;
- vertigo;
- earache and discharge;
- viral prodrome;
- trauma.

Examination

- Look for facial asymmetry—young children can be asked to copy facial movements.
- Complete or partial weakness—partial sparing of the forehead muscles is indicative of a central lesion (📖 p.299).
- Older children can identify diminished sensation on the face.
- Evidence of tearing when crying.
- Examine ear and parotid region.
- Look in throat.
- Look for evidence of head injury.

Investigations

- Hearing test—age-appropriate.
- CT scan if suspect fractured petrous temporal bone.
- Electrophysiological testing not required acutely ***except*** in cases of trauma and recovering brain injury to establish if complete transection of facial nerve has occurred.

Treatment

Tailored to diagnosis.

- Protect eye—artificial tears and lubricating ophthalmic ointment at night. Consider eye pad and taping eye at night. If child reports grittiness or pain, get ophthalmology review.

ⓘ Bell's palsy

Most common diagnosis—10% recurrent. Children tend to have spontaneous recovery.

- Rapid onset over days to 3 weeks—may have mild viral prodrome.
- Can be associated with pain and diminished sensation ipsilateral face/head/ear.
- Hearing normal.
- Exclude acute otitis media and herpes zoster.

Role of steroids Evidence in adults equivocal and there has been no study specifically looking at the benefits of steroids in children. Therefore only used for patients with complete paralysis and/or severe pain within the 10 days of illness. Prescribe 1 week course prednisolone 1–2mg/kg.

ⓘ Herpes zoster

- Rapidly progressive facial nerve palsy.
- Severe pain.
- Hearing loss and vertigo.
- Vesicles in ear canal and on pinna; also sometimes in throat.

Role of steroids and acyclovir No studies in children; some evidence in adults. However as 30–50% patients have persistent weakness, treat with a 10 day course of prednisolone and 2 weeks of acyclovir.

ⓘ Acute otitis media

Usually occurs when the bony canal covering the facial nerve in the middle ear is dehiscent.

N.B. Signs and symptoms of the acute infection may be masked if the patient is already on antibiotics.

Start IV antibiotics, e.g. augmentin, and refer to ENT for myringotomy.

ⓘ Chronic otitis media

Usually associated with a cholesteatoma.

- History of smelly otorrhoea and hearing loss.
- Look for presence of keratin (often appears as a white pearl) in a pocket or perforation superior or postero-superior ear drum ± pus.

If suspicious, ask for ENT review as patient will need surgical decompression (mastoidectomy).

Chapter 18

Orthopaedics

Assessment

Paediatric orthopaedic assessment follows the normal pattern of history, examination, and investigation. Most ED presentations follow a recent injury—try to obtain a precise description, e.g. fell hurting ankle. Did the child fall over towards the little toe or big toe? At risk of avulsion of distal tibial epiphysis, but eversion = medial fracture; inversion = lateral fracture.

Remember that many structures refer pain elsewhere, e.g. hip pathology presenting as knee pain.

Examination

Look

The whole patient should be examined, e.g. looking for systemic signs of infection, as well as the presenting localized area. Record any:

- clinical deformity—swelling, bruising;
- degree of angulation of distal fragment (Fig. 18.1);
- describe % of displacement where 100% = off-ended, as well as the plane of displacement lateral vs. medial, dorsal vs. volar.

Compare the affected side with the normal side.

Feel It is important to have a structured, systematic approach to examination with attention to bony landmarks and surface anatomy. For example, in the knee, palpate along the superior border of the tibia to elicit any joint line tenderness. Knee effusions can be elicited by stroking downwards on one side of the patella, then the other.

Pay particular attention to the neurovascular status of a limb/periphery.

Move Before moving a painful joint, observe the child at play. Note the ability to weight bear and the active range of motion and function, then assess passive range of joint motion. When in doubt, compare movement with the normal joint.

Hips Check for dislocation—Barlow–Ortolani in children under 6 months (see box); compare knee height in older children. Document movement in all planes—flexion, extension, abduction/adduction, internal and external rotation.

Barlow–Ortolani tests

These are two separate tests. Lie the baby on its back and place your index and middle fingers along the greater trochanter with your thumb along the inner thigh. Flex hip to 90°, and hold the leg in neutral rotation. Be gentle—no force is required.

With **Ortolani**, the hip is gently abducted while lifting the leg anteriorly. With this manoeuvre, a 'clunk' is felt as the dislocated femoral head reduces into the acetabulum.

With the **Barlow** test, position the baby as above with hips flexed to 90°. The leg is gently adducted while posteriorly directed pressure is applied to the knee. A palpable clunk or sensation of movement is felt as the femoral head exits the acetabulum posteriorly.

Knees Movement: flexion and extension. Assess lateral stability by flexing the knee to 30° and applying varus and valgus stresses. Test ACL with anterior drawer test—child lies supine with knee flexed to 90°; fix foot by gently sitting on it and pull forwards on the tibia. Compare with other side.

Older children may injure menisici and need McMurray's test—child lies on abdomen with feet in the air. Push down whilst rotating foot from side to side, noting any tenderness. Alternatively, ask the child to squat and walk 'like a duck', i.e. on feet with knees bent.

Patella apprehension—perform last! Move patella gently from side to side—this is tender if there is any knee joint pathology and the patient will often intervene.

Investigation The history and clinical examination should direct investigations such as radiographs, blood tests, bone scans, and CT/MRI. The old adage of 'x-ray the joint above and below' can limit missed diagnoses because of referred pain.

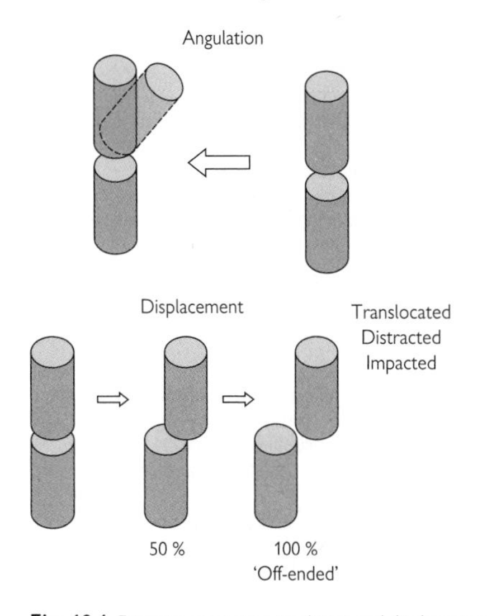

Fig. 18.1 Diagram comparing angulation and displacement.

ⓘ Limp

Limp is a common presenting complaint in orthopaedics. It can be an acute or chronic event and is usually associated with pain. Remember that pain may be referred, e.g. appendicitis, UTI, pelvic inflammatory disorder.

Causes

- Soft tissue—trauma, foreign body, neighbouring lymphadenitis.
- Muscle—trauma (sprain), myositis.
- Bone—trauma (consider NAI); osteomyelitis (📖 p.331); malignancy, e.g. leukaemia, osteosarcoma; metabolic bone disease, e.g. rickets; haematological (sickle cell anaemia, thalassaemia).
- Joint—trauma; infection (📖 p.330); Henoch–Schönlein purpura (📖 p.258); inflammation (juvenile idiopathic arthritis (📖 p.334)); secondary to GI disease, e.g. Crohn's, ulcerative colitis; haematological (haemophilia, leukaemia).

History

Determine whether the limp is an acute or chronic event. Most children will have suffered falls in the days preceding presentation, so obtain a precise description of any accidents that caused pain. If pain is present, ask whether the pain is:

- constant or intermittent, e.g. after certain movements;
- in the same location, e.g. flitting arthropathy of rheumatic fever;
- worse at certain times of day, e.g. morning in JIA; night in malignancy.

Ask if the limp improves during the day, e.g. musculoskeletal, JIA, or worsens, e.g. bone pain. Associated symptoms of abdominal pain, fever, and rashes may be relevant.

Examination

- Note temperature, rashes.
- Abdomen—exclude appendicitis, inflamed inguinal lymph nodes, etc.
- Spine.
  - Look for scoliosis, hair overlying spina bifida occulta.
  - Palpate for tenderness—discitis, metastases, fracture. There may be paraspinal muscular spasm.
  - Limitation of flexion/extension/rotation—fracture, spondylolisthesis (one vertebral body slips forward on the body lying caudal to it).
- Inspect and palpate lower limb skin, muscle, and tendons. Exclude limb length discrepancy.
- Examine hip and knee.
- Foot—inspect skin for foreign bodies; check toenails and shoes.

Investigations

- X-ray—may need to image joints above and below. Sprain is a diagnosis of exclusion!
- FBC, CRP, ESR, blood culture even if not febrile.
- Consider urine analysis—UTI, HSP.

Children who have been limping for over a month may need a rheumatological opinion as well as an orthopaedic one.

Infection

Prompt treatment of musculoskeletal infection is essential. Infection can be direct, e.g. open fractures, or by haematogenous spread, especially in immunocompromised patients. Underlying sepsis can be difficult to distinguish from the everyday bony injuries sustained by children.

Septic arthritis

The consequences of untreated septic arthritis can be devastating. Pus within a joint can destroy the articular surface within hours. Longer-term sequelae include subluxation/dislocation, physeal growth arrest, deformity, and degenerative joint disease.

The hip is the most common site in infants; the knee is the most common site in children.

Clinical features

- Pyrexia.
- Pain especially on joint movement; patient often holds the limb in a 'fixed position'.
- Limp/inability to weight bear.
- Swelling, redness, warmth.

It is important to note that the presentation can be very varied. Inability to weight bear with increased temperature, WCC, and CRP is 95% specific for septic arthritis, but, even if only one of these parameters is raised, 10% will have septic arthritis.[1]

Investigations

- FBC, CRP, ESR, blood cultures—inflammatory markers raised. CRP normalizes before ESR.
- Plain x-rays—increase in joint space, subluxation. Periosteal reaction visible after 10–14 days (90% abnormal by 28 days).
- USS and aspiration can be performed.
- Aspirate with aseptic technique under sedation. Send for Gram stain, microscopy and culture. *Staphylococcus aureus* most common.
  - >50 000 WCC/mm^3 with 90% polymorphs is highly suggestive.
- Bone scan may be necessary to distinguish from osteomyelitis.

Treatment

- Urgent referral to orthopaedic team for open arthrotomy and washout of the affected joint.
- IV antibiotics, e.g. flucloxacillin and benzyl penicillin, until cultures known and clinical response.
- Request long line insertion as weeks of IV antibiotic therapy necessary.

N.B. Septic arthritis is akin to appendicitis, i.e. if in doubt it is better to open the joint and find it normal, than ignore a possible sepsis.

1 Kocher, M.S., Mandiga, R., Zurakowski, D., Barnewolt, C., and Kasser, J.R. (2004). Validation of a clinical prediction rule for the differentiation between septic arthritis and transient synovitis of the hip in childern. *J. Bone Joint Surg. Am.* **86-A** (8),1629–35.

⑦ **Transient synovitis** Post-viral phenomenon, usually in boys. Commonly involves the hip or knee. Movement is limited by pain but usually no effusion is present. May have raised inflammatory markers as recent infection. Resolves with bed rest and NSAIDs.

⑦ Osteomyelitis

Osteomyelitis is common in children due to their rich metaphyseal blood supply and thick periosteum. Diagnosis in the neonate can be difficult and pyrexia is not a constant clinical feature. *Staphylococcus aureus* is the most common pathogen in all age groups, with *Haemophilus influenzae b* decreasing since vaccination began. However an organism is only identified in approximately 50% of cases.

Investigation

- Baseline FBC, ESR, CRP—usually all raised.
- Blood cultures ***before*** commencing antibiotics. At least two sets from different sites.
- Plain x-ray (N.B. 10–14 days before changes appear).
- Consider USS/MRI/isotope bone scan.
- Aspiration and culture using aseptic technique.

Treatment

- IV antibiotics, e.g. flucloxacillin 50mg/kg/dose qds + benzyl penicillin 30mg/kg/dose tds. Always be guided by your local antibiotic regimen. Neonates and young infants will need IV antibiotics for the entire course of treatment. Consider long line placement.
- Limb splintage in position of safety, non-weight bearing.
- Surgical debridement if:
  - failure to respond to IV antibiotics;
  - frank pus on aspiration;
  - presence of a sequestered abscess.
- When fever and pain resolve, and inflammatory markers normalizing, convert to oral antibiotics. Treat for a minimum of 4–6 weeks with progress monitored by temperature, WCC, CRP, ESR.

Complications

- Septic arthritis.
- Recurrence within 1 year after treatment (<4%).
- Chronic osteomyelitis (<5%).
- Growth arrest secondary to physeal damage.

⑦ **Discitis** Infection of intervertebral discs, possibly secondary to vertebral osteomyelitis. Can present with back pain or discomfort when walking or sitting. The diagnosis should be considered in any child with PUO or an abnormal gait. Palpation of the spine reveals localized tenderness. Bone scan will confirm suspicions and spinal MRI will distinguish from vertebral osteomyelitis.

ⓘ Joint pain

The key features of the history are whether the pain is acute or chronic; and whether one joint or multiple joints are involved. Further questions include the following.

- History of trauma.
- Recent febrile illness:
  - bone infection (📖 p.330);
  - rheumatic fever (📖 p.187);
  - JIA (📖 p.334).
- Rashes:
  - Henoch–Schönlein purpura (📖 p.258);
  - rheumatic fever;
  - JIA (Still's disease).
- Medications, e.g. cephaclor.

Examination should clarify whether the pain is from the:

- Joint—joint line tenderness, effusion ± palpable warmth;
- Neighbouring bone, e.g. trauma, osteomyelitis, malignancy.

The age of the patient influences differential diagnoses (Table 18.1). But for all acute presentations, infection and trauma need to be excluded.

Perform FBC, ESR, CRP, blood cultures and request x-ray: AP, lateral, and joint-specific views

The conditions mentioned in Table 18.1 are discussed on the following pages. Causes of chronic pain can affect any joint and, although they are discussed separately from joint-specific conditions, they must be considered when formulating the differential diagnosis.

Table 18.1 Differential diagnoses of acute joint pain in children by age*

	Pre-school	**5 to 10 years**	**Over 10 years**	**Specific x-ray**
Back	Discitis (📖 p.331) Vertebral osteomyelitis (📖 p.331) Tumour Scoliosis	As pre-school	Spondylolisthesis Scheuermann's disease (📖 p.336) Acute prolapsed intervertebral disc	Consider early MRI
Hip	Transient synovitis (📖 p.331) Septic arthritis of the hip (📖 p.330) Late presentation of developmental dysplasia of the hip Infection (📖 p.330) Perthe's disease	Infection (📖 p.330) Perthe's Juvenile idiopathic arthritis	Slipped upper femoral epiphysis Infection (📖 p.330) Juvenile idiopathic arthritis	Frog's leg lateral
Knee	Toddler's fracture Leukaemia Juvenile idiopathic arthritis Haemophilia	As pre-school ***plus***: Ewing's Rheumatic fever	As previous ***plus***: ACL injuries STDs causing septic arthritis, reactive arthritis Patellar tendon injuries	Tunnel

* N.B. In all age groups, trauma and infection must be excluded by FBC, CRP, ESR, blood culture, and x-ray AP and lateral.

Chronic joint pain

Chronic or recurrent joint pain is suggestive of haematological and rheumatological conditions, e.g. haemophilia, JIA. Nocturnal pain is suggestive of malignancy.

① **Haemophilic arthropathy** Spontaneous haemarthrosis is common in severe haemophilia (<1% of factor VIII or IX activity). Presentation is usually after 6 months as the baby becomes more active. The joints most commonly involved are knee, elbow, ankle, shoulder, and hip. Presentation can resemble that of septic arthritis.

① Juvenile idiopathic arthritis

A group of diseases characterized by persistent non-infectious arthritis in one or more joints, lasting more than 12 consecutive weeks (Table 18.2).

Check FBC, ESR, CRP, antinuclear antibodies, rheumatoid factor.

- **Pauciarticular**—Girls, under 5 years, usually knee.
  - Need ophthalmic review to exclude uveitis.
- **Still's disease.** Systemic involvement—fever, rash, splenomegaly, lymphadenopathy ***plus*** relapsing polyarthritis. Pericarditis often present.
  - Investigations to exclude malignancy, and infection, e.g. serology for *Mycoplasma*, viruses, e.g. rubella.
  - Dipstick urine for proteinuria. If positive = renal involvement.
- **Polyarticular** >5 joints involved, e.g. knee, ankles, small joints of hand and feet, jaw, cervical spine.
  - Investigations should include HLA B27.

⑦ **Reactive arthritis** Post-viral phenomenon. Often in adolescent boys, who are HLA B27 positive.

① Neoplasm

Associated with nocturnal pain and systemic symptoms, such as fever, malaise, and weight loss. Spinal tumours may cause nerve root compression.

Primary bone malignancies

- Osteogenic sarcoma—distal femur or proximal tibia.
- Ewing's—can arise in femur, tibia, fibula, humerus, pelvis, scapula, or ribs; then metastasize rapidly.

Secondary malignancies

- Leukaemia.
- Neuroblastoma.

Table 18.2 Juvenile idiopathic arthritis (JIA) sub-types

	Subtype of JIA			
	Pauciarticular JIA (<6 joints)	**Polyarticular JIA (>5 joints)**	**Systemic onset JIA**	**Enthesitis (subgroup of pauci-articular)**
% of all JIA	50	30–40	10–15	<5
Sex	2F : 1M	3F : 1M	M = F	M > F
Age	2–3 years (rarely >10 years)	2–5 and 10–14 years	Any	Especially teenagers
Joints	Any; Rare in hips	Any; Rarely starts in hips	Any	Hip, ankle, back
Systemic manifestations	No	No	Salmon-pink rash, persistent fever, lymphadenopathy, hepatosplen-omegaly ± pericarditis	No
Uveitis	20% especially if ANA positive	Rare	Rare	If ANA positive
Leucocytosis	No	No	Yes	No
Anaemia	No	Mild anaemia	Normochromic, normocytic	No
ESR	Normal	May be raised	Usually high	Normal
ANA	30% positive, mainly female	Sometimes in younger	Negative	Sometimes positive, often HLA B27 positive
Rheumatoid factor	Negative	Often in girls with small joint disease	Common in >10 year olds	Negative
Destructive arthritis	Rare	>50%	>50%	Uncommon

Joint-specific conditions

⑦ Back pain

Back pain in children is cause for concern as many have an underlying cause, other than musculoskeletal trauma.

Differential diagnosis of acute severe back pain:

- trauma—fracture, ligament injury;
- infection—discitis, vertebral osteomyelitis;
- malignancy—primary and secondary;
- systemic disease.

Adolescents may also develop the following.

- **Spondylolisthesis**—anterior displacement of L5 vertebra relative to S1. Assess for neurological compromise, e.g. incontinence; loss of perineal sensation.
- **Scheuermann's disease**—non-flexible thoracic kyphosis, which seldom has neurological compromise.

Note any spinal deformities, loss of mobility, paraspinal muscle spasm and assess neurological function thoroughly.

All acute back pain should be referred to the orthopaedic team.

Hip pain

⑦ *Late presentation of developmental dysplasia of the hip*

Despite neonatal checks, some dislocated hips are missed. By 2–3 months, the 'clunk' of Barlow–Ortolani is lost. There may be asymmetry of thigh skin folds. If the feet are placed together and the flexed knees are compared, there will be loss of height. Hip x-ray shows superior and lateral displacement of the femur (relative to Perkins and Hilgenreiner's lines, Fig. 18.2); with acetabular hypoplasia and loss of femoral head.

Refer to orthopaedics clinic for ongoing management.

⑦ *Slipped upper femoral epiphysis*

Disorder of the proximal femoral epiphysis, resulting in posterior slippage of the superior part. Most common in obese, adolescent boys (10–16 years), often with a positive family history. 25% of cases are bilateral. Pain can be felt in the hip, thigh, or groin and referred pain from the knee is common. Classically, the child walks with feet externally rotated. If under 10 years, endocrine work-up is mandatory—hypothyroidism, growth hormone, type 2 diabetes.

Classification

- Stable slip: weight bearing possible with or without crutches.
- Unstable slip: weight bearing impossible due to severe pain.

Treatment

- Non-weight bearing.
- Refer to on-call orthopaedic team for treatment.
- N.B. 50% of unstable slips develop avascular necrosis of the femoral head.

Perthe's disease

Idiopathic avascular necrosis of femoral head. Presents with chronic pain and limp, boys 4:1 girls, commonly 4–10 years. X-ray of pelvis shows flattening of the femoral head and widening of joint space between head of femur and acetabulum.

Discuss with orthopaedic team to arrange follow-up.

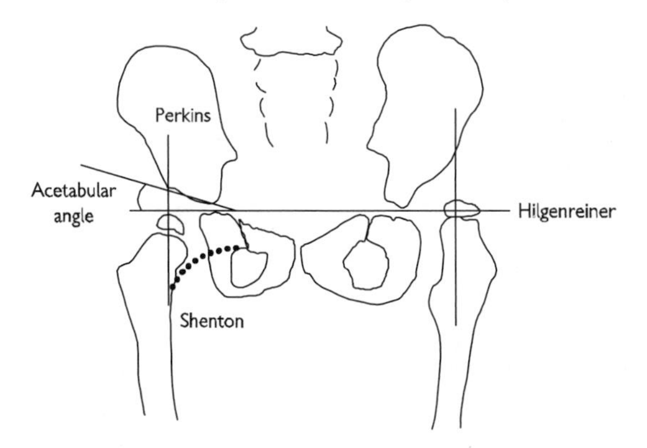

Fig. 18.2 Schematic representation of AP x-ray of pelvis showing developmental dysplasia of left hip and relevant radiographic lines.
Hilgenreiner, horizontal line between the two triradiate cartilages. Acetabular angle, created by line along the superolateral and inferomedial borders of the acetabulum and the Hilgenreiner line. The acetabular angle is 28° at birth and lessens with age; however it will be increased in DDH.
Perkins, perpendicular to Hilgenreiner at the outer border of the acetabulum. Divides the hip joint into quadrants. The femoral head should lie within the lower medial quadrant.
Shenton, a smooth arc between the medial femoral metaphysis and the inferior border of the superior pubic ramus. Loss of the continuous arc is suggestive of DDH or fracture of the pubis.

ⓘ Knee pain

A frequent source of pain in young children as often involved in falls! Bear in mind that pain may be referred from nearby joints, e.g. hips, and that the knee is a common site of involvement in systemic diseases, e.g. leukaemia, rheumatic fever. Adolescents suffer knee injuries similar to those of adults.

- **Toddlers' fracture**—spiral fracture of the tibia after an apparently innocuous stumble. Treat in long leg cast and refer to orthopaedics as growth plate damage can occur.
- **Patellar tendon injuries**—seen in sporty adolescents. Tendon can be avulsed from the tibia acutely, causing pain and sudden inability to bend the knee. Or the trauma can be repetitive resulting in anterior knee pain whenever exercise begins (Osgood–Schlatter's—traction apophysitis).

If x-ray reveals avulsion of the tibial tuberosity, surgery is necessary. The management of Osgood–Schlatter's involves rest until the tuberosity ossifies. Some patients benefit from patellar tendon supports.

ⓘ Elbow pain

This is commonly secondary to trauma, such as pulled elbow and supracondylar fracture. Both can be sustained whilst playing with siblings so a clear description of mechanism of injury may not be obtained. If the diagnosis is not clear after examination, perform x-ray before attempting manipulation—analgesia may be necessary to ensure that a good lateral view can be obtained.

> In a 'good' lateral view, the humeral lateral condyle above the capitellum should resemble an '8'

Reduction of a pulled elbow will hurt so warn the parents and child. Hold the arm at the hand and the elbow, pronate and supinate the arm as you flex the elbow. A 'pop' should be felt with resolution of pain. If there has been a delay in presentation, oedema develops which may limit the success of reduction. If unsuccessful, place the arm in a sling. Ask the parents to return for reassessment, if the child is still not moving the arm by the following morning.

Chapter 19

Ophthalmology

Ocular anatomy

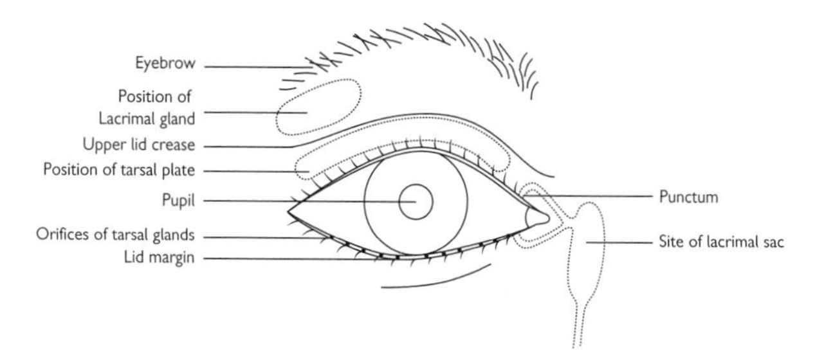

Fig. 19.1 External anatomy of the eye

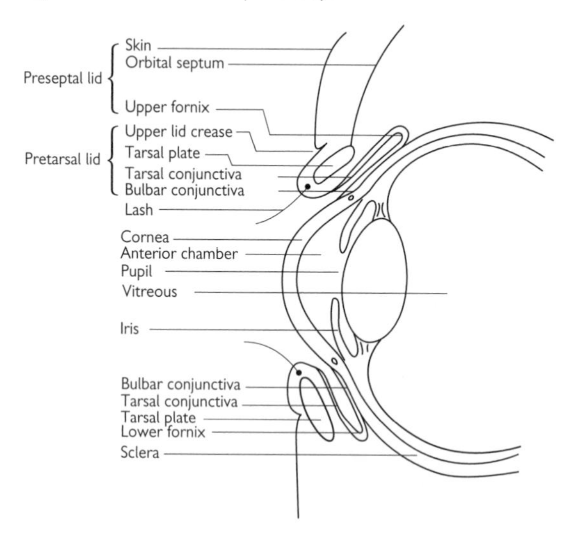

Fig. 19.2 Cross-section of the eye. (Figure kindly provided by Dr. T. Sleep.)

Assessment

History

Take a thorough history, unless immediate first aid is needed, e.g. chemical burns (📖 p.344). The history should include prenatal and postnatal events, e.g. CMV exposure; ophthalmological history (glasses? lazy eye? surgery?); and family history, e.g. cataracts.

Normal visual milestones

- Steady fixation: 6 weeks
- Fixing and following: 2 months
- Visually directed reaching: 4 months
- Detailed hand–eye coordination: 1 year
- Ocular motor fusion (i.e. straight eyes, no squint): 3–6 months
- 6/6 vision with recognition tasks by 3–4 years

Parents' assessment of whether their child is visually normal is valuable. Uniocular or gradual visual loss usually goes unnoticed in young children.

Examination

Pupils

- Check direct and consensual reaction.
  - Quickly swing a bright, focused light from directly in front of one pupil to the other and back. Watch to see if there is dilatation, or failure to constrict on either side.
  - Both responses should be equal. If consensual response is greater than direct response, a relative afferent pupillary defect (RAPD) is present, i.e. major retinal or optic nerve pathology.
- Pupils should also constrict to sustained accommodation.

Extraocular structures

- Evert the lid when looking for foreign bodies.
- Ask patient to follow a pen torch to test extraocular movements.

Globe

- If there is pain on opening the lids, apply topical anaesthetic, e.g. proxymetacaine drops.
- Fluorescein stains corneal or conjunctival epithelial defects and fluoresces green under cobalt blue light from a pen torch or slit lamp.
- Ideally, examine the anterior segment and lens using the slit lamp, but the direct ophthalmoscope on a +4 to +10 setting at a close distance can be used to magnify the surface of the globe.

Visual axis

- Elicit the red reflex with a bright direct ophthalmoscope set to 0 from 30cm. The red reflex should be bright and equally illuminated across the pupil in both eyes. Then come in very close to examine the optic nerve, the macula, and the blood vessels.
- Visual fields can be performed in children, using a toy, e.g. finger puppet, brought into the peripheral field, whilst they fix on a toy straight ahead.

Troubleshooting

How do I persuade the child to open the eye?

- Involve the parents in soothing the child before approaching
- If at all possible, do not touch the child. Provide interesting noisy toys to look at and give them a really good chance to open the eye themselves. Hold the lids open as a last resort only as it will probably be the last thing they will let you do!
- Explain to the parent and child what you are going to
- Use your finger or a cotton bud to elevate the lid, applied very close to the lashes, and then press against the superior orbital rim to keep elevated
- Before applying anaesthetic drops, warn that they may sting. Proxymetacaine drops sting least if at room temperature

How do I evert the lid?

- Use a local anaesthetic drop
- Tell the child to look down, and that you are going to pull on their lashes, but that it won't hurt if they keep looking at their toes
- Hold the upper lid lashes firmly as the child looks down, and pull the lid away from the globe with your left hand
- Push towards the globe and down with a cotton bud just above the tarsal plate (i.e. at the top of the eyelid)
- Then as the lid flips over, use your left thumb to press the lash's lid margin towards the globe to hold it steady whilst you look

How can I examine the retina?

- Use mydriatics, e.g. tropicamide 1%, cyclopentolate 1% (0.5% if premature)
- Warn the child that their vision will be blurred for at least an hour and that they will be sensitive to light

How can I assess acuity if the child cannot read?

Paediatric ophthalmic charts have everyday objects, e.g. toys, animals as silhouettes. Alternatively, point to a letter and ask the child to identify the letter from a selection in front of him.

If the child cannot do this, ask them to pick up a coloured 'hundred-and-thousand' at 6/9 vision. Ultimately, ask whether the light from an ophthalmoscope is on or off.

Trauma

Chemical burn

Chemicals may not only scar the cornea or conjunctivae, but some, especially alkalis, can penetrate the globe and cause uveitis, glaucoma, and cataract. Irrigation takes priority over further history and exam.

- Drop of local anaesthetic such as proxymetacaine.
- Copious irrigation (saline or Ringer's).
  - Irrigate fornices—use a speculum; evert upper eyelid.
  - Sweep fornices for particles. N.B. Plaster, which continues to burn if left. Irrigate for as long as possible, 30 minutes ideally.
  - Check pH with litmus paper 5 minutes after irrigation. If not neutral, continue to irrigate.
- Emergency ophthalmological assessment. Topical or systemic treatment and admission may be needed if severe.

Blunt injury

Ruptured globe

If suspected, minimal examination.

- Wound may be obvious—prolapse of brown/red uveal tissue through the sclera or cornea; soft eye; shallow anterior chamber compared to the other side.
- Corneal wound may self-seal, but leak may be seen with fluorescein.
- Vitreous haemorrhage (no view of the retina).

Management NBM, shield, no pad, urgent referral for EUA and repair.

Hyphaema

- Blood in the anterior chamber, either settled or circulating.
- Additional signs include uveitis, raised pressure, cloudy cornea, dilated pupil (traumatic mydriasis), posterior segment trauma.

Management Aimed at preventing rebleeds, which can cause long-term glaucoma.

- Exclude ruptured globe.
- Bed rest—consider admission.
- Topical steroids with mydriatics, e.g. dexamethasone 1% drops qds, and atropine 1% drops tds.
- Refer to ophthalmology.

Blow-out fracture

Follows blunt injury by an object fitting into the orbit, e.g. squash ball.

Signs Sunken or proptosed eye, limited up gaze with diplopia, numbness over cheek (infraorbital nerve), surgical emphysema of the lids or over zygoma. If significant enophthalmos and diplopia, surgery needed.

Management

- Instruct not to blow nose.
- Systemic broad spectrum antibiotics, e.g. co-amoxiclav.
- Request CT orbit.
- Consult with ophthalmology and maxillofacial surgeons.

⑦ ***Foreign body***

The child may report a sensation of something under the lids or else that it hurts whenever they blink. It may help to apply amethocaine drops prior to the examination. The foreign body may be visible on eversion of the lid and can be removed by a moistened cotton bud or by irrigation. Apply fluorescein to check for a corneal abrasion (📖 p.346). Apply chloromycetin drops before discharge.

Lacerations and abrasions

⑦ ***Eyelid laceration*** Urgent referral to ophthalmology for repair, especially if through the lid margin or medial ends of lids through canalicular system.

⑦ ***Conjunctival laceration*** Usually do not need repair. Exclude other ocular injuries; use chloramphenicol ointment for comfort.

⑦ ***Corneal abrasion*** See 📖 p.346.

The red eye

Conjunctivitis

☼ *Ophthalmia neonatorum*

Conjunctivitis in the newborn, acquired from the birth canal. Needs conjunctival swabs, urgent microscopy. N.B. *Chlamydia* requires specific swab and culture medium. Check if mother has had vaginal swabs performed. If STD confirmed (see Table 19.1), remember to treat both parents. If other bacteria isolated, treat with broad-spectrum systemic and topical antibiotics such as Chloromycetin.

ⓘ *Bacterial/viral conjunctivitis in the child*

Bilateral diffuse redness, worse in the fornices, with normal vision. Bacterial infection tends to cause a purulent discharge, whereas viral is watery. It is advisable to apply fluorescein to avoid missing a corneal abrasion or an evolving dendritic ulcer.

Swab and treat on results. If asymmetric or resistant think *Chlamydia*, and refer to GU clinic. Strict hygiene.

ⓘ Corneal ulcer

- White infiltrate or branching lesion that may stain with fluorescein.
- Unilateral, painful, photophobic, watery or sticky eye.
- Vision affected either by lesion or hypopyon—pus in the anterior chamber.

Management Urgent referral to ophthalmology for corneal scrapes and empirical treatment based on appearance.

ⓘ Uveitis/iritis

- Vision affected slightly to severely.
- Unilateral redness around limbus; pupil small, irregular, immobile.
- Photophobic, watery, hypopyon if very severe.

N.B. Uveitis is common in JIA and may cause minimal symptoms. But late complications include band keratopathy, cataract, and glaucoma.

Management Urgent referral to ophthalmology; cycloplegic and steroid eye drops. Exclude systemic disease. If severe, post-trauma, post-surgery, or with systemic illness, consider ☼ **endophthalmitis** (intra-ocular infection). Endophthalmitis necessitates emergency referral for vitreous biopsy and intravitreal antimicrobial agents.

ⓘ Corneal abrasion

- Unilateral, painful, photophobic, watery, swollen lids.
- History of trauma; finger nail injury common.
- Staining corneal lesion without infiltrate.

Management Check for foreign body under lid. Chloramphenicol drops or ointment qds. Local anaesthetic drops and also dilating drops, e.g. cyclopentolate tds may help. A pad can be used for comfort but is contraindicated if contact lenses usually worn (*Pseudomonas* can ulcerate).

Table 19.1 Treatment of ophthalmia neonatorum secondary to STDs

	Appearance	Treatment
Gonorrhoea	Purulent conjunctivitis in first 48h; profuse discharge. May cause corneal ulcer and perforation	Irrigation of eyes to remove pus qds IV benzyl penicillin 10mg/kg/dose tds ***plus*** topical erythromycin 2 hourly
Chlamydia	Mucopurulent discharge, between days 5 to 12 of age	Oral erythromycin 12.5mg/kg/dose qds ***plus*** topical tetracycline ointment qds
Herpes	Conjunctivitis ***without*** discharge. May have corneal ulcer or stromal keratitis (non-staining corneal opacity)	IV and topical acyclovir

Lids

Lid lesions can become an emergency in paediatrics if the visual axis is occluded. Deprivational amblyopia develops very quickly and may be untreatable if left untreated for a significant period.

⑦ Ptosis

Aetiology

- Congenital—poor lid crease, lid 'hung up' on downgaze.
- Horner's syndrome—congenital or acquired, mild ptosis.
- Third nerve palsy—congenital or acquired.
- Neuromuscular—myasthenia, botulism, ADEM (acute disseminated encephalomyelitis).
- Marcus Gunn jaw wink ptosis—lid height varies with action of the masseter or pterygoid muscles, i.e. chewing, sucking, protruding jaw.
- Mechanical—a lump.

A chin-up posture is a sign that the child is attempting to use the occluded eye or eyes. If this is lost, the ptosis may have become too severe to overcome and will need urgent surgery to lift lid out of visual axis. Prompt referral to ophthalmology required, along with cranial MRI.

Masses that may cause ptosis

- **Chalazia**—firm round lump in the tarsal plate. Common; may be associated with preseptal cellulitis. Usually settle with antibiotics and warm compresses; may leave a discrete lump that needs incising.
- **Capillary haemangioma**—often enlarge rapidly in the first few weeks of life. May require intralesional or systemic steroids to halt enlargement and clear the visual axis. Doppler USS and/or CT scanning needed if deep to distinguish from solid malignancies, e.g. rhabdomyosarcoma.
- **Rhabdomyosarcoma**—initially a discrete lump, then rapidly progressing ptosis and proptosis. Tissue diagnosis required.

⑦ Congenital lid abnormalities

Symblepharon Fusion of the eyelids by a pedicle of skin at birth. They are usually easily divided, and this should be done promptly.

Lid coloboma A gap involving the lid margin. May be found with other ocular abnormalities, e.g. microphthalmia; coloboma of the iris, lens, or retina. Other associations include facial clefts.

Exposure of the globe can result in corneal scarring, in which case early surgical repair warranted. If seen at neonatal check, use lubricating eye drops and ointment until assessed.

Lid laceration See 🕮 p.345.

Orbital disease

Orbital disease may present with proptosis, pain, lid swelling or redness, or with a normal globe with restricted eye movements and double vision.

ⓘ Preseptal cellulitis

Inflammation anterior to the orbital septum. Risk factors in the history include: cysts, skin infections, dacrocystitis, lid trauma, insect bites, URTI.

Signs

- Lids red, swollen and hot. N.B. Allergy causes swollen, and oedematous lids but not inflammation or induration.
- White eye, or very minimal injection, no proptosis.
- Eye movements, vision, and pupillary reactions normal.

Management

- Older, well children with mild inflammation: oral antibiotics with a review within 12h after presentation, to ensure no progression.
- Others: admit under joint care of paediatricians and ophthalmologists, IV antibiotics.

Investigations Swabs from conjunctival sac. If unwell, FBC, blood cultures; consider CT scan orbit and sinuses.

Best guess antibiotics IV Flucloxacillin 50mg/kg/dose qds (if over 5) or IV cefotaxime 50mg/kg/dose tds (if under 5). Consider Gram-negative cover after trauma.

☠ Orbital cellulitis

Inflammation extends behind the orbital septum. Usually secondary to sinusitis, dacrocystitis, or orbital trauma.
Signs as above, plus signs of orbital disease:

- proptosis, restricted eye movements;
- injected eye with chemosis;
- reduced acuity.

Management Admit, joint care of paediatricians, ophthalmologists, and ENT.

Investigations As above but CT scanning mandatory. Any collections require surgical drainage or debridement.

Antibiotics Admit for IV flucloxacillin 50mg/kg/dose qds (if over 5) or IV cefotaxime 50mg/kg/dose tds (if under 5). Anaerobic cover may be necessary.

☠ Cavernous sinus thrombosis Presents as a severe orbital cellulitis, with worsening of signs despite treatment. Contralateral signs may develop, with oculomotor nerve palsies and facial numbness. Requires emergency referral to neurology/neurosurgery.

Proptosis in childhood Vascular tumour (capillary haemangioma/lymphangioma), rhabdomyosarcoma, neuroblastoma, leukaemia/lymphoma, thyroid eye disease, other orbital inflammation. Urgent referral and scanning is mandatory.

Leucocoria and corneal opacity

ⓘ Leucocoria—the white pupil

Usually detected during the baby check, but urgent whenever seen. Opacity in the visual axis may lead to irreversible deprivational amblyopia within days. Some causes are life-threatening.

Best appreciated with a bright direct ophthalmoscope set on 0 at a distance of 30 to 45cm, illuminating both pupils simultaneously. Any asymmetry or a white/yellow reflex needs urgent referral.

Causes

- Congenital or childhood cataract.
- Retinoblastoma.
- Retinal disease—Coat's disease (massive lipid exudation from retinal vessels seen as yellow subretinal lesions), infection, inflammation, retinal detachment secondary to retinopathy of prematurity, trauma, or other cause
- Congenital abnormality—persistent hyperplastic primary vitreous—(seen as a white anterior vitreal mass, usually also with cataract); myelinated nerve fibres; retinal coloboma.

Management Take thorough maternal, family, and medical history. Urgent ophthalmology referral for full examination is necessary. Cataracts will usually need urgent surgery—within 6 weeks of birth if bilateral. Paediatric consultation is also recommended for exclusion of systemic disorders such as galactosaemia, congenital rubella, Lowes syndrome.

ⓘ Corneal opacity

Cloudiness of the cornea may be diffuse or discrete in patches.

Diffuse opacity

- **Congenital glaucoma.** Rare—cloudy, large cornea with a watery eye and photophobia, emergency referral.
- **Others**, e.g. metabolic disorders such as mucopolysaccharidoses, cystinosis; fetal alcohol syndrome; congenital infection, e.g. rubella; birth trauma. Rare but need investigation and urgent referral.

Discrete opacity

- **Corneal ulcer** (📖 p.346)—red painful eye, white ulcer staining with fluorescein, hypopyon, emergency referral.
- **Congenital infection**—interstitial keratitis, e.g. secondary to congenital syphilis. Central opacity, no staining, painful red eye, urgent referral.
- **Band keratopathy**—white band of calcium deposit across cornea, usually non-staining. May be a late sign of a chronic asymptomatic uveitis; needs urgent referral.
- **Congenital abnormality**, e.g. Peter's anomaly (posterior corneal defect, with adhesions to iris or lens). Appears as central opacity without staining; needs urgent referral.

Squints and neuro-ophthalmology

Squint: a misalignment of the visual axes

Cover test: ask the patient to look at a target. Cover one eye at a time. If, when one eye is covered, the other eye moves to re-adjust fixation, the uncovered eye has a squint.

Squints may be intermittent, e.g. fatigue, or of gradual onset. However the sudden onset of a constant squint is an ophthalmic emergency, as it is more likely to be secondary to intracranial or retinal pathology. In addition, the squinting eye will become lazy. Urgent assessment by ophthalmology, optometry and orthoptics is necessary.

Cranial nerve palsies see Fig. 19.3.

Result in an incomitant squint, i.e. size of squint varies with position of gaze. Unless the cause is known, CT scan is necessary along with urgent ophthalmological assessment.

Third nerve palsy Ptosis—either ipsi- or contralateral, mydriasis (dilated pupil), eye deviated down and out with limitation of elevation, depression, and adduction.

Causes Congenital, head injury, brain tumour, meningitis, migraine, post-infectious, idiopathic.

Fourth nerve palsy Head tilt to unaffected side, oblique or vertical double vision if head straight.

Causes Congenital, head injury, posterior fossa mass, post-viral.

Sixth nerve palsy Convergent squint. Limited abduction. Diplopia reduced by turning face.

Causes Congenital, raised ICP, basal skull fracture, brain tumour, meningitis/other infection, drugs, post-infectious, idiopathic.

IIIrd nerve palsy

Look ahead

Down and out

IVth nerve palsy

Head tilt to opposite side to level gaze

VIth nerve palsy

Look to the right

Look to the left

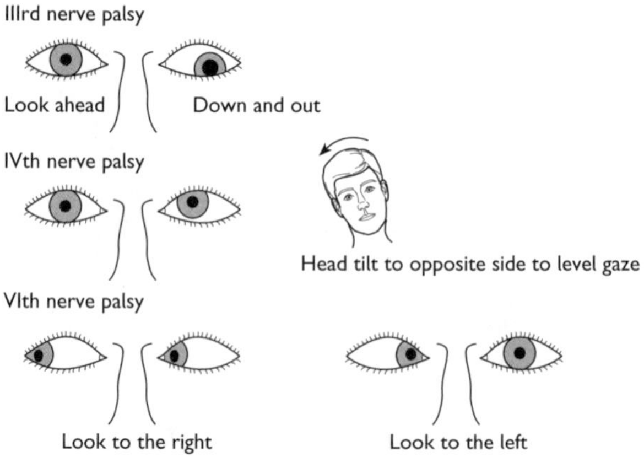

Fig. 19.3 Ocular nerve palsies. Left eye affected in all cases.

⑦ Anisocoria

Unequal pupils.

Causes

- **Physiological**—present from birth, difference equal in light and dark.
- **Horner's syndrome**—small pupil, mild ptosis—urgent investigation.
- **Third nerve palsy**.
- **Pharmacological**—fixed dilated, e.g. contact with atropine-like substance, nebulized iptratropium
- **Blunt trauma** to the eye causing mydriasis.
- **Tonic pupil**—dilated pupil, accommodates but slow light reaction. Usually caused by Adie's syndrome (tonic pupil with reduced deep tendon reflexes ± mild blurring of vision). Often post-viral.

⑦ Nystagmus

Rapid to and fro movements of the eyes.

- Congenital idiopathic nystagmus—onset shortly after birth.
- Strabismus.
- Poor vision.
- Intracranial pathology—horizontal = cerebellar; vertical = brainstem.
- Drugs, e.g. phenytoin.

New cases need urgent ophthalmological and neurological assessment.

Papilloedema

Swollen optic nerves caused by increased ICP. Blurring of vision is a late symptom. Fundoscopic appearances include:

- optic nerves look raised, with whitish blurred edges;
- the blood vessels over the disc may be obscured;
- retinal splinter haemorrhages may be present.

Urgent head CT should be performed, followed by ophthalmological assessment to exclude other causes of swollen nerves. Neurosurgical consultation may also be required.

⑦ Optic neuritis

Arises due to inflammation or demyelination of the optic nerve. An extremely rare complication of viral illness, but may be the first manifestation of MS in adolescents.

Classically it develops over days with:

- visual loss ranging from mild to severe. Loss of vision may vary with temperature or exercise;
- colour vision impairment;
- any pain is exacerbated on eye movements.

There is a relative afferent pupillary defect (📖 p.342) and optic nerves look swollen, resembling papilloedema. Ophthalmology/neurology referral is needed to elucidate cause.

Useful lists

Causes of sudden loss of vision with white eye

- **Uveitis** (toxoplasma, pars planitis): blurred vision, floaters, white retinal lesions (📖 p.346).
- **Optic neuritis** (📖 p.353).
- **Retinal vascular disease**: uniocular sudden onset, painless visual loss.
- **Retinal detachment**: uniocular, sudden onset, floaters, flashing lights, visual field defect, relative afferent pupillary defect, detachment visible on ophthalmoscopy.
- **Cerebral vascular event**: bilateral sudden onset of painless visual loss or field defect. Rare but exclude embolic event, e.g. arrhythmia.
- Sudden discovery of **chronic visual loss** (cataract, retinal pathology).
- **Functional** visual loss.

Causes of eye pain

- **Foreign body** (📖 p.345).
- **Preseptal cellulitis/orbital cellulitis**/dacrocystitis (📖 p.349).
- **Corneal abrasion/ulcer** (📖 p.346).
- **Endophthalmitis** (📖 p.353).
- **Optic neuritis** (📖 p.353).
- **Dry eye.**
- **Acute iritis/uveitis** (not conjunctivitis) (📖 p.346)—uniocular, with blurred vision and photophobia. Perilimbic redness and a constricted pupil with a sluggish response to light.
  - **Management.** Atropine 1% eyedrops and prednisolone one drop bd for 5 days. Investigate for auto-immune illness, such as JIA.
- **Scleritis**—severe pain with radiation to the head. Eye deep red; refer.
- **Myositis**—pain on movement, red over extra ocular muscles; refer.
- ☼ **Acute glaucoma.** Rare, usually a delayed presentation after trauma. Painful eye, with marked visual impairment. Corneal clouding with perilimbic redness.
  - **Management.** Start IV mannitol 250mg/kg, keep NBM, and request urgent ophthalmology opinion.

ⓘ Vulvovaginitis

Vaginal redness is a cause of significant distress to parents, who fear that their child may have been sexually abused. Fortunately, there are often benign causes.

The child may be distressed by the pain, especially on micturition. Be very gentle and reassuring as you conduct the examination. Any evidence of trauma necessitates senior review ± forensic examination.

N.B. *Candida* seldom arises in the pre-pubertal child (📖 p.358).

Poor perineal hygiene

Usually presents when the girl is just starting self-toileting. Introitus appears swollen and inflamed and there may be a mucoid discharge.

Emphasize importance of wiping from front to back. Recommend cotton underpants and avoidance of bubble baths. Wash the area with a mild soap and allow to air dry. Severe cases may require topical hydrocortisone 1% for 3 days.

Lichen sclerosus et atrophicus

Found in girls under the age of 4 when oestrogen levels tend to be low. Skin pale and waxy and may extend from either side of the vagina to perianally ('hourglass' appearance). Skin often friable and can bleed.

Treat with topical high potency steroid cream, e.g. betamethasone valerate. Often easier to attach sanitary towel to underpants and apply cream to towel, rather than directly on to child.

Pinworms

May be associated with perianal itching, particularly at night. If no worms visible, apply Sellotape® to skin and then stick on to a glass slide and send for microscopy for entrobial ova.

Treat with oral mebendazole. Emphasize importance of hand washing. Siblings and pets may also require treatment.

Intercurrent URTI

Bacteria may be introduced digitally, e.g. *Streptococcus* can cause linear ulceration and requires a course of penicillin.

Herpes causes vesicles, then discrete shallow ulcers. The vesicles are often found on the peripheries of the lesion. Although commonly arising after digital contact with cold sores, the possibility of sexual abuse, whether from orogenital or genito–genital contact, must be considered.

Confirm by sending swabs for viral culture. Treat with oral acyclovir. Young children may not be able to manage tablets and require admission for IV treatment.

ⓘ Vaginal bleeding

Generally, this results from trauma in the prepubertal girl and menstruation in adolescents. In adolescents, it is imperative to exclude pregnancy as bleeding can herald life-threatening conditions for the mother and fetus (📖 p.364).

Other causes are easily identified during assessment.

History

- Any vaginal discharge? If malodourous, presume foreign body or infection (📖 p.359).
- Any other bleeding points? Mucosal bleeding, e.g. nose, is indicative of platelet disorders (📖 p.378).
- If post-menarche, obtain menstrual history—usual cycle, duration of bleed, any associated pain or clots.
- If sexually active, think of reasons why a pregnancy test is not indicated. If pregnancy confirmed, obtain an estimation of gestation.
- Medications—exclude overdose of anticoagulant or OCP.

Examination

- ☠ If shock, think ectopic pregnancy, placental abruption, DIC.
  - ABC, fluid resuscitation, summon senior help.
- Any abdominal masses palpable?
  - Pregnancy—measure fundus (pubis symphysis to apex); distance in cm equates to gestation in weeks. Note any fundal tenderness.
  - Uterine duplication associated with partial vaginal septae with accumulated menstrual blood. Uterus may be tender (📖 p.358).
  - Tumours are extremely rare.
- Obtain urinary β-HCG, arrange USS. Consult with gynaecology.
- Gynaecological examination—internal assessment as indicated.

Causes

Trauma Typically arising after a straddle injury. However, sexual abuse should be considered if the injury is unexplained. Hymenal injuries heal spontaneously, but surgical opinion should be sought for vaginal lacerations.

Menstruation disorders

Dysfunctional uterine bleeding is either heavy ('menorrhagia') or painful ('dysmenorrhoea').

Menorrhagia Typically, the girl has an erratic cycle with a heavy, prolonged menstrual bleed that is painless. Once pregnancy excluded, start Provera 10mg daily for 5 days. Arrange GP review to discuss regular Provera at the start of each menstruation, or else OCP.

Dysmenorrhoea Pain associated with menstruation is not unusual and often arises 6 to 18 months after menarche. It usually responds to topical heat and NSAIDs, such as ibuprofen or naproxen. If not, discuss starting OCP.

Pain that precedes menstruation or starts within 6 months of menarche raises the possibility of endometriosis, which necessitates a referral to gynaecology.

Pregnancy complications (📖 p.364)

First trimester

- Ectopic pregnancy.
- Threatened abortion.

Third trimester

- Placenta praevia.
- Placental abruption.

Contraindications for starting the OCP

- The patient is not mature enough to make decision without parental consent
- Pregnancy
- Hypertension
- Pre-existing liver disease
- Predisposition to thromboembolic disease, e.g. sickle cell anaemia; family history of DVT
- Previous cerebrovascular or coronary artery disease, e.g. Kawasaki
- Breast or endometrial malignancy

? Sexually transmitted diseases

These should be considered in every adolescent girl who presents with any of:
- vaginal discharge;
- abdominal pain;
- joint swelling.

The diagnosis provides the opportunity to check that the girl is not a victim of coercive sex, to emphasize the importance of safe sex practices, and to screen for diseases such as HIV and hepatitis B.

The following three diseases are discussed because, if untreated, there are implications for the patient and, potentially, her children. If one disease is suspected, many would advocate screening for all three, with concomitant treatment.

Swabs should be taken from endocervix ± rectum and pharynx.

Chlamydia

The detection of *Chlamydia* is important because it can cause PID with subsequent impaired fertility. Unfortunately, up to 80% of women with the disease may be asymptomatic. Symptoms include a yellow-green purulent vaginal discharge, dysuria, and possible cervical tenderness, noted on penetration.

Confirm by swab—non-wooden handle—and request specific culture medium from microbiology lab. Urine can also be screened for *Chlamydia* PCR.

Treat with single dose azithromycin 20mg/kg (maximum 1g).

Gonorrhoea

Prepubertal girls tend to present with a profuse yellow vaginal discharge, whereas adolescents may have cervicitis and abdominal pain from salpingitis. Other complications include:
- PID;
- arthritis, either poly or mono especially of the wrist, ankle, or knee;
- febrile illness with tender pustular rash. Occasionally can resemble meningococcaemia as both *Neisseria*.

Confirm by culture of swab ± FBC, blood culture if evidence of disseminated disease.
- If uncomplicated, treat with single dose ceftriaxone IM 125mg.
- If disseminated disease, admit for daily IV ceftriaxone 50mg/kg (maximum 1g) for 7 days.

Syphilis

Has three distinct stages of which the first two can resolve spontaneously. Diagnosis may be missed as the primary stage may not manifest and the secondary stage has non-specific features.
- Primary. Painless genital ulcer with indurated edges. Appears 3 weeks after exposure and can resolve within 3 to 6 weeks.
- Secondary. Starts 9 to 15 weeks after exposure. Malaise with fever, sore throat, and headaches. On examination, generalized lymphadenopathy and rash that originates on trunk and flexor surfaces,

then spreads to palms and soles. Rash typically dull red and papular but has other appearances.

- Tertiary. Neurological and cardiovascular complications arise many years after initial exposure, so unlikely to be seen in children unless congenitally acquired.

Confirm by taking blood for VDRL, TPHA. Treponemes may be visible on microscopy from swabs of primary and secondary lesions.

Treatment is single dose IM benzathine penicillin G 1.8g.

Remember

- ALL of these diseases are notifiable (📖 p.156)
- Don't forget that your patient's partner will need treatment
- Arrange follow-up in a specialist unit

Pregnancy

Many teenage pregnancies are concealed, which may compromise the health of the mother and the fetus. The possibility of an undisclosed pregnancy should always be borne in mind when arranging abdominal x-rays or prescribing medications, such as trimethoprim, that may potentially harm a fetus.

When treating pregnant adolescents, your responsibility is to your patient and not her parents. Assess her maturity (or 'Gillick competence', 📖 p.356) as to whether she can make important decisions independently. Discuss with her whether her parents are to be informed and encourage her to involve a trusted adult in her care.

Diagnosis of pregnancy

Determine the gestation from the LMP. Try to ascertain paternity in order to exclude sexual abuse. On examination, record the following.

- Weight.
- BP.
- Abdominal examination—fundus palpable after 12 weeks. Is size consistent with dates?
- Arrange follow-up with your patient's preferred medical practitioner within the next 48 hours. It is better that she discusses continuation of the pregnancy with a doctor she knows well.

☼ Pre-eclampsia

Teenagers are prone to hypertensive disease of pregnancy. If untreated, hypertension will impair fetal growth and, ultimately, place the mother at risk of hypertensive seizures and intracranial bleeds (eclampsia).

- If BP >140/90, screen for pre-eclampsia:
  - FBC, UEC, LFT, urate;
  - dipstick urine for proteinuria.

Discuss with obstetrician and admit.

☼ Bleeding

Bleeding in pregnancy must be assessed carefully as the life of the mother and fetus could be jeopardized. Painful bleeding is a worrying symptom, but painless bleeding does not exclude the following conditions.

First trimester: ectopic pregnancy

Usually in association with abdominal pain, which can radiate to the shoulder and back if bleeding is retroperitoneal. The pain is usually continuous but can be colicky, reflecting intermittent blood flow from the ruptured pregnancy. Blood loss can be so precipitous that the patient suffers haemorrhagic shock.

- ABC including BP.
- Abdominal tenderness, especially in adnexae. Mass palpable in <50%.

Treatment

- If shock, apply oxygen and summon senior assistance.
- Obtain immediate IV access.
  - Take blood for FBC, cross-match.
  - If shock, give bolus of 20ml/kg 0.9% saline.
- Obtain urgent USS and gynaecological opinion.
- Give anti-D.

First trimester: threatened abortion

Painful bleeding does not preclude a viable pregnancy.

- ABC with BP.
- Palpate the fundus—note any tenderness and whether the size is consistent with dates.
- Inspect cervix via speculum—cervical dilatation means abortion is inevitable. If any products of conception visible, remove with forceps as this will limit bleeding.

Treatment

- If shock, apply oxygen; obtain immediate IV access.
  - Take blood for FBC, cross-match.
  - Give bolus of 20ml/kg 0.9% saline.
  - Start oxytocin infusion
- If inevitable abortion, perform FBC, cross-match as D & C may be necessary.
- If threatened abortion, admit for bed rest. In a third of cases, the pregnancy will reach term.
- Request gynaecological opinion.

Third trimester These conditions may be difficult to distinguish clinically so the management is the same.

- **Placenta praevia**. Painless bleeding due to placenta lying near the os. Bleeding can be so profuse as to cause haemodynamic shock.
- **Placental abruption**. Heavy bleeding secondary to placental detachment. Usually painful but occasionally abruption can be concealed. Risk factors include pre-eclampsia and blunt abdominal trauma.

Treatment

- If shock, apply oxygen; obtain immediate IV access.
  - Take blood for FBC, cross-match.
  - Give bolus of 20ml/kg 0.9% saline.
- Palpate fundus—tenderness = abruption necessitating emergency caesarean section.

Do not perform internal examination for fear of dislodging placenta praevia

- Arrange USS to confirm position of placenta.
- Start CTG monitoring of fetus—fetal distress mandates emergency Caesarean section.
- Obtain urgent obstetric opinion.

Chapter 21

Haematology

Anaemia

Anaemia arises when the haemoglobin falls below normal range for age (see Table 21.1).

Anaemia is usually of gradual onset, presenting with non-specific malaise and lethargy, but acute crises, e.g. haemolytic, or aplastic, can arise. The latter are more common if the marrow is under stress, e.g. haemoglobinopathy, acute leukaemia. There are also some rare bone marrow disorders, e.g. Diamond Blackfan, that result in isolated anaemia or Fanconi's giving rise to pancytopenia.

History and examination

A thorough systems review is important. Include the following.

- Possible sources of blood loss—obvious and occult, e.g. GI tract.
- Duration of symptoms.
- Recent infection.
- Dietary review, e.g. red meat intake, 'milk-aholics' (iron-deficiency anaemia); ingestion of beans, mothballs (!) (G6PD).
- Medication, e.g. chloramphenicol.
- Neonatal history noting any jaundice.
- Ethnic group.
- Family history.

Symptoms

- Lethargy.
- Tiredness.
- Shortness of breath.

Signs

- Pallor, jaundice.
- Bruising, active bleeding.
- Lymphadenopathy.
- Hepatosplenomegaly.
- Dysmorphic features, e.g.:
    - radial/thumb anomalies (thrombocytopenia/absent radius (TAR)); Diamond Blackfan (triphalangeal thumb);
    - frontal bossing—marrow expansion, e.g. haemoglobinopathy.

Remember to inspect the stool for occult blood loss.

Alarming signs include:

- active bleeding—suggestive of coagulopathy (p.378);
- signs of cardiac failure—cardiac compromise due to profound anaemia.

Investigations

- Full blood count and film.
- Reticulocytes (expect >2% if normal bone marrow response).
- Mean cell volume (MCV).
- Direct Coombs' test—to look for haemolysis.
- UEC.
- LFT including unconjugated and conjugated bilirubin.

Table 21.1 Normal haematology values

Age	Hb (g/dl)	Haematocrit	MCV (fl)	WCC ($x10^9/l$)	Neutrophils	Lymphocytes	Eosinophils	Basophils	Platelets	Reticulocytes
Birth	15–23	0.45–0.75	100–125	10–26	2.5–14	2–7	0–0.9	0–0.1	150–450	110–450
2 weeks	13–20	0.4–0.65	88–110	6–21	1.5–5.5	3–9	0–0.9	0–0.1	170–500	10–80
6 months	10–13	0.3–0.4	73–84	6–17	1–6	3–11	0.5–0.9	<0.2	210–560	15–110
12 months	10–13	0.3–0.4	70–80	6–16	1–8	3–10	<0.9	<0.13	200–550	20–150
2–5 years	11–13	0.3–0.4	72–87	6–17	1.5–9	2–8	<1.1	<0.12	210–490	50–130
5–12 years	11–15	0.3–0.4	76–90	4–14	1.5–8	1.5–5	<1	<0.12	170–450	50–130
>12 years										
Female	12–15	0.35–0.45	77–95	4–13	1.5–6	1.5–4.5	<0.8	>0.12	180–430	50–130
Male	12–16	0.35–0.5	77–92	4–13	1.5–6	1.5–4.5	<0.8	>0.12	180–430	50–130

- Sample for group and save ± cross-match.
- G6PD.
- Virology—specifically request parvovirus serology.
- Urine dip—haemoglobinuria or bilirubin suggests haemolysis.
- Stool—occult blood.

Management

If shock, apply oxygen via face-mask and obtain immediate IV access. Give bolus of 20ml/kg 0.9% saline. Consider:

- haemoglobinopathy: see sequestration (p.374); sepsis as functionally asplenic ± aplastic crisis (p.375);
- acute haemolysis. The rate of fall of haemoglobin directs management;
  - insert sampling cannula;
  - obtain Hb and reticulocyte count every 2 hours;
- major blood loss, e.g. in trauma.

The presence of hypotension indicates a 25–30% blood volume loss. Blood should be given in 10ml/kg boluses of packed red cells mixed with normal saline warmed to body temperature. This will aid speed of transfusion and warm the patient. Boluses should be repeated until systemic perfusion is satisfactory

Need to check clotting regularly and aim to normalize PT/APTT with FFP 12–15ml/kg as packed cells contain little clotting factors.
Aim also to keep platelets above 100.

All newly diagnosed blood dyscrasias, i.e. leukaemia, red cell aplasia, should be discussed with the on-call haematologist. The management of newly diagnosed leukaemics is covered on p.386.

The other forms of anaemia can be subdivided according to their MCV (Fig. 21.1).

Hypochromic microcytic anaemia MCV <70fl under 6 years, <75fl in >5 year olds.

Take blood for ferritin level ± haemoglobin electrophoresis to exclude a haemoglobinopathy (p.372), as well as transferrin saturation. As iron stores drop, there is initially only a drop in ferritin (N.B. ferritin is an acute phase protein, so can be falsely normal/high). Further reduction in stores causes a decrease in transferrin saturation. A drop in MCV follows and eventually there will be concomitant anaemia.

If iron deficiency is confirmed, do the following.

- Provide dietary advice, e.g. increase consumption of red meat, limit cows' milk intake.
- If necessary, add an iron supplement. Ferrous gluconate is the most palatable but can cause either diarrhoea or constipation. Iron supplements will increase Hb by 1g/dl a week.
- Arrange follow-up with GP so that Hb rise can be confirmed.

Normochromic normocytic anaemia MCV 70–90fl. If the unconjugated bilirubin is increased and there is a reticulocytosis, this suggests haemolysis may be present.

Macrocytic anaemia Rare in children, secondary to folate and B_{12} deficiency. Due to malabsorption, congenital deficiencies, or drugs (phenytoin, methotrexate, trimethoprim).

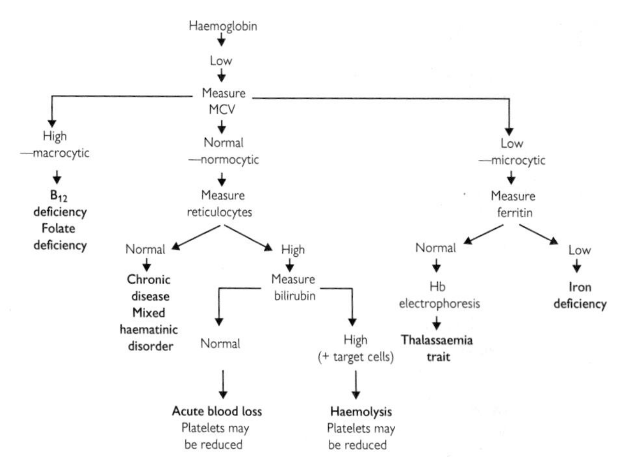

Fig. 21.1 Investigation of anaemia.

Haemoglobinopathies: sickle cell anaemia

Sickle cell anaemia is mostly seen in children of African descent. HbSS becomes deformed when in conditions of relative hypoxia or acidosis, e.g. venous stasis, dehydration. The erythrocytes aggregate resulting in impaired perfusion and ischaemia, further exacerbating the sickle crisis.

N.B. These children tend to have low Hb and MCV. Do ***not*** transfuse these patients because of a low Hb alone, as this can precipitate a crisis

Four distinct clinical complications of sickle cell anaemia exist:

1 vaso-occlusive crises:
- bony crisis;
- acute chest syndrome;
- acute abdominal pain;
- acute CNS event;
- priapism.

2 acute sequestration crisis.
3 aplastic crisis.
4 infection.

Most centres will have protocols on how to treat emergencies in these patients. It is important to remember that these patients can become very unwell and, if in doubt, senior input must be sought.

Vaso-occlusive crises

These are very painful as the intravascular sickling results in tissue infarction.

The mainstay of treatment for vaso-occlusive crises is as follows,
- Avoid dehydration—IV maintenance.
- Avoid hypoxia—oxygen.
- Treat pain stepwise—simple oral, diclofenac, IV opiates.
- If temperature over 38°C, start antibiotics, e.g. ceftriaxone + erythromycin.

ⓘ *Painful bony crisis*

- Local tenderness, erythema, and swelling.
- May have increased WCC and fever.
- Difficult to distinguish between crisis and osteomyelitis.

Sites involved

- Common sites.
  - L/S spine.
  - Knee.
  - Shoulder.
  - Elbow.
  - Femur.
- Rare sites.
  - Sternum.
  - Ribs.
  - Clavicles.
  - Mandible.
  - Maxilla

N.B. Dactylitis:

- Involvement of small bones of hands and feet.
- Under 5 years of age.
- Fingers and toes are swollen and painful.

Treatment As per vaso-occlusive treatment (see box opposite).

Acute chest syndrome

Infection, fat emboli, and infarction are all implicated in the aetiology of acute chest syndrome.

Clinical features

- Chest pain.
- Fever.
- Cough.
- Pleural rub/effusion.
- Hypoxia.
- Increased WCC.
- New infiltrate/effusion on CXR.

Management

- As per vaso-occlusive treatment (see box opposite).
- But also:
  - antibiotics—ceftriaxone and erythromycin;
  - blood transfusion/exchange—depends on unit policy;
  - involve senior early as patient can deteriorate rapidly.

ⓘ *Acute abdominal pain*

Thought to be due to mesenteric infarction, which may resemble an acute surgical abdomen. N.B. Intra-hepatic sickling may be confused with biliary colic, or acute cholecystitis.

Management

- As per vaso-occlusive treatment (see box opposite).
- Also:
  - abdominal USS—to assess gallstones;
  - surgical opinion.

☠ *Acute central nervous system event*

7% of children with HbSS have a CVA. Symptoms include: hemiplegia, seizures, coma, visual disturbance. Some children may fully recover but the mortality rate is high at 20%.

Management

- Immediate involvement of senior colleagues.
  - Involve haematology consultant and PICU.
- Resuscitate and stabilize patient.
- Admit to ICU, neuro HDU.
- Intubate if GCS <8.
- Hourly neurological observations.
- Exchange transfusion (📖 p.466)—aiming to decrease HbS to less than 30%.
- Urgent cranial imaging—MRI optimal.
  Once over acute event:
- long-term transfusion programme to keep HbS less than 25–30 % and Hb between 10 and 14;
- middle cerebral artery Doppler flow rates help predict patients at high risk of CVA.

ⓘ *Priapism*

Usually multiple short episodes, but can last over 24 hours increasing the risk of future impotence.

Treatment

- As per vaso-occlusive treatment (📖 p.372).
- Involve senior colleague as important to prevent long-term problems, e.g. impotence.
- Corporeal aspiration, if prolonged priapism, requiring specialist urologists.

☠ Acute sequestration crisis

Sudden massive enlargement of the spleen from trapping of the red cell mass with resultant acute drop in haemoglobin.

Clinical features

- Weakness.
- Dyspnoea.
- Rapidly increasing abdominal girth.
- Left-sided abdominal pain.
- Hypovolaemic shock.

Treatment

- Immediate venous access and cross-match of packed red cells.
  - Aim to transfuse Hb to normal levels for that patient.
  - Bolus 20ml/kg until adequately resuscitated.
  - Discuss with local and/or regional paediatric haematologist.

ⓘ **Aplastic crisis** Usually associated with parvovirus B19 infection. Spontaneous recovery is normal, but may need support with blood products, for a number of weeks.

Infection Most common cause of death in child less than 2 with sickle cell anaemia. Recurrent splenic infarcts render the child functionally asplenic and susceptible to encapsulated bacteria (*Streptococus pneumoniae*, *Haemophilus. influenzae*, *Salmonella*). All children should have up to date vaccination with Prevenar® (7-valent pneumococcal vaccine) and be on prophylactic penicillin.

It may be difficult to distinguish clinically between infection and bony crises or acute chest syndrome. Moreover, the latter two can have an apparent neutrophilia on machine-generated FBC, secondary to nucleated reticulocytes. A blood film will confirm. When in doubt, start antibiotics

Treatment

- Immediate IV ceftriaxone 50mg/kg/dose **bd** (maximum 4g/day) until culture results known.
- Check vaccination status.
- If catch-up vaccination required, emphasize importance of immunization to parents. Give single dose of Prevenar® and notify GP that further dose required, according to schedule.

Haemoglobinopathies: thalassaemia

Thalassaemia is a term encompassing a wide spectrum of diseases from thalassaemia minor to intermedia and major.

? **Thalassaemia minor** Often asymptomatic and only discovered in routine blood tests, where the MCV ± MCH are found to be low. The blood film may be normal.

? Thalassaemia intermedia

- Huge number of genotypes giving rise to one phenotype.
- Varying degree of anaemia.
- Have hypochromic microcytic indices.
- May require transfusion but not RBC dependent.

! Thalassaemia major

- These patients are transfusion-dependent.
- Without treatment they get:
  - extramedullary haemopoiesis, with frontal bossing;
  - LVF secondary to anaemia;
  - hepatosplenomegaly;
  - short stature.

These patients normally require treatment by the age of 5 years.

Treatment includes the following.

- 3–4 weekly blood transfusions.
  - Aim for Hb around 12g/dl.
  - Pre-transfusion Hb should not go below 9–10g/dl as this helps prevent extramedullary haemopoiesis.
- Reduction of iron overload from repeated transfusion.
  - Monitor serum ferritin.
  - Start desferrioxamine infusion given with transfusion to keep ferritin around 1000mcg/l.
  - Iron overload can predispose to *Yersinia* infection in the gut. **Warn parents to always report diarrhoeal symptoms.**

ⓘ Bleeding and bruising

Bruising in childhood is common. A coagulopathy should be considered either if bruises are in unusual areas, e.g. abdomen (but consider NAI), or else arise in conjunction with active bleeding.

A coagulopathy is either because of problems with platelets or clotting factors.

Platelet dysfunction

Associated with mucosal bleeding. Either platelets are insufficient (thrombocytopenia) or ineffective (thrombasthenia).

Thrombocytopenia either arises by decreased production, e.g. acute lymphoblastic leukaemia, aplastic anaemia; or by increased destruction, e.g. ITP, hypersplenism.

Thrombasthenia Low or normal count but reduced activity, e.g. von Willebrand's disease—technically a clotting factor deficiency, but the lack of vWF impairs platelets forming haemostatic plugs.

Clotting factor disorders

Associated with joint bleeds. Mainly due to reduced or abnormal production.

Congenital

- Haemophilia A—factor VIII deficiency (📖 p.382)
- Haemophilia B—'Christmas disease' or factor IX deficiency (📖 p.382).

Acquired

- Vitamin K deficiency:
  - neonatal;
  - malabsorption—small bowel ± bile salt disorders, CF;
  - liver disease;
  - drugs, e.g. warfarin, broad-spectrum antibiotics.
- DIC.

Assessment

When faced with a child with a potential coagulopathy, the important haematological conditions to exclude are:

- ALL;
- ITP;
- haemophilia;
- vitamin K deficiency.

History

A history should include the following points:

- history of trauma.
- bruising in unusual places, i.e. other than shins/legs in toddlers.
- recurrent mucosal bleeding, e.g. nose bleeds.
- swollen painful joints.
- recent viral infection.
- GI symptoms, e.g. diarrhoea, liver compromise.

- Previous history of bleeding after operation/dentist.
- Medication.
- Family history.
- Maternal history is relevant, e.g. heavy menses, recurrent miscarriages.

Examination

- Skin—pallor, petechiae, purpura, stigmata of liver disease.
- Palpate for lymph nodes—neck, axillae, groin.
- Palpate abdomen for liver and spleen.
- Note any joint swelling.

Investigations

- FBC and film—bone marrow failure, isolated decrease in platelets.
- Reticulocytes.
- Clotting screen (see Table 21.2 for normal values).
  - PT—measures factors II, V, VII, X.
  - APTT—measures factors II, V, VIII, IX, X, XI, XII.
  - Thrombin time—measurement of fibrinogen quantity or function; prolonged by heparin (cf. reptilase which is not affected by heparin) and presence of FDPs or fibrin.
  - Fibrinogen.
- FDP if suspect DIC.

Table 21.2 Clotting indices

Coagulation tests (mean values)	1–5 years	6–10 years	11–18 years
PT	11	11.1	11.2
INR	1	1	1
APTT (seconds)	30	31	32
Fibrinogen (g/l)	2.75	2.8	3
Bleeding time (mins)	6	7	5

Treatment of thrombocytopenia

Platelet transfusion may be given if there is:

- active uncontrolled bleeding;
- platelets below 10×10^9/l;
- febrile neutropenia and platelets are below 20×10^9/l;
- platelets below 50×10^9/l and needs a procedure e.g. LP for intrathecal medication;
- suspected decreased platelet production.

Give 5 units of platelet over 30 minutes.

ITP

ITP is usually self-limiting and does ***not*** require treatment. Platelets are ***not*** normally given in this condition.

The exceptions are:

- mucosal bleeding (hard palate);
- fundal bleeding;
- haematuria;
- intracranial bleed.

If persistent bleeding with ITP, discuss management with haematologist. A bone marrow aspirate may be necessary and subsequent treatment options are:

- short course of steroids (1mg/kg/day);
- immunoglobulin IV 1g/kg/day for 2 days.

Treatment in congenital factor deficiencies See 📖 p.383

Treatment in vitamin K deficiency

- Give IV Vitamin K 300mcg/kg/day (maximum 10mg) ***slowly***.
  - Possibility of anaphylaxis—have resuscitation drugs/equipment readily accessible.

Treatment of DIC

Combination of low platelets and abnormal clotting (see Table 21.3).

- Involve a senior colleague early.
- Treat underlying cause, e.g. septic shock.
- Platelets 5 units over 30 minutes, then re-check.
  - Aim to keep platelets over 50 or more.
- FFP 10ml/kg over 30 minutes.
- Discuss use of cryoprecipitate with haematologist.
- Give FFP if DIC confirmed and clinically bleeding.

Table 21.3 Differentiation between bleeding disorders*

Disorder	PT	APTT	Fibrinogen	FDPs†	Thrombin time	Platelets	Reptilase	Other
Haemophilia A (Factor VIII deficiency)	→	↑↑	→	→	→	→	→	Factor VIII <50%
Haemophilia B (Factor IX deficiency)	→	↑	→	→	→	→	→	Factor IX reduced
Thrombocytopenia	→	→	→	→	→	↓	→	
Vitamin K deficiency	↑↑	↑ or →	→	→	→	→	→	Reduced vitamin K-dependent factors II, VII, IX, X
Von Willebrand's	→	↑	→	→	→	→	→	Reduced vWF
Heparin in sample	↑	↑	→	→	↑↑	→	→	
DIC	↑	↑	↓	↑	↑	↓	↑	
Liver disease	↑	↑	↓	→	Variable	↓		

* →, Normal; ↑, raised; ↓, reduced.
† FDPs can be raised for a number of reasons and isolated raised FDPs does not indicate the presence of DIC unless the other clotting factors are also deranged.

Haemophilia

In haemophilia A there is factor VIII deficiency (80–85% of cases). In haemophilia B it is factor IX that is deficient.

There are numerous genotypes and phenotypes, but severity is determined by level of clotting factors:
- Mild disease: factor levels 6–40%;
- Moderate disease: factor levels 2–5%;
- Severe disease: factor levels <1%.

Presentation
- Intracranial haemorrhage at birth.
- Increased bruising/joint bleeds when start to mobilize
- Most diagnosed once become mobile (30% have no family history).

Management
Delivery of child to known carrier[1]
- Vaginal delivery but early LSCS if difficulties.
- No high or rotational forceps.
- No Ventouse.
- No IM vitamin K.
- Cord blood sample to lab.
- No NSAIDs.
- Avoid venepuncture if possible.
- If need to do heel prick, apply pressure for 5 min.

Involve haemophilia centre antenatally and delivery at affiliated hospital. Early involvement of haemophilia centre is mandatory.

Prevention of bleeding
- Regular check-ups.
- No NSAIDs.
- ***No*** contact sports.
- All immunizations subcutaneous.
- Factor concentrate replacement prior to invasive procedures.
- Prophylactic factor concentrate in severe patients.

Management of bleeding
- Resuscitate with blood, if necessary.
- All bleeds should be treated with factor replacement as soon as possible (ideally within 2 hours of onset).
- Discussion with usual haemophilia centre important.
- Site of bleed important in determining amount of factors required and will be calculated by haemophilia centre or haematologist.

1 Kulkami, R. and Lusher, J. (2001). Perinatal management of newborns with haemophilia. *Br. J. Haematol.* **112,** 264–74.

Dosing

The site of the bleed influences the dose and duration of therapy (Table 21.4). The table is a general guide but individual cases must be discussed with the treatment centre.

Haemophilia A

$$\text{Factor VIII (units)} = \frac{\text{weight in kg} \times \text{\% rise in factor VIII desired}}{2}$$

Haemophilia B

$$\text{Factor IX (units)} = \text{weight in kg} \times \text{\% rise in factor IX desired}$$

Table 21.4 Relation of site of bleed to therapy

Distribution of bleed	Desired factor level (%)	Duration of therapy (days)
☠ Throat/neck	80–100	1–7
☠ CNS/head	80–100	1–7
Then maintenance	50	8–21
Joint/muscle	40–60	1–2
Gastrointestinal	80–100	1–6
Renal	50	3–5

Further information

World Federation of Haemophilia (2005). *Guidelines for the management of haemophilia.* World federation of Haemophilia, Montreal. Can be accessed at *www.wfh.org*

Chapter 22

Oncology

Acute leukaemia

Acute leukaemia occurs when a single progenitor cell undergoes a malignant transformation in the bone marrow. This results in multiplication of immature blasts replacing the normal bone marrow cells and appearing in the peripheral blood.

There are two main lineages:
- acute lymphoblastic leukaemia (ALL)—commonest in childhood;
- acute myeloblastic leukaemia (AML).

Clinical features

A full history and examination is essential. Ask specifically about immunization status and previous exposure to VZV.

Some of the common symptoms and signs are listed in the box.

Some signs and symptoms of acute leukaemia

Symptoms
- Tiredness
- Lethargy
- Bone pain
- Recurrent fever

Signs
- Pallor
- Bruising
- Petechiae
- Bleeding
- Hepatosplenomegaly
- Lymphadenopathy
- Mediastinal mass and associated symptoms

Palpate thoroughly for lymph nodes—not only neck and groin but also axillae, supraclavicular region and also around bones such as the olecranon. Also palpate long bones and spine for localized bony tenderness. Perform fundoscopy to exclude retinal haemorrhages or papilloedema.

Investigations for newly diagnosed leukaemia

- FBC and film—commonly anaemia with thrombocytopenia. WCC can be high or low.
- UEC, LDH, urate.
- Coagulation—DIC may occur in AML.
- Viral serology for hepatitis B,C; HIV; CMV; VZV; measles.
- Blood group ± cross-match as subsequent CVL insertion probable.

Do not transfuse until viral serology obtained

- CXR—to look for mediastinal mass.
- Bone marrow aspirate and trephine for morphology, cytogenetics, and immunophenotyping.
- Lumbar puncture to diagnose CNS disease.

The latter two may be deferred and performed under GA, along with central line insertion.

Transfusion indicated if:
- Hb <7g/dl **except** if WCC >50 × 10^9/l (see Hyperviscosity below);
- child symptomatic e.g. bleeding. If breathless, exclude hyperviscosity;
- procedure needs to be performed and Hb <8 × 10^9/l.

Give 20ml/kg of blood over 4 hours.

Platelet transfusion may be given if there is:
- active uncontrolled bleeding;
- platelets below 10 × 10^9/l;
- febrile neutropenia and platelets are below 20 × 10^9/l;
- platelets below 50 × 10^9/l and needs a procedure e.g. LP for intrathecal medication.

Give 5 units of platelets over 30 minutes.

Complications

The five complications listed may present shortly after diagnosis, prior to or during induction treatment.

Infection It is important to remember that any child presenting with acute leukaemia is functionally neutropenic. Most of the white cells in the peripheral blood at presentation are blasts and do not function as mature neutrophils. Treat as febrile neutropenia (📖 p.388).

Obstruction secondary to mediastinal mass see 📖 p.389.

Tumour lysis syndrome 📖 p.390.

Hyperviscosity

High risk patients are those presenting with a high white cell count of >100 × 10^9 per ml. The complications are caused by stasis of the blood.

Clinical signs
- Hypoxia and dyspnoea due to pulmonary leucostasis.
- Poor peripheral circulation.
- Retinal haemorrhages.
- Papilloedema.
- CNS depression due to cerebral infarcts.
- Focal CNS abnormalities.

Management
- Rehydrate with 3l/m^2/day 0.9% saline (📖 p.517).
- Correction of coagulation defects and thrombocytopenia.
- ***Avoid*** blood transfusion to correct anaemia as transfusing packed cells will increase risk of stasis.
- Consider exchange transfusion and involve an experienced senior colleague.

Disseminated intravascular coagulation (DIC)

Characteristic of M3 AML.

If bleeding is controlled, there is no need to normalize blood results unless child about to have procedure, e.g. CVL insertion, BMA, LP. Otherwise give FFP, platelets ± cryoprecipitate to control active bleeding (📖 p.380).

Febrile neutropenia

Neutropenic patients with fever may have a potentially life-threatening infection. These patients must always be assessed promptly and treated as a medical emergency.

Neutrophils <1.0 x 10^9
and Fever >38.0°C on two occasions 4 hours apart
or Fever >38.5°C once

Assessment

History should include:
- current treatment including recent chemotherapy, prophylactic antibiotics, GMCSF, etc;
- duration of fever;
- rigors—may suggest line infection;
- abdominal pain. (N.B. Steroid treatment may mask signs.)

Examination must be thorough and should include inspection of any central line site, mouth (for mucositis), ENT, and skin, including the peri-anal area. The blood pressure and peripheral circulation must be documented as they may be the only signs of septic shock.

Investigations

- FBC, UEC, CRP, blood cultures taken centrally if line *in situ.*
- Urine for M,C & S.
- CXR—routine in some units; only if symptoms in others.
- Stool sample if diarrhoea present. Send for M,C & S, virology ± *Clostridium difficile* toxin if recent course of antibiotics.

Management

Empirical antibiotic therapy must be commenced within 2 hours of presentation, if the child appears septic or neutropenia is confirmed. If in doubt, involve a senior colleague at an early stage, and discuss all patients with oncology. Medications and fluids can safely be given via the CVL, even if line infection is suspected.
- ***Fluid resuscitation.*** If the child is showing signs of shock, give bolus of 20ml/kg 0.9% saline. If there is little improvement, consult with PICU as inotropes may be required.
- ***Antibiotics.*** Broad spectrum intravenous antibiotics according to local policy, e.g. ceftriaxone 50mg/kg daily and gentamicin 7mg/kg daily (reduced dose if renal function impaired).
    - Add vancomycin or teicoplanin if suspected line infection.
- Consider antifungal if fever persistent.
- If there is evidence of central line infection or if high-risk organisms such as *Staphylococcus aureus, Escherichia coli* or *Pseudomonas* have been isolated in the blood cultures, discuss possible central line removal with oncology.

Superior vena cava compression

Compression of the superior vena cava by an anterior mediastinal tumour or thrombosis; often associated with tracheal compression.

Causes

- Acute lymphoblastic leukaemia—mainly T-cell.
- Non-Hodgkin's lymphoma.
- Hodgkin's lymphoma.
- Neuroblastoma.
- Thrombosis of SVC.

Clinical features Onset varies, can be gradual or acute.

Symptoms and signs of SVC compression

Symptoms	*Signs*
• Cough	• Stridor, wheeze
• Shortness of breath	• Dyspnoea
• Orthopnoea	• Plethora, facial cyanosis
• Chest pain	• Facial oedema
• Headaches due to raised ICP	• Distended veins on chest and neck
• Syncope	• Papilloedema
	• Hypertension
	• Pulsus paradoxus

Investigations

- FBC and film—may show leukaemia.
- UEC—raised potassium suggestive of high tumour bulk.
- Ca, PO_4, urate, LDH.
- Urinary catecholamines.
- CXR PA and lateral. May show widened mediastinum, pleural effusions, or pericardial effusion.
- CT chest. N.B. This needs careful evaluation as the patient is at considerable risk during the procedure if orthopnoea is present.
- Biopsy. There is a very high risk of anaesthetic/sedation-related problems due to mediastinal mass. It may be possible to obtain diagnostic material under local anaesthetic, e.g. bone marrow aspiration, pleural aspiration, or lymph node biopsy.

Ensure you discuss case with oncology and senior colleagues before proceeding with biopsy

Treatment

- If the mass is identified, treat with current recommended treatment protocol.
- If not, start empiric treatment to reduce obstruction and alleviate symptoms, e.g. steroids or radiotherapy. Once treatment started, monitor for improvement so biopsy can be performed as soon as possible. Watch for tumour lysis syndrome (p.390).

Tumour lysis syndrome

A combination of metabolic abnormalities and renal dysfunction that arises as a result of tumour cell death, which may be spontaneous or treatment-related.

Can occur in leukaemia and lymphoma. Most at risk if WCC is high or bulky disease present. Mainly seen in:

- T-cell ALL;
- T-cell NHL;
- B-cell NHL.

Metabolic abnormalities

- **Hyperkalaemia**. Potassium release can be rapid and very dangerous. At risk of arrhythmias and cardiac arrest (p.446).
- **Hyperuricaemia**. Increase in uric acid due to release of purines from nuclei of dying cells. May deposit in kidneys and cause acute renal failure due to urate nephropathy. Risk is increased if physiological pH is acidic, i.e. sepsis, leucostasis.
- **Hyperphosphataemia**. Phosphate released from dying lymphoblasts, which contain four times as much phosphate as normal cells.
- **Hypocalaemia**. Secondary to hyperphosphataemia.

Management

- Assess the risk.
- Examination including weight.

Investigations

- Baseline bloods—FBC, UEC, urate, LDH, Ca, PO_4, Mg.
- CXR.

Treatment

- Hyperhydration. 0.45% saline with 2.5% dextrose at $3l/m^2/d$ (p.517).
  - This should be commenced at least 12 hours prior to chemotherapy.
  - Do not add potassium to fluids.
- Allopurinol $100mg/m^2$ tds PO or IV rasburicase 0.2mg/kg over 30min.
- Notify oncology and PICU.

Once treatment has commenced, careful monitoring is vital. The following observations and investigations should be undertaken.

- Repeat electrolytes 4 to 6 hourly, particularly to monitor K^+ and PO_4.
- Accurate fluid balance with hourly input/output recordings.
- Weight bd.
- Four hourly observations of pulse, BP, and RR.

Consider diuretics if urine output decreases below 1ml/kg/h or weight increases.

Management of hyperkalaemia

Initially can be treated with increasing fluids to maximum of 4.5 to $5l/m^2$. Need careful fluid balance monitoring. If K^+ levels rise above 5.5mmol/l, see 📖 p.446 for management options.

- Contact PICU and senior colleagues.
- Consider renal dialysis.

Management of hyperphosphataemia

- Increase hydration.
- If necessary, use phosphate binders, e.g. calcium carbonate suspension.

Spinal cord compression

Either due to local tumour extension or tumour metastases compressing spinal cord. Main causes are neuroblastoma and soft tissue Ewing's sarcoma (PNET).

Presentation There is often a delay in diagnosis, but once identified it requires rapid treatment.

Symptoms and signs of spinal cord compression

Symptoms
- Back pain
- Weakness
- Sphincter dysfunction
  - Retention of urine
  - Constipation
- Sensory deficits
- Gait disturbances

Signs
- Localized tenderness of spine
- Motor weakness
- Paraesthesia

Investigations

If the tumour has not been identified:
- FBC and film;
- UEC
- LDH;
- germ cell tumour markers;
- urinary VMA.

Urgent imaging is necessary. MRI is the gold standard but, if not available, obtain CT with contrast.

Management

- If there is a high suspicion of spinal cord compression, give IV dexamethasone 1mg/kg over 30 minutes. This can be given prior to scanning or performance of diagnostic biopsy.
- Obtain senior decision regarding ongoing treatment. This may include immediate surgery, chemotherapy, or radiotherapy. The treatment chosen depends on the extent and speed of onset of the neurological problems and the anticipated response to chemotherapy and radiotherapy.

Chapter 23

Dermatology

Assessment

A history should include:

- preceding illnesses;
- recent drugs—prescribed and alternative;
- a family history;
- any recent foreign travel.

Then describe accurately the morphology and distribution of the lesions.

- **Primary**
  - Macule—non-palpable lesion <1cm diameter.
  - Papule—palpable lesion <0.5cm diameter.
  - Nodule—palpable lump >0.5cm diameter.
  - Vesicle—blister <0.5cm (containing clear fluid).
  - Bulla—blister >0.5cm.
  - Pustule—papule containing pus.
- **Secondary**
  - Excoriation—scratch mark.
  - Lichenification—thickening of skin caused by rubbing.
  - Necrosis.
  - Scarring.
  - Erosion—partial loss of epidermis.
  - Ulcer—full thickness loss of epidermis.

Care should then be taken to examine the nails, scalp, and oral mucosa, which may provide important diagnostic clues.

Purpura

Purpuric lesions are non-blanching skin haemorrhages, and range from tiny 'petechial' purpura to large 'ecchymoses'. Vasculitis is likely if the purpuric lesions are painful and palpable.

Other causes include:

- infections—meningococcaemia must be excluded;
- thrombocytopenia;
- clotting disorders;
- Henoch–Schönlein purpura (HSP)—with arthralgia, abdominal pain ± nephritis;
- autoimmune disease;
- drugs.

Management will be dictated by the clinical context of the purpura, but standard investigations include:

- full blood count ± blood film;
- blood cultures;
- clotting studies.

If HSP likely, check BP, perform a urine dipstick, and take blood for above plus UEC and ASOT (📖 p.258).

Blistering

Acute generalized blistering in children needs immediate assessment and emergency management, in collaboration with a dermatologist.

☼ **Staphylococcal scalded skin syndrome (SSSS)** Extensive exotoxin-mediated erythema, blistering, and erosions, usually with a febrile illness. There is no mucous membrane involvement. Bacterial swabs of the skin are necessary prior to IV anti-staphylococcal antibiotics (flucloxacillin or erythromycin) and opiate analgesia.

☼ Toxic epidermal necrolysis (TEN) and Stevens–Johnson syndrome (SJS)

Both conditions are usually drug-induced, e.g. anticonvulsants, antibiotics, and NSAIDs. TEN carries a higher mortality.

Both result in:

- epidermal detachment—>30% in TEN; <10% in SJS.
- mucous membrane inflammation, e.g. mouth ulcers, conjunctivitis.

A successful outcome depends on rapid cessation of the causative drug and nursing in a burns unit or in intensive care (if necessary) with careful fluid support and analgesia. Evidence favouring the use of intravenous immunoglobulin therapy (IVIg) in TEN remains weak.

ⓘ **Epidermolysis bullosa (EB)** EB is caused by a genetic deficiency of proteins linking the epidermis to the underlying dermis. All main types of EB can cause severe congenital blistering, with skin 'sheeting off' within hours of birth.

Neonates should be coated in 50/50 liquid and white soft paraffin ointment, with nothing taped to the skin.

The local dermatologist should contact the clinical nurse specialist for EB at Great Ormond Street Hospital (020 7405 9200) or Birmingham Children's Hospital (0121 333 8224) who will come out to counsel the parents, take the skin biopsies, and advise the nurses on dressings.

Other causes of neonatal blistering

- Herpes viruses—likely to be very unwell. Start IV acyclovir; arrange EEG ± MRI and ophthalmological review.
- Bacterial infection.
- Mastocytosis—an excess of mast cells in the skin and other organs. Degranulation can result in anaphylaxis.
- Miliaria crystallina—vesicles caused by superficial obstruction of sweat ducts.
- Incontinentia pigmenti—an X-linked dominant syndrome of blistering, warty and pigmented skin lesions, with associated eye, skeletal, and neurological abnormalities.
- Bullous congenital ichthyosiform erythroderma—congenital blistering and erythroderma caused by keratin 1 and 10 mutations.
- Placental transfer of maternal pemphigoid auto-antibodies.

Generalized pustular rashes

Generalized pustulosis is unusual and, in children under the age of 2, the possibility of immunodeficiency should be considered.

⑦ Neonatal generalized pustulosis

- Transient neonatal pustulosis.
- Toxic erythema of the newborn.
- Incontinentia pigmenti (📖 p.396).
- Bacterial folliculitis.
- Congenital herpes.
- Candidiasis.
- Congenital syphilis.

⑦ **Bacterial folliculitis** The pustules only arise from hair follicles. The lesions should be swabbed and managed with topical antiseptics, or systemic antibiotics if severe.

⑦ **Generalized pustular psoriasis** Characterized by generalized sterile pustules on a background of erythema. There will usually be a past history of psoriasis, often treated with topical or systemic steroids, which have triggered the pustulation. Pustular psoriasis carries a significant mortality, and needs urgent admission.

⑦ **Acute generalized exanthemic pustulosis (AGEP)** In AGEP, the pustules are triggered by a drug or viral infection, and resolve within days or weeks with no specific treatment.

Immunodeficiency Young children with recurrent pyoderma (pustules, abscesses) should be screened for phagocyte dysfunction. The commonest phagocyte disorder is chronic granulomatous disease; 66% of cases are X-linked. FBC is normal and the diagnosis is confirmed by nitroblue tetrazolium test (NBT).

ⓘ Erythroderma

The causes of generalized red skin (erythroderma) vary with different age-groups of children. In older children, eczema, psoriasis, and drug reactions predominate (e.g. glandular fever and ampicillin).

In neonates, causes of erythroderma also include:

- bullous congenital ichthyosiform erythroderma;
- non-bullous congenital ichthyosiform erythroderma;
- urticaria pigmentosa;
- staphylococcal scalded skin syndrome (📖 p.396);
- candidiasis;
- Netherton's syndrome—a rare autosomal recessive syndrome of erythroderma, 'bamboo hair', ichthyosis, and atopy.

In addition to contacting the local dermatologist to make an accurate diagnosis, treatment of all types of erythroderma should include specialized nursing care, with careful fluid and temperature management and early emollient use to limit desquamation.

? Exanthems

Exanthems are acute viral rashes and are common in young children (📖 p.146). They usually comprise pink macules and, as a general rule, these eruptions fade as rapidly as they came and no specific investigation or treatment is necessary.

? Atopic eczema (atopic dermatitis)

Atopic eczema is typically flexural (antecubital fossae, neck, and behind knees) but commonly arises on the face in younger children. Severe flares of longstanding eczema can lead to generalized dry and itchy skin.

Eczema is frequently complicated by bacterial infection (impetigo; see below) and, more rarely, super-infection with herpes simplex (eczema herpeticum; see below).

Treatment

- Topical emollients applied at least four times a day, during and in between flares. Choice of emollient varies between individuals, so a variety should be tried and tested. A bath oil should also be considered.
- Topical steroids should be used for short sharp courses for flare-ups. For example, betamethasone valerate 0.1% ointment for the body and 1% hydrocortisone cream for the face, applied twice daily for up to 2 weeks. The duration of topical steroid use depends on the age of the child, and the site being treated (📖 p.494).
- If the eczema appears infected (impetiginized), bacterial swabs should be taken. Consider oral anti-staphylococcal/streptococcal antibiotics, e.g. flucloxacillin and penicillin, or erythromycin if penicillin-allergic.
- Severe cases necessitate admission.
- Antihistamines can be prescribed to alleviate itch and ease sleep.

New steroid-sparing treatments such as tacrolimus ointment can be used in children older than 2 years. However, the lack of long term safety data suggests that they should be used only when the combination of emollients and topical steroids fails to achieve control, and in collaboration with a dermatologist.

ⓘ ***Treatment of impetigo*** This highly contagious staphylococcal or streptococcal skin infection causes blistering and yellow crusting. It requires bacterial skin swabs followed by topical antibiotics, e.g. mupirocin cream, or systemic antibiotics, e.g. flucloxacillin or erythromycin, if severe.

ⓘ ***Treatment of eczema herpeticum*** Rapidly spreading vesicles on an erythematous base. The patient usually needs admission for IV acyclovir, following viral culture of skin lesions. The response to antiviral therapy is usually rapid, but the patient will also require additional treatment of the atopic eczema as described above. Any lesions near the eye necessitate ophthalmological review to exclude herpetic keratitis or a corneal ulcer (📖 p.346).

Urticaria and angioedema

? Urticaria

Urticaria ('hives' or 'nettle rash') is an itchy eruption of transient pink swellings with central pallor ('wheals').

The usual trigger is a recent viral infection, but other possibilities include drugs, food allergy, streptococcal infection, and intestinal worms. A detailed food history should be obtained, and consideration given to whether a full blood count (for eosinophils) and stool samples (for intestinal parasites) should be taken.

The choice of antihistamine will depend on the child's age, but chlorpheniramine is an appropriate first-line agent.

Angioedema is swelling of deeper layers of skin. Severe angioedema resembles anaphylaxis, causing respiratory obstruction or shock, and is treated with steroids and adrenaline (p.62). Otherwise triggers and management are similar to those in urticaria. A family history should be taken to exclude hereditary angioedema, due to C1 inhibitor deficiency. This results in recurrent episodes of angioedema without urticaria. A C4 complement level should be the initial investigation.

Infantile haemangiomas

Many types of haemangioma affect children. The capillary haemangioma ('strawberry naevus') may rapidly proliferate within weeks or months of birth, but the majority will involute slowly over several years.

Complications of infantile haemangiomas include pain, bleeding, infection, obstruction of vision, and sequestration of platelets (Kasabach–Merritt syndrome). Such cases necessitate dermatological review for discussion of therapeutic options, e.g. topical, intralesional, or systemic steroids; laser surgery. Stridor in an infant with haemangiomas raises the possibility of tracheal compression and must be actively excluded (MRI and/or bronchoscopy).

Disseminated neonatal haemangiomatosis (DNH) is characterized by multiple cutaneous and visceral haemangiomas. It usually presents in neonates and has a high mortality rate.

Fungal kerion of the scalp

This is a painful, boggy, and pussy mass on the scalp and is an acute form of tinea capitis. Plucked hairs and scrapes of scale should be sent for mycology (in special mycology envelopes).

The only licensed systemic antifungal for children is griseofulvin, used at a dose of 10mg/kg daily. Higher doses (20mg/kg) may be required if *Trichophyton tonsurans* is cultured. Oral terbinafine may be used for tinea capitis in children, but is not licensed.

Chapter 24

Endocrinology

Diabetic ketoacidosis

Can present with any combination of:
- vomiting, abdominal pain;
- polyuria, polydipsia—ask specifically;
- weight loss;
- Kussmaul (deep sighing) respiration;
- smell of ketones;
- reduced conscious level (10–20%).

Confirm DKA with:
- blood glucose >15mmol;
- pH < 7.3;
- blood ketones >3mmol/l;

Resuscitate if necessary—see Fig. 24.1.

Management

Fluid management Aim is to rehydrate slowly over 48 hours, which minimizes risk of cerebral oedema (📖 p.507).

IV fluid type
- Use 0.9% saline for at least the first 6 hours.
- Once glucose down to 12mmol/l:
  - if during first 6 hours, add 5% dextrose to 0.9% saline, then change at 6 hours to 0.45% saline + 5% dextrose;
  - if after first 6 hours, change to 0.45% saline + 5% dextrose (📖 p.506).

Insulin Rehydration will lower blood glucose. Do not start insulin until fluids have been running for at least an hour. Insulin should be given as a continuous intravenous infusion.

Insulin infusion
- Draw up 50 units soluble insulin, and make up to 50ml with 0.9% saline (1 unit/ml) and run at 0.1 units/kg/hour.
- If blood glucose falls too low, increase the dextrose concentration of the fluid.

Do not reduce the insulin below 0.05 units/kg/hour until pH > 7.3

Table 24.1 Maintenance fluid volumes

Age (years)	Fluid requirement (ml/kg/24h)
0–2	80
3–5	70
6–9	60
10–14	50
>15	30

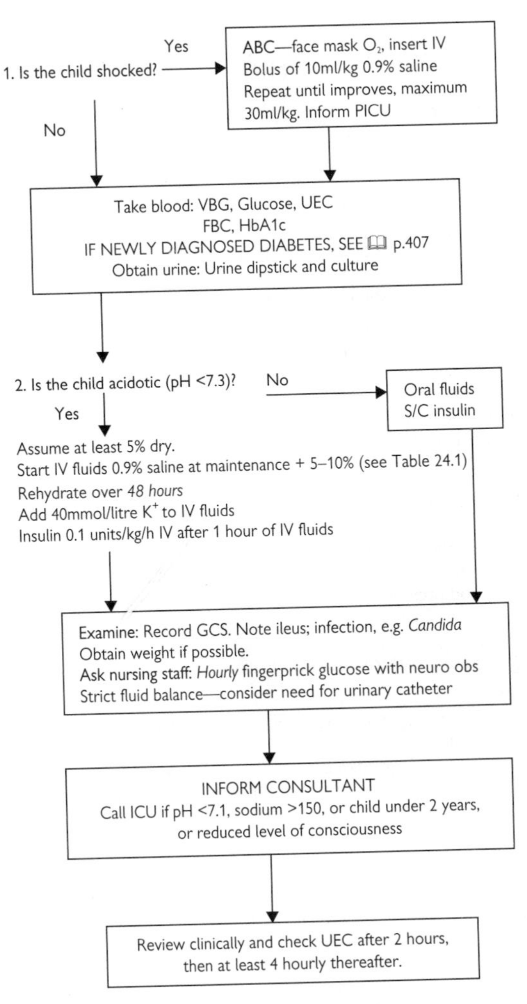

Fig. 24.1 Algorithm for treating diabetic ketoacidosis.

Continuing management

Aim for gradual resolution of acidosis, with normalization of glucose and potassium.

Observations to be carried out

- Repeat blood gas and electrolytes at 2 hours and then at least 4 hourly.
  - A sampling cannula can be helpful.
- Nursing staff should be asked to report:
  - any change in conscious level;
  - any drop in heart rate or BP, even if transient;
  - any headache.

These may all indicate cerebral oedema and need urgent review.

Subcutaneous insulin can be started once:

- child feeling like eating/drinking;
- acidosis resolved;
- blood glucose normal.

No need to wait for urine ketones to resolve. Use usual regime of your department and stop any IV insulin 60 minutes after first subcutaneous dose given.

Complications: cerebral oedema

Consider if:

- reduction in conscious level;
- fall in heart rate;
- increase in blood pressure;
- headache;
- convulsion;
- irregular respiratory pattern, respiratory arrest.

Management

- IV mannitol 0.5g/kg = 2.5ml/kg mannitol 20% over 20 minutes.
- Inform senior staff.
- Restrict IV fluids to 2/3 maintenance.
- Move to ICU—intubation may be necessary.

Newly diagnosed diabetes

The majority of children will not be acidotic on presentation. In Europe, most newly diagnosed diabetics have type 1. However, with the increasing prevalence of obesity, type 2 diabetes is also a possibility. To distinguish, perform:

- fasting insulin;
- C-peptide levels;
- measure islet cell and GAD auto-antibodies.

When in doubt, it is safer to commence on insulin, and each centre should have guidelines for starting.

If advice is not available, whether from guidelines or a paediatrician, then start insulin at a total daily dose of 0.5 units/kg if prepubertal, and 0.7 units/kg if in puberty.

Use NPH/isophane (intermediate-acting) insulin, or a biphasic mixture twice daily, 3/5 in the morning and 2/5 before the evening meal. For example, a 7-year-old child weighing 25kg will require 8U NPH/isophane in the morning and 5U NPH/isophane before evening meal. Short-acting insulin can be added in due course, dependent on blood glucose levels over subsequent days. Multiple daily injections can be started from diagnosis but require intensive education.

Involvement of a dietician is important to discuss how to maintain a reasonably constant daily intake of food, with consideration of the glycaemic index of foods. Until the child sees a dietician, advise them to eat a normal diet, ensuring that there is a snack in between meals.

Before discharge

- Ensure child/parents are able to draw up insulin and administer safely.
- Ensure child/parents can recognize symptoms and signs of hypoglycaemia and know how to manage (📖 p.408).
- Arrange for them to be reviewed within a few days by local paediatrician, dietician, and diabetes educator or community nurse.
- Give them a 24 hour phone number for advice—paediatric registrar or diabetes educator.

Hypoglycaemia in the diabetic child

The child may report feeling hungry and then become tremulous, sweaty, and pale. Neuroglycopenia can cause headache, irritability, confusion, and seizures.

Confirm with finger prick blood glucose <4mmol/l.

If unconscious/fitting

- ABC.
- Obtain IV access.
- Give 2–5ml/kg of 10% dextrose intravenously and check blood glucose levels as above.
- If cannot obtain IV access, use IM glucagon (see below). Glucagon may cause vomiting.
- Continue to repeat blood glucose measures until child feeling well enough to eat/drink.

If conscious

- Offer 100ml fruit juice or 2–3 dextrose tablets or 6 small jelly beans.
- Check blood glucose 10 minutes later.
- If increasing, give long-acting carbohydrate, e.g. biscuit/toast; otherwise repeat.

If conscious but refusing food/drink

- Use GlucoGel® in side of mouth—½ tube in all ages. Repeat if no clinical improvement in 10 minutes.
- If GlucoGel® not tolerated, use IM or SC glucagon:
  - 500mcg if <10 years;
  - 1mg if >10 years.
- Check blood glucose 10 minutes later to confirm rise. Once recovering, give long-acting carbohydrate.

If not improving

- Consider alcohol overdose—glucagon is unlikely to work.
- Insert IV cannula. Give 2–5ml/kg of 10% dextrose intravenously and, if no response, consider infusion at 0.05ml/kg/min (5mg/kg/min).

After treatment

- After treatment, assess reason for the 'hypo' and consider alteration in usual insulin dose, or review food/exercise regimen.
- Refer to endocrinology.

Adrenal crisis

Usually in a child with chronic adrenal insufficiency subjected to additional stress, e.g. illness, trauma, or surgery.

Suspect if:

- vomiting;
- dehydration;
- hypotension;
- abdominal pain/fever;
- history of weakness/tiredness;
- pigmentation;
- seizures secondary to hypoglycaemia;
- hypoglycaemia ± hyponatraemia, hyperkalaemia.

Causes

Primary

- Congenital adrenal hyperplasia (CAH; 📖 p.412).
- Congenital adrenal hypoplasia.
- Autoimmune adrenalitis (Addison's disease).
- Adrenoleucodystrophy—X-linked, associated with developmental delay arising when boy over 6 years.
- Unresponsiveness to ACTH.

Secondary

- Hypopituitarism of any cause.
- Long-term glucocorticoid therapy e.g. asthmatics on fluticasone propionate >400mcg/day

Management

- Obtain IV access.
- Investigations must be performed ***before*** glucose/fluids given. Lab will require notification:
  - UEC;
  - blood glucose.
- And, if underlying diagnosis not established, these can still be taken immediately after fluids/glucose given:
  - cortisol, 17 hydroxyprogesterone;
  - renin and aldosterone;
  - ACTH.
- If cause uncertain, perform other investigations for hypoglycaemia (📖 p.413).
- Resuscitation may be necessary—IV bolus 0.9% saline 20ml/kg.
- If hypoglycaemic, give IV 2–5ml/kg 10% dextrose.
- IV hydrocortisone.
  - 50mg if under age of 5; 100mg if over age 5. Give 4 hourly or by continuous infusion.
  - Reduce over 2 days to maintenance 4–5mg/m^2 tds (5–6mg/m^2 tds in CAH).

- Consult with endocrinology:
  - consider oral 9 α fludrocortisone 150mcg/m^2/day;
  - infants may require sodium chloride supplementation;
  - arrange short Synacthen® test;
  - discuss need for stress doses of hydrocortisone (See box).

Stress doses of hydrocortisone may be required to avert an adrenal crisis during a future illness.The following protocol is suggested.
- If mildly unwell with raised temperature, double the dose of hydrocortisone
- If unwell with diarrhoea, systemic illness, or high temperature, triple the dose of hydrocortisone
- If the dose is vomited, repeat the increased dose 30 minutes later
- If still not tolerated, give IM hydrocortisone (age-dependent dose; see 📖 p.410)

Check that parents:
- are familiar with protocol
- always have a dose of IM hydrocortisone available
- have written instructions for doctors treating their child

Congenital adrenal hyperplasia (CAH)

Suspect if:
- virilized female genitalia, e.g. 21 hydroxylase deficiency, 11β hydroxylase deficiency;
- ambiguous genitalia in both sexes, e.g. 3β hydroxysteroid dehydrogenase deficiency;
- salt wasting crisis in newborn period;
- signs of virilization in older children, i.e. features of the following: early pubic hair (<8 years in girls, <9 years in boys), advanced skeletal maturity, rapid growth, ± phallic or clitoral enlargement.

Record:
- BP—may be elevated in some forms;
- exact description of external genitalia;
- pubertal development—Tanner staging.

Investigations

- UEC, glucose—hyponatraemia, hyperkalaemia ± hypoglycaemia.
- 17-OH progesterone levels, adrenal androgens, and testosterone.
- Urinary steroid profile.
- Karyotype.
- USS of internal genitalia.

Management

Acute

- Hypoglycaemia—IV 10% dextrose 2–5ml/kg; then continue dextrose infusion at 0.05ml/kg/min (5mg/kg/min). Adjust according to glucose response.
- Salt-losing crisis—IV 0.9% saline to rehydrate and raise sodium.
- IV hydrocortisone 25mg 6 hourly IV (or continuous infusion) until improved.
- Admit under endocrinology with referral to specialist surgeons if indicated. Short Synacthen® test may be necessary.

Maintenance

Treatment will involve oral hydrocortisone, 9α fludrocortisone, and, during first 1–2 years of life, sodium chloride. Stress doses of hydrocortisone will be required in future illnesses (📖 p.411).

Hypoglycaemia in the non-diabetic child

Can arise in normal children after period of starvation, e.g. gastroenteritis. It can also be a manifestation of a metabolic disorder, e.g. hyperinsulinism. Presentations include:
- afebrile convulsion;
- decreased level of consciousness;
- 'near miss' sudden infant death.

Investigations
- Finger prick glucose <3.0mmol/l. ***Must*** confirm with laboratory blood glucose estimation (<2.6mmol/l) before treatment
- Discuss with biochemistry lab to get correct bottles for hypoglycaemic screen. Some will need to be placed on ice after collection.

Hypoglycaemic screen must be taken at time of hypoglycaemia or immediately after a dose of IV dextrose

- Insert IV cannula.
- Take blood for:
  - true blood glucose, UEC, LFT;
  - beta-hydroxybutyrate, free fatty acids, carnitine profile;
  - insulin, C-peptide;
  - amino acids;
  - cortisol, ACTH;
  - growth hormone;
  - ammonia, lactate (pyruvate);
  - alcohol, toxicology screen.
- Place urine bag (dipstick for ketones); send for urinary metabolic screen.

Management
- Give 2–5ml/kg 10% dextrose.
- Check finger prick glucose after 5 minutes. If glucose not rising, give further bolus of dextrose.
- If blood glucose does not remain normal, start dextrose infusion—0.05ml/kg/min (5mg/kg/min).
- If no cannula possible then use GlucoGel® gel: ½ tube all ages.
- Glucagon not always effective, e.g. glycogen storage disorders.
- Refer to endocrinology/metabolic teams.

Acute diabetes insipidus

Lack of ADH. Seldom seen in ED, but may follow trauma, e.g. head injury. Suspect if:

- producing more than 2.5ml/kg/h of urine;
- hypernatraemia;
- urine osmolality <750mOsm/l ***plus*** plasma osmolality >295mOsm/l.

Management

- Insert IV cannula for sampling.
- 4–6 hourly plasma, urinary electrolytes, and osmolality.
- Strict fluid balance—catheterize if necessary.
- Daily weights.
- IV fluids—0.45% saline + 5% dextrose (plus K^+ requirement) (see 📖 p.506).
  - Rate = previous hour's urine output + 0.5ml/kg (insensible losses).
- Consult with endocrinology ± ICU.
  - Discuss need for DDAVP if plasma Na > 150mmol/l; or osmolality >300mOsmol/l and urine osmolality <750mOsmol/l.

> - DDAVP must be given with caution because of risk of water overload
> - DDAVP is prescribed as single doses, until effect on diuresis is gauged.

  - Discuss need for cortisol replacement—if inadequate, unable to excrete water load.
- Measure urgent electrolytes and osmolality if not improving:
  - urine output >2.5ml/kg/hour in 3 consecutive hours;
  - or weight loss >5%;
  - or cumulative fluid deficit in 48 hour period >30ml/kg.

Thyrotoxic storm

Seldom seen as hyperthyroidism usually has a gradual onset. Causes include:

- hyperthyroidism with other precipitant, e.g. acute infection, trauma;
- concurrently with diabetic ketoacidosis;
- secondary to ingestion of thyroxine, e.g. adolescents to aid weight loss;
- neonates whose mothers have Graves' disease.

Suspect if:

- tachycardia;
- fever;
- restlessness, lethargy;
- in neonate—poor feeding, poor weight gain;
- confusion;
- nausea, vomiting, profuse diarrhoea.

Investigations

- Free T4; free or total T3 (high).
- TSH (suppressed).
- ECG.

Management

- Insert IV cannula.
- Supportive treatment:
  - cooling;
  - intravenous fluids;
  - sedation if necessary.
- Discuss ongoing treatment with endocrinology.

Neonates' regimen

- Lugol's iodine 1–2 drops daily.
- Propranolol 0.25–0.75mg/kg 8 hourly. N.B. Risk of hypoglycaemia, bradycardia.
- Propylthiouracil 0.5–1.5mg/kg/day single daily dose.
- Prednisolone 2mg/kg/day.

Children's regimen

- Intravenous sodium iodide 1–2g daily.
- Propranolol 0.2–1.5mg/kg every 8 hours.
- Propylthiouracil 200–300mg 6 hourly.
- Dexamethasone 1–2mg 6 hourly.

Chapter 25

Psychiatry

Introduction

In the emergency department, child psychiatric emergencies are any community-based behaviours that reach crisis point before ordinary mental health services, social services, or the criminal justice system become involved. Designating a behaviour as a psychiatric emergency is not purely based on clinical assessment of the behaviour itself, but reflects the resources available within the community. So expect anything!

The range of emergency presentations within the hospital is restricted but includes acute confusional states (delirium), psychosis, and self-harm. Emotional problems can present in the guise of physical ones, e.g. somatizing disorders and anorexia.

Given the wide range of possible presentations it is helpful to have a system for determining the degree of urgency (see box).

Rosenn's classification[1]

Class I	'Potentially life-threatening emergency', e.g. suicidal and homicidal behaviour
Class II	'States of heightened disturbance requiring urgent intervention', e.g. significant agitation or aggression, witnessing or experiencing violence or rape
Class III	'Serious conditions requiring prompt but not immediate intervention', e.g. verbal threats of suicide or violence, child unmanageable but not dangerous
Class IV	'Situations in which intervention is requested but not necessarily warranted', e.g. chronic antisocial behaviour, ignorance of appropriate care pathways, consumer frustration

This chapter will cover a variety of situations that may fall between Rosenn's classes I and III and some class IV situations, where referral should be prioritized.

Remember to inform the GP of any presentations!

Be aware that emotional and behavioural disturbance is anxiety-provoking for all staff. This means that you may be called on to act more rapidly than the situation demands. Remember to use the hierarchy in the box. On some occasions a simple referral to appropriate community services will be all that is required.

1 Rosenn DW (1984). Psychiatric Emergencies in Children and Adolescents. In *Emergency Psychiatry: Concepts, Methods and Practices* (Bassuk EL, Biek AW, eds), pp. 303–49. Plenum, New York.

To date, there are no randomized controlled trials determining the optimal drugs and dosages for children with acute psychiatric problems, requiring immediate medication. The drugs mentioned in this chapter may differ from your own hospital's regimens. The doses quoted are for adolescents 50kg and over and tend to be high, presuming that you have only one opportunity to medicate the child! The doses in brackets are for younger children, and may need to be titrated to achieve sedation without respiratory compromise.

Assessment and mental state examination

Assessment should be based on observation of behaviour as well as information given by carer and child. If you have been busy, ask other staff how the child has behaved since arrival. Is behaviour variable or consistent? Are they the same with staff, parents, and other children? Speak to the young person alone as well as with their carer. A chaperone is advisable if you are talking to a teenager, or if you are concerned about safety.

Central aspects of history taking are:

- **history of presenting complaint**—the behaviour or emotional state and its impact;
- **developmental history**—the underlying level of function;
- **family and social history**—the family context including potential triggers and inheritable conditions.

Don't be scared of taking a **behavioural history**—the principles are those of a pain history. Focus on a specific behaviour, e.g. aggression, and ask the following:

- How bad is it?
- Has it happened before?
- Is it episodic or persistent?
- When did it start?
- Did it come on quickly or slowly?
- Does anything help?
- Does anything make it worse?
- Is it different in different situations?
- What has it stopped you/them from doing?

Mental state examination (MSE)

This follows the same general format as in adult psychiatry but with a far greater emphasis on appearance and behaviour, as young people can struggle to describe more complex internal states.

Appearance Prevailing facial expression, overall body language, signs of neglect, hygiene, size for age.

Behaviour Level of motor activity (restlessness, fidgetiness, stupor); co-ordination, tics, posturing; eye contact (quality and quantity); rapport, co-operation, and compliance, observed conduct problems; social style, e.g. reserved, aloof, expansive, disinhibited, cheeky, precocious, teasing, negativistic, shy, confident, surly, manipulative, odd.

Language Comprehension, articulation, mutism, speech spontaneity, and quantity.

Affect Emotional responsiveness; predominant mood, e.g. irritable, angry, aggressive, sad, tearful, desperate, apathetic, perplexed, confused, anxious, elated; discrepancy between described and observed mood.

Thoughts Worries, fears, obsessions, guilt, negative cognitions, abnormal beliefs (persecutory ideas, self-reference, grandiosity).

Perceptions Visual hallucinations (usually organic (📖 p.424)); auditory hallucinations (📖 p.426).

Cognition Test orientation (time, place, person) and attention, e.g. days of week, months of year, addition, serial 3s from 20. Check premorbid level with carer—deterioration suggests organic cause (📖 p.424).

Hints on psychiatric interviewing

- Find somewhere quiet and try to avoid interruptions.
- Try to adopt a friendly, relaxed manner even if you don't feel it.
- Explain who you are and the purpose of the interview.
- Sit down so that you are at the same level as the child.
- Start with a neutral topic before moving on to the more emotive.
- Try to talk with, not down to.
- Remember that punitive critical interviews do not reduce self-harm!
- Remember that speaking to children can be fun!

Children

- Children pick up on other people's emotions especially those of their parents. If you can defuse parental/carer anxiety, you will reduce the child's own anxiety.
- Use simple words and stick to the immediate and concrete.
- Drawings can sometimes help communication when words are not enough.
- Pre-empting, e.g. predicting that a child may not wish to speak but giving permission for this.
- Offer a range of choices for how they might feel, e.g. sad, fed up, cross.

Adolescents

- Always offer the chance to speak without carer present.
- Feel able to intervene if carer and teenager start arguing.
- If alone explain that what they say is 'private' and you would not tell their carer unless it affected their health or safety (see box on 'Confidentiality').
- Use normalizing comments,—e.g. 'Some teenagers whom I see, who feel sad, think about hurting themselves. What about you?'
- Ask if they want to be here. Usually they do not, but at least it is then acknowledged!
- Try to empathize but avoid 'I remember when I was your age …' It is too much for them to imagine that you ever could have been!

Confidentiality

If we expect young people to discuss sensitive or painful matters with us then we need to offer them some privacy even from their parents. However, it is likely that we will later wish to share some or all of the information with other members of the medical team. If there is a disclosure of abuse, then it becomes a professional duty to inform a statutory agency (police or social services). In offering the opportunity to talk we need to offer confidentiality but point out its limits. This then avoids 'secrets' within the team and losing the child's trust in you or other professionals.

Delirium and acute confusional states

These are among the commonest of all psychiatric disorders in general hospitals, though often not the main reason for presentation. Clouding of consciousness is linked to a wide variety of physical causes (📖 pp.142, 290). Florid delirium is obvious to most clinicians, but more subtle forms are frequently missed. In children the onset is usually rapid, but subacute onset does occur, and a fluctuating course can complicate the diagnosis. Usually the presence of physical illness is obvious.

Clinical features All may vary in severity over time.

- Reduced ability to focus, shift, or sustain attention.
- Reduced, heightened, or mixed level of arousal.
- Other disturbances of cognition—orientation, memory, visuospatial skills, language. ***Missed if not tested!***
- Reduced awareness due to fluctuating level of consciousness.
- Perceptual disturbance, e.g. misperceptions, hallucinations usually visual.
- Emotional lability, especially fear, anxiety, irritability, apathy.
- Sleep cycle disturbance.
- Improvement with treatment of underlying physical cause.

Causes

Substrate deficiency

- Electrolyte disturbance, e.g. dehydration, burns, renal disease.
- Hypoxia/anoxia, e.g. pulmonary failure, cardiac failure, CO poisoning.
- Hypoglycaemia—inborn errors (📖 p.413); iatrogenic.
- Vitamin deficiency, e.g. B_{12}, niacine, thiamine in IBD.
- Endocrinopathies, e.g. adrenal, thyroid, parathyroid.

Delivery problems

- Anaemia.
- Haemoglobinopathies.
- Hypotension, e.g. cardiac failure, 2° to medication.
- Cerebrovascular disorders, e.g. stroke, vasculitis, haemorrhage.

Interference with cerebral metabolism

- Systemic infections, e.g. endotoxin release, competition for metabolic fuels, fever.
- Acid/base disturbances.
- Endocrinopathies, e.g. glucose, adrenal, thyroid, parathyroid.
- Toxins, e.g. solvents, pesticides, heavy metals.
- Drugs—prescription, ethnic, and recreational.

Functional or structural cerebral impairment

- Trauma.
- Cerebral infection, e.g. encephalitis, meningitis, abscess, parasites.
- Hydrocephalus.
- Intracerebral tumour.
- Drug withdrawal, e.g. alcohol, benzodiazepine.
- Epilepsy, e.g. non-convulsive status, post-ictal.
- Migraine, e.g. confusional or basilar migraine.
- Neurodegenerative disorders, e.g. adrenoleucodystrophy.

Examination

- Full MSE. Look out for:
  - appearance: dishevelled, glazed eyes 'off with the fairies'
  - behaviour: talking to self; responding to unseen stimuli; paranoia may also manifest as a silent, apprehensive child. Persecutory beliefs, social withdrawal, and refusal to eat are alarming and require urgent psychiatric review;
  - affect: rapid changes in emotional state.
- Full physical examination including neurological system looking for focal deficits and primitive reflexes. Cerebellar signs are suggestive of intoxication.
- Pulse, BP, temperature.
- Height and weight.

Investigations guided by history and examination.

- Bloods: UEC, glucose, LFT, TFT, FBC, ESR, CRP.
- Blood cultures.
- Pulse oximetry.
- Arterial blood gases (ABGs) ± carboxyhaemoglobin.
- Urinalysis (protein, nitrites, glucose).
- CXR.
- Cranial CT or MRI scan.
- EEG.
- Urine drug screen—specify the drugs you suspect.

Treatment

- Find and treat the underlying cause.
- Review medication for likely causes or aggravating factors.
- Remember children report delirium to be terrifying.
- Try to balance need for orientation against overstimulation.
- 1:1 supervision (nurse or parent) providing reassurance and reorientation.
- Nurse in well-lit area and restrict visitors/examiners.
- Silence monitor alarms if clinically appropriate.
- Consider medication after above steps in place. N.B. Doses quoted are for children 50kg and over with these for children <50kg in brackets.
  - Low dose **haloperidol** 0.25–0.5mg oral (75mcg/kg/day) every 6–8 hours. N.B. Risk of acute dystonia (📖 p.431).
  - If agitation not controlled by haloperidol, adjunctive use of **lorazepam** 0.5–1mg (0.05mg/kg/dose) 6–8 hourly may be useful.
  - If night-time agitation is a particular problem, **chloral hydrate** 250mg to a maximum of 1g (25–50mg/kg/dose) can help with sleep.
- Physical restraints usually agitate patients. If necessary for patient safety or life support apparatus, use only during episodes of agitation and remove during periods of calm.

If patient aggressive and assaultative, see 📖 p.431.

Hallucinations

Hearing voices or seeing visions are significant symptoms that worry parents and professionals alike. It is worth checking that they are distressing to the child or adolescent themselves. They are far more concerning if this is the case.

Organic causes

- **Delirium:** typically visual but also auditory hallucinations and illusions (sensory misperceptions).
- **Hypnogogic and hypnopompic hallucinations:** vivid visual and auditory hallucinations experienced settling to and waking from sleep.
- **Epilepsy:** epileptic auditory and visual hallucinations are usually transitory, brief, simple 'elemental' sights (flashes, colours, and zigzags) or sounds (buzzing and ringing). Seeing faces or hearing voices is relatively unusual especially as isolated epilepsy symptoms.
- **Migraine:** aura is not usually confused with visual hallucinosis.

Non-organic causes

Children commonly experience 'voices', e.g. imaginary friends, and these do not necessarily represent child psychiatric disorder. There is not a clear cut-off between normal experience and psychosis but the characteristics in Table 25.1 help with distinction:

Other causes

- **Autistic spectrum disorder:** affected children experience brief non-psychotic hallucinations when highly anxious. May also label own thought processes as 'voices' or have conversations with imaginary friends. Requires specialist assessment if first occasion.
- **Post-traumatic stress disorder:** may hear voice of abuser or hostile critical comments.

Table 25.1 Range of experience of auditory hallucinations

Characteristic	Normal	Psychotic*
Voice location	Within the head or mind	Outside, in real space
Whose voice?	Imaginary friend	Unknown person or people
Form of voice	Voice of conscience or own thoughts	Commentary or discussion between voices (often derogatory)
Emotional response	Accepting, not distressed	Frightened and/or puzzled
Behavioural response	No obvious change in behaviour	Observed responding to voices or distracted May follow commands

* Psychosis requires urgent assessment from psychiatric services.

Suicidal behaviour and deliberate self-harm

Young people may harm themselves for many different reasons, e.g. as a coping strategy, to communicate distress, or as a deliberate attempt to end their lives. In the emergency situation the focus is usually on the assessment and treatment of the physical damage that they have caused. However, it is important to have some way of establishing the immediate risk and likely severity of future self-harm in order to manage them safely both inside and outside of the hospital. Some knowledge of habitual self-harm like 'cutting' will also help you to manage the anger and rejection that this behaviour engenders in parents and professionals alike.

Suicide Completed 'successful' suicide is rare in young people. In the UK, the incidence in the under 14 year old population is ~1 per million. This rises to ~15 per million in the 15–19 year group. Suicide is most common in young men, which is linked to their preference for violent, irrevocable methods (e.g. hanging, firearms).

Deliberate self-harm (DSH) While definitions for DSH vary, it is one of the commoner reasons for presentation to casualty. The majority attend for self-poisoning. The prevalence of DSH in teenagers may be up to 8% if cutting is included, though not all will attend an emergency department. Male:female ratio is 1:3. DSH should be taken seriously and requires admission and further assessment, as there is a significantly increased risk of later suicide particularly in the first year.

Risk factors

- **Mental illness.** Found in only 30% of young people: usually conduct disorder; depression; alcohol and drug abuse.
- **Family.** Parental depression and personality disorder; inconsistent but rigid parenting style; poor intrafamilial communication.
- **Social.** Bereaved; identification with self-harm subculture; runaway; accommodated by social services.
- **Previous history.** 10–17% will repeat self-harm.
- **Physical health.** Pregnancy and chronic ill health.
- **Triggers.** Relationship crisis; disciplinary crisis (home or school); bullying (start of school term); exams; undisclosed sexual abuse.

Assessment

Determine the likely presence of major mental illness and the risk of repetition.

- **Details of attempt.** Extent of planning; attempts to avoid discovery; dangerousness of self-harm; person informed, e.g. suicide note; timings.
- **Child's expectation of lethality.** More relevant than clinician's view.
- **Precipitating circumstances.** Why now? Involvement of alcohol?
- **Current suicidal intent.** Do they still wish to die? Do they regret failing?
- **Previous emotional/behavioural problems.** Especially depression.
- **Family relationships and social networks.** Whom could you go to for help if you felt like this again?

The risk of future self-harm and suicide is significantly increased by:
- evidence of planning and attempts to avoid discovery;
- continuing suicidal intent and hopelessness;
- presence of mental illness (depression, conduct disorder, alcohol);
- male gender and violent method of self-harm;
- accommodation by social services.

Management

In the UK, the Royal Colleges of Psychiatrists and Paediatrics and Child Health have an agreed policy to admit all young people, who are suicidal or who have self-harmed. This applies regardless of the physical severity of the act. An overnight stay allows for a period of reflection and respite, as well as recovery from the effects of the overdose and/or alcohol. A member of the local mental health team will then further assess the young person before discharge.

If the young person chooses to refuse treatment of their self-harm, this may require treatment under parental authority. If a young person wishes to leave hospital while there is significant concern about their risk then they may be detained under parental authority or pending a mental health act (MHA) assessment under section 5(2) of the 1983 MHA (📖 p.439).

'Cutting'

Cutting or 'delicate cutting' as it is known in the USA is a form of DSH. It is more common in women and is typically performed privately and kept secret. Surveys suggest that up to 50% of cutters have been sexually abused. Only a minority of cutters will get as far as the emergency department and usually unwillingly. Cutting has a habitual, addictive quality and serves to reduce tension for many. It is best viewed as a coping strategy.

> 'I hurt myself to feel better not to annoy others or be seen as attention-seeking.'
> 'You don't cut to die, you cut to ease the pain that life is bringing you.'
>
> Typical comments from cutters

Possible reasons for cutting include:
- rapid reduction in physiological and psychological tension;
- no other effective coping strategies—self-injury usually follows interpersonal conflict;
- limited communication of internal state;
- tendency to impulsiveness and rapid mood fluctuation;
- experience of the behaviour within peer group or through media.

Cutters are often angry about their hospital experiences (they hear comments like 'Why don't you do it properly, next time!') and often avoid accessing appropriate medical help as a result. How you treat them can make a difference.

Aggression and the assaultative patient

Aggressive behaviour includes verbal hostility, threats, and intimidation and overt physical violence. It is the endpoint of a variety of events and different mental states. Aggression is a primitive behavioural response that can arise when more complex emotions, e.g. fear, anger, or sadness, cannot be articulated or managed internally. Chronic aggression can develop in families where aggression is the preferred communication style or where violence succeeds in resolving conflict.

No matter what the cause, the principles of the acute management are the same. The triggers and maintaining factors can be tackled after the patient, staff, and other young people are all safe.

The identification of potential aggression is an essential first step. The prevention and de-escalation of aggression is far easier than the direct management of assaultative behaviour.

Assessment Look out for the following.

- **Signs of arousal**: pallor; sweatiness; wide-eyed gaze; scanning eye movements; restlessness; shouting.
- **Disinhibition:** history of alcohol or drug intoxication; previous head injury; attention deficit hyperactivity disorder (ADHD); and conduct disorder.
- **Impaired communication**: global learning difficulties; speech and language delay; autistic spectrum disorder.
- **Pain**: preverbal children may be in pain; check ears and teeth.
- **Previous aggression**: check with carers and hospital records.
- **Risk**: physical size of patient; possibility of weapons.

Management

Continue down the list until you have contained the situation. Following this, transfer the patient to a more appropriate environment (if available). Some of the later steps will only be necessary if there is actual violence.

1 Maintain your safety and that of the patient, carer, and others

- If possible, remove others from the area.
- Younger patients may be more anxious without carer present.
- Teenagers may be more volatile with carer present.
- Do not be alone with the patient.
- Ensure your colleagues know where you are and bring your panic alarm.
- Use a large room and ensure an escape route for yourself and colleagues.

2 Attempt to talk to the young person and to calm them down

- Maintain a good distance and go to their eye level to minimize their perception of threat.
- Explain what is happening—talk calmly and avoid confrontation.
- Avoid sustaining direct eye contact.
- Ask what they want and meet their needs if possible.

3 If physical restraint is required
- Assemble sufficient staff to do so safely.
- Enlist security guards and porters if necessary.
- Do not be afraid to summon the police if necessary.
- Remember that more people will increase the patient's anxiety and potentially their aggression. So act quickly once assembled.

4 Consider use of medication (rapid tranquillization)
- Given the small evidence base for the safety and effectiveness of rapid tranquillization (RT) in young people, this should be the final step not the first.
- Ensure you have sufficient people for safe administration of IM medication if oral refused.
- Continue to monitor the physical state after RT.

Rapid tranquillization of teenager[1]

N.B. Doses quoted are for children 50kg and over; for children who weigh <50kg use doses in brackets.

A Offer oral treatment
- Use either of:
  - haloperidol 2–5mg (0.15mg/kg/day) ± lorazepam 1–2mg (0.1mg/kg/dose);
  - risperidone 0.5–2mg (0.02–0.04mg/kg) ± lorazepam 1–2mg (0.1mg/kg/dose).
- Repeat every 45–60 minutes if no response or inadequate.
- N.B. Lorazepam can be be disinhibiting in young people so do not repeat if the behavioural disturbance worsens.
- Move to step B if 3 single or combined doses fail or patient refuses.

B Consider IM treatment
- Use either of:
  - haloperidol 2–5mg ± lorazepam 1–2mg;
  - promethazine 25–50mg (0.5mg/kg/dose).
- N.B. Lorazepam IM should be diluted 1:1 with water.
- Promethazine has a slower onset of action.

C Contact an expert who may consider the following
- IV diazepam 5–10mg (0.05 to 0.2mg/kg) over 5 minutes. Be ready with flumazenil as risk of respiratory arrest.
- IM amylobarbitone 100–250mg (respiratory depressant).

Monitoring
- Lorazepam can cause respiratory depression and antipsychotics can cause arrhythmias. After any parenteral administration, monitor respiratory rate, pulse, BP, temperature every 5–10 minutes for first hour; then half-hourly until patient ambulatory.
- If asleep or unconscious, patient requires 1:1 nursing and pulse oximetry till conscious.

Haloperidol can cause **acute dystonia** (including oculogyric crisis)—treat with procylidine 5–10mg (0.1mg/kg/dose IV/IM).

1 Taylor, D., Paton, C., and Kerwin, R. (2003). Acutely disturbed or violent behaviour. In *The Maudsley prescribing guidelines* pp. 236–8. Martin Dunitz, London.

Acute psychological trauma

Traumatized children are more likely to present to paediatric emergency settings than anywhere else. The trauma may be the direct result of physical injury, acute first presentation of physical illness, or exacerbation of chronic medical conditions. Unfortunately, staff may inadvertently worsen the traumatic response by their treatment of these life-threatening clinical problems. In addition, emergency departments may be the site of first presentation for physical abuse and domestic violence involving or witnessed by young people.

Psychological trauma may be best understood as overwhelming, unexpected danger that cannot be effectively mentally processed or resolved by 'fight or flight'. There is significant variation in individual resilience, which means that events experienced as traumatic by one child may not be so for another.

Long-term psychological responses to trauma cover a range of symptoms and syndromes from post-traumatic stress disorder (PTSD) and phobic disorders to anxiety, depression, and personality change. The most important aspect in the acute context is identifying those children who will require referral to psychiatric or psychological services.

Risk factors for later traumatic response

- **Event factors**. Physical proximity to event, emotional proximity, social disruption, and physical displacement (e.g. loss of home).
- **Individual factors**. Physical injury particularly with disfigurement or disability, prior trauma, prior and current psychiatric history, familial and social support, age (younger children are more dependent on carers).
- **Acute response**. Three possible appearances:
  - autonomic hyperarousal, e.g. overactivity, exaggerated startle, hypervigilance;
  - dissociation—poverty of speech and movement and blunted affect;
  - profound avoidance and withdrawal.

This last group has been shown to be highly predictive for later PTSD. In one study of paediatric road traffic accidents, 28% of children had severe symptoms, of whom 50–80% went on to develop PTSD.

Management

Given that most emergency departments do not have resident child and adolescent psychiatrists, the priority is acute management and appropriate referral.

- **Assessment and full MSE**. Look out for above risk factors.
- **Acute symptoms**. Anxiety management strategies are preferred to anxiolytic medications. Refer on to child and adolescent mental heath services (CAMHS) as risk of future problems is high.
- **Consider safety**. Will the child remain at risk if they return home?
- **Education of carers**. Advise of possibility of long-term effects and need to access CAMHS in future.

Child abuse

While child abuse is not, strictly speaking, a child psychiatric disorder, it can be the cause of significant psychiatric morbidity, both immediate and in later life. It is a culturally determined concept that varies by place and time. The margins may be blurred but severe physical abuse by parents or carers is a serious problem and has an annual mortality of 1 in 10 000 in the UK.

There are four main types of abuse:

- non-accidental injury or physical abuse;
- child sexual abuse;
- neglect;
- emotional abuse.

Children may experience harm by any of these, and they may be concurrent. A specific variety of abuse is '**fabricated or induced illness**' (previously called '*Munchausen's syndrome by proxy*'). It is a form of both physical and emotional abuse. While uncommon, it is particularly relevant for healthcare professionals and will be covered separately (📖 p.436).

Causes

The causes of abuse are multifactorial and may only be inferred, but a profile of risk factors has emerged.

- **Child factors**. Under 3 years for physical abuse; first born; difficult temperament, e.g. uncontrollable crying, non-compliance. Gender ratio equal for all abuse, except sexual where girls predominate.
- **Abuser factors.** Young parents; biological parent's partner; experience of abuse as children; substance misuse especially alcohol; low self-esteem; poor impulse control. Actual mental illness rare.
- **Social/family factors.** Domestic violence; poverty; social isolation.

But remember: abuse occurs in all social classes and cultures

History

Try to get a clear description of what has happened from both parents as well as from the child. Carefully document the accounts. Delays in presentation, inconsistencies, or unusually vague accounts are common in abuse.

If the child is old enough to be interviewed separately, do so. Avoid leading questions but queries like 'Is anyone hurting you or forcing you to do things that you do not want to do?' will occasionally yield useful answers.

Remember to discuss confidentiality limits (📖 p.422).

Examination If abuse is suspected then the examination may form part of a child protection investigation and should be performed in a planned fashion by a senior paediatrician. If sexual abuse is suspected, attempt to limit the examination to once only to minimize the child's trauma, as well as preventing contamination of forensic evidence.

Clinical signs

Physical abuse Finger-tip bruising, cigarette burns, adult bite marks (📖 p.120), bruising of different ages, torn tongue frenulum, multiple fractures of different ages, unexplained retinal haemorrhages or subdural haematoma, fearfulness of parents.

Sexual abuse Pregnancy; encopresis; recurrent UTI, STDs; local trauma. Specialist colposcopy may be required.

Neglect Recurrent attendance for accidents, failure to thrive (height and weight centiles); poor hygiene; language delay; head-banging; rocking; 'frozen watchfulness'.

Investigations

Consider:

- clotting profile: FBC, PT, APTT, TT, fibrinogen;
- skeletal survey (for previous fractures);
- bone scan for recent rib fractures;
- ophthalmology review;
- CT head ± abdominal ultrasound if suspicion of trauma;
- medical photography.

Remember that these may be used as court evidence and that there should be an unbroken chain of identity.

Management of suspicion

- Involve a senior colleague early on.
- Follow your hospital's child protection procedure which will include the following.
    - Full documentation of injuries including photographs and diagrams.
    - Senior paediatrician will inform parents and child of medical concerns and of intention to involve local social services.
    - Referral to local social services department.
    - Admission of child to hospital.
    - If parents refuse, UK law allows for application for an emergency protection order (📖 p.439).

Fabricated and induced illness (FII)

There is a spectrum of parental attitudes towards their children's health needs, which may or may not coincide with the doctor's view. At one extreme, parents neglect their children's health needs, while at the other they push for more intervention. In FII, carers, usually mothers, repeatedly present their children for medical assessment, usually resulting in multiple medical procedures. With increasing severity, they may invent descriptions of illness about their children, falsify physical signs, or actually cause illness, e.g. by poisoning or suffocation. The condition is serious because of the immediate physical danger (10% mortality) and the long-term psychological harm to the child.

In the emergency situation, the priority is treatment of the acute physical problem. However, 'thinking the unthinkable' may allow for earlier identification and prevention. Look out for the following risk factors:
- unusual condition that only occurs when mother present;
- symptoms improve with separation;
- maternal healthcare background;
- inconsistencies;
- recurrent admissions;
- sibling with similar pattern or early death.

Admit the child for careful observation, minimizing time that the child is alone with the carer. Involve a senior paediatrician as soon as possible and consider using child protection procedures.

Somatizing and conversion disorders

The way in which children present with illness varies with their family, culture, and previous experience. Some children can remain stoical, while others are dramatic or highly anxious. This can hamper the assessment of the severity of the physical condition. The impact of a child's emotional state on their physical state can range from 'psychological overlay' to stress-related exacerbations of chronic conditions, e.g. asthma, migraine, to conversion disorders like pseudoseizures and 'hysterical' paralysis.

The diagnosis of conversion disorders rests with exclusion of physical pathology, which is not always possible. With acute presentation, an obvious trigger may be found, such as recent bullying or sexual abuse. In more chronic cases, the 'sick role' may be beneficial: increased adult attention; reduced parental expectation; family harmony; and school avoidance. Another useful concept is that of young people using illness as an unsophisticated type of communication to resolve a difficult predicament. It may be impossible to uncover the predicament in the emergency situation.

Assessment

- **History**. Clear account of development of symptoms; recent stressors at home and school; level of impairment; contact with anyone with similar symptoms; variation with company or by school day; families with chronic sickness; inconsistencies (best functioning vs. worst); educational difficulties.
- **Examination**. Can symptoms be brought on by suggestion? Does the pain or dysfunction follow dermatome? Do the physical signs change with distraction strategies?
- **MSE in full**. Usually unremarkable but look for anxiety, depression, apparent indifference to symptoms, perfectionistic personality traits, problems expressing emotions.

Management

- Remember that in most cases the child is not trying to deceive you.
- Restrict investigations to a minimum, but do the important ones early.
- Avoid confrontation no matter how certain you are that the symptoms are not organic.
- Acknowledge the validity of the symptoms. The pain is genuine; the leg will not move!
- Engage the parents, ensuring they understand the child is not 'faking'. Use models like stress-related headache.
- Allow 'escape with honour'. A course of physiotherapy can be very helpful for rehabilitation. Plan for early return to school.
- Children can be very suggestible. Predict rapid improvement but ensure close monitoring.
- Suggest referral to a specialist if symptoms not improved within a week.

Eating disorders

Anorexia nervosa is a rare condition in which deliberate weight loss causes undernutrition. It is defined as being <85% of expected weight for height, along with specific thinking and behaviour patterns, e.g. avoidance of fatty foods, distorted body image, self-induced vomiting, or excessive exercise. It predominantly affects young women whose menstruation is affected. It has significant morbidity—osteoporosis and infertility—and mortality, secondary to suicide and physical complications, e.g. cardiac arrhythmias. (see also **Bulimia** 📖 p.237).

Certain physical complications require immediate admission. These include:

- bradycardia or hypotension: HR <40bpm or BP <90/60mmHg;
- electrolyte imbalance, e.g. K^+<3mmol/l;
- dehydration;
- hypothermia;
- muscle weakness;
- hepatic/renal or cardiovascular impairment.

Assessment

- **History**. Development of physical symptoms and low mood; date of loss of periods; details of food restriction and exercise; food label interest; current daily intake of food and fluid; use of laxatives.
- **Physical examination**. Cachexia; dry skin; lanugo hair; dry mucosae; ketotic breath; acne; peripheral cyanosis; cold extremities; pubertal status (Tanner staging); enamel erosion from teeth (2° to recurrent vomiting); burns or cuts from self-harm.
- **MSE in full.** Baggy clothing; quiet speech; bizarre food beliefs, e.g. water is fattening; body image disturbance; fear of fatness; objective and subjective low mood.

Investigations

- Plot height and weight on centile chart. Calculate BMI (📖 p.517).
- Pulse, BP—note any postural drop. ECG.
- UEC: urea, Na^+, K^+ ↑ due to dehydration. K^+ can be ↓ due to vomiting or abuse of diuretics or laxatives.
- LFT: ALT, AST, and ALP ↑; GGT sometimes ↑.
- Cholesterol ↑.
- FBC and ESR: normal.
- Endocrine: cortisol ↑, T_3↓.
- Anti-TTG IgA antibodies, plus total IgA (to exclude coeliac disease).

Management

- This may be against the patient's wishes but with parental consent (📖 p.439). Consider need for psychiatric inpatient treatment.
- Correction of dehydration and electrolyte disturbance.
- Consider nasogastric feeding with the psychiatry team. Involve dietician.

Medico-legal aspects

By their very nature psychiatric emergencies generate all sorts of ethical and legal questions. Treating a young person against their wishes is a difficult step for all health professionals. The management after disclosure or suspicion of abuse is equally complex, balancing confidentiality and risk. There are significant national variations in the legal aspects to these situations but the focus here, will be on the law in England and Wales.

Common law is the term given to a set of general legal principles that are derived from specific cases. There have been no successful cases of prosecution for assault of medical professionals undertaking life-saving emergency treatment against a minor's wishes. While we prefer to work with young people's consent, courts understand and will support a doctor treating in the best interests of a child, in an emergency. It is up to the doctor to consider the degree of urgency and the probability of successful treatment and to attempt to gain the parent/carer's agreement.

Parental consent Under British law, parents are responsible for all healthcare decisions of their children under 18. In an apparent legal anomaly, competent minors can give consent for a medical treatment but not refuse it. Thus, it is legally possible to give any medical treatment provided you have the parent's agreement. In practice, forcing treatment on young people may be harmful to the doctor—patient relationship and jeopardize future care, so it is only justified in extreme situations.

1983 Mental Health Act This applies to children and adults with mental disorder. Under the act, two doctors (one with special expertise) and an approved social worker may compulsorily detain patients in a psychiatric hospital for up to 1 month (section 2) or 6 months (section 3). In a general hospital setting, any doctor can use section 5(2) of the act to detain an admitted patient for up to 72 hours, pending a specialist mental health assessment. This may be useful for suicidal or psychotic young people but cannot be used in the emergency department. A specific form should be available, which is then passed on to the hospital manager.

1989 Children Act The basic principles of this legislation are as follows.

- The welfare of the child is paramount.
- Children should be brought up and cared for within their own family wherever possible.
- Children should be safe and protected.

When parents harm their children or cannot protect them from harm, there can be conflict between these principles. This may lead to the use of court orders, which are applied for by social workers:

- **Emergency protection order**. Following a successful application, the court will direct that the child be protected in a place of safety for a maximum of 15 days.
- **Police protection**. This grants the police the power to remove a child who is suffering or likely to suffer significant harm. Lasts 72 hours.
- **Care order**. Gives the local authority parental responsibility for a child.

Chapter 26

Biochemistry

Glucose

Hyperglycaemia

Fingerprick glucose >7mmol/l if starved; >11.1mmol/l if not.

- Diabetes mellitus (🕮 p.404).
- Stress response, especially if on steroids or inotropes.
- Acute pancreatitis (🕮 p.250).
- Hyperadrenalism (Cushing's syndrome). Check BP, growth.
- Hyperthyroidism (🕮 p.415).

Hypoglycaemia

Fingerprick glucose < 4mmol/l. Exclude shock.

Check for ketones (smell breath, dipstick urine). If not ketotic, work quickly as no substrates for cerebral metabolism!

For hypoglycaemia in diabetes mellitus (See 🕮 p.408).

Non-diabetic causes

- Ketotic.
  - Endocrine: hypoadrenalism; panhypopituitarism; growth hormone deficiency.
  - Glucagon storage deficits.
  - Ketotic hypoglycaemia of infancy.
- Non-ketotic.
  - Fatty acid oxidation deficits; amino acid and organic acid disorders; mitochondrial cytopathies.
  - Hyperinsulinaemia—endogenous or exogenous.
  - Gastrointestinal, e.g. liver failure (🕮 p.248); dumping syndrome after fundoplication.
  - Medication, e.g. alcohol (🕮 p.168), aspirin (🕮 p.161), beta blocker overdose, insulin (consider Fabricated or induced illness 🕮 p.436).

Sodium

Hypernatraemia Sodium > 145mmol/l.
Secondary to water loss exceeding loss of sodium. Develop weakness, and appear confused before possible seizures or coma. Older children will complain of thirst. History of diarrhoea or polyuria. Causes include the following.

- **Gastroenterological**—osmotic diarrhoea, e.g. bottle-fed infants with gastroenteritis; carbohydrate malabsorption; lactulose overdose.
- **Renal**—osmotic diuresis, e.g. diabetes mellitus, diabetes insipidus; loop diuretics.

Investigations

- Blood—UEC, glucose, plasma osmolality (normal = 275–295mOsm/kg).
- Urine—dipstick and osmolality. If <750mOsm/kg, concurrent with plasma osmolarity >295 mOsm/kg, this is diagnostic of diabetes insipidus (📖 p.414).

Treatment

- Rehydrate over 48 hours, using ORF or IV fluids. For example, for a 12kg child with 5% dehydration:
  - maintenance fluids = 1100ml/24h;
  - deficit = 5% of 12000g = 600ml;
  - replace deficit over 48 h: (1100 + 1100 + 600ml) = 2800ml in 48 hours, i.e. 58.3ml/h.
- Check UEC every 4 hours. Aim to reduce sodium by no more than 10mmol/l every 24 hours.

Hyponatraemia Sodium < 135mmol/l.
May complain of nausea, headache, lethargy with progression to confusion. Seizures occur if sodium falls below 120mmol/l.

Usually secondary to water gain or sodium loss, resulting in a hypotonic hyponatraemia. Causes include the following.

- **Water gain.** Syndrome of inappropriate ADH secretion (SIADH; see box); oedema, e.g. CCF, liver failure; oliguric renal failure, e.g. acquired; excessive IV rehydration; psychogenic polydipsia (very dilute urine ***and*** dilute plasma).

SIADH

- Low serum sodium (and often urea and creatinine)
- Plasma osmolarity <280mOsmol/kg
- Inappropriately concentrated urine >100mOsmol/kg
- Elevated urine sodium >20mEq/l

- **Sodium loss.** Diarrhoea; burns; adrenal failure including CAH, hypothyroidism; thiazide diuretics.

Very rarely, sodium loss may be exceeded by excessive water loss—polyuric renal failure such as congenital renal failure, or an osmotic diuresis, e.g. diabetes mellitus—resulting in a hypertonic hyponatraemia.

Management Stop any IV fluids until cause known—usually easy to distinguish conditions clinically or from bedside tests, e.g. urinary dipstick.

Investigations
- Blood—UEC, glucose, plasma osmolality (normal = 275–295mOsm/kg).
- Urine—dipstick (expected specific gravity >1.005) and osmolality (expected >750mOsm/kg); 24 h urinary collection for urinary sodium.

Treatment
- **Shock**—20ml/kg IV 0.9% saline; fingerprick glucose, e.g. adrenal failure; severe dehydration (10%).
- **Dehydration**—rehydrate over 48 hours with IV 0.9% saline (or can calculate and replace deficit—see box).

Dose of Na (mmol) = weight (kg) x 0.8 x (140 – current serum Na^+)

- **Seizures**—discuss with ICU. Hypertonic saline (3%) may be useful. Risk of central pontine myelinolysis (quadriparesis with lower face weakness ± 'locked in') if sodium replacement too rapid.
- **SIADH**—fluid restrict to 2/3 maintenance, using 0.45% saline.

Potassium

Hyperkalaemia Potassium >5.5mmol/l.

Cardiac effects usually precede symptoms of tingling and weakness. Causes include the following.

- Spurious, e.g. difficulty obtaining blood sample (haemolysed).
- Dietary excess, e.g. liquorice—rare if normal renal function.
- Increased cellular release:
  - increased cellular destruction—tumour lysis, rhabdomyolysis;
  - acidosis—metabolic >respiratory;
  - hereditary—malignant hyperthermia.
- Impaired excretion:
  - adrenal failure;
  - acute renal failure, renal tubular disease;
- Drugs—cyclosporin, ACE inhibitors, spironolactone, digoxin.

Management

- Stop IV fluids containing K^+ or any contributory medications.
- Start cardiac monitoring—VF, asystole (📖 p.70, p.74).

Investigations

- Urgent UEC, glucose, VBG (excludes acidosis and provides rapid, confirmatory K^+ result). If possibility of increased tissue destruction, add CK, uric acid, PO_4, Ca.
- ECG—peaked T waves,↑ PR interval, flattened P wave, widened QRS.

Treatment

In order of speed of action. Urgent if ECG changes, digoxin toxicity.

- Treatments can be combined.
  - Salbutamol: **either** nebulized 2.5mg <5y; 5mg >5y;
  or IV 4mg/kg over 20 minutes.
  - $NaHCO_3$: IV 1–2mmol/kg. Excellent in acidosis, as promotes uptake of K^+ into cells.
  - Calcium gluconate 10%: IV 0.5–1mg/kg (first line if associated with hypocalcaemia or symptomatic arrhythmia (to stabilize myocardium)).
  - Glucose ± Insulin: IV glucose 0.5g/kg ± Insulin 0.1U/kg. Requires close monitoring, not recommended for children under 1 year.
  - Resonium: oral or rectal 1g/kg. N.B. hours before effect.
- Discuss with renal team—loop diuretics, dialysis.

Hypokalaemia $K^+ < 3.5$mmol/l.

May complain of cramps and weakness. Most frequently seen secondary to diarrhoea; other causes include the following.

- GI—laxative abuse in eating disorders; chemotherapy-induced.
- Renal—renal tubular disorders, e.g. RTA, Barrter's; drug toxicity such as aminoglycosides, amphotericin; diuretic excess; hyperaldosteronism, e.g. Cushing's, CAH, renal artery stenosis; metabolic alkalosis.
- Iatrogenic—IV fluids with β agonists or aminophylline.

Management Check BP: exclude hypertension.

Investigations

- ECG—flattened T wave, ST depression, U wave presence.
- UEC, VBG ± 24 hour urinary collection for K^+ if cause uncertain.

Treatment

- If symptomatic or ECG changes, give IV 0.2mmol/kg (maximum 40mmol/l). If more required, obtain central access and give 0.5mmol/kg with ECG monitoring. If symptomatic, give as a slow bolus; otherwise infuse over 1 hour.
- Oral supplements 2mmol/kg can be given but seldom palatable!

Calcium

Serum calcium levels influenced by binding to albumin. Ionized calcium, i.e. 'free calcium', obtained from arterial blood gas, will clarify abnormal results.

Hypercalcaemia Serum calcium >2.7mmol/l or ionized >1.4mmol/l. Symptomatic when calcium >3mmol/l. Symptoms include the following.
- GI—nausea, vomiting, anorexia, abdominal pain, constipation.
- CVS—hypertension, bradycardia, shortening of QT (📖 p.193).
- PNS—weakness, proximal myopathy.
- CNS—confusion, ataxia, psychosis, coma.
- Ectopic calcification, e.g. nephrocalcinosis.

Causes include the following.
- Endocrine: hyperparathyroidism, Addison's.
- Renal: renal failure, thiazide diuretics.
- Intake: excess vitamin D, excess vitamin A, phosphate deficiency.
- Other: malignancy, immobilization, William's syndrome.

Investigations
- UEC, calcium, PO_4, magnesium, albumin, LFT, alk phos, glucose.
- ABG for ionized calcium.
- PTH; 25 hydroxy vitamin D; 1,25 dihydroxy vitamin D.
- Urinary calcium, PO_4, creatinine.
- ECG ± imaging e.g. x-ray hands, wrists; renal USS.

Treatment
- Hyperhydration, e.g. IV 0.9% saline at 3000ml/m^2/day (📖 p.517). N.B. Use with caution if renal disease; monitor electrolytes.
- Once hydrated, frusemide 1mg/kg/dose qds PO.
- Discuss with endocrinology—bisphosphonates may be useful.

Hypocalcaemia Serum calcium <2mmol/l, ionized calcium <1.0mmol/l. ***Symptoms*** include the following.
- Stridor secondary to laryngospasm—may need intubation.
- Seizures, particularly in neonates.
- Neuromuscular, e.g. tingling—in hands, around mouth; carpopedal spasm. Chvostek's sign—tap VIIth at external auditory meatus (positive in 10% normocalcaemic patients); Trousseau's—inflate BP cuff 20mmHg over systolic BP to elicit spasm. N.B. Unpleasant test to perform on child.

Causes include:
- Dietary—poor intake; malabsorption involving fat-soluble vitamins.
- Endocrine: hypoparathyroidism; pseudohypoparathyroidism; vitamin D deficiency (lack of sunlight, medications, e.g. phenytoin, renal disease).
- Calcium sequestration—acute pancreatitis, rhabdomyolysis.

Investigations As for hypercalcaemia.

Treatment Urgent if symptomatic or in neonate: IV Ca gluconate 10% 0.5ml/kg (diluted 1 in 10), given over 2–3 minutes, ideally via long line or else via major vein.
- Any hypomagnesaemia should correct as Ca^{2+} rises. If not see 📖 p.450.
- Long term: discuss with endocrinology ± renal.

When in conjunction with hypoalbuminaemic states, correct serum calcium by 0.1mmol/l, for every 5g/l reduction in serum albumin under 40g/l.

Magnesium

Seldom seen in ED, but magnesium not routinely tested!

Hypermagnesaemia

Magnesium >1.0mmol/l. Extremely rare as any dietary excess corrected by normal renal function. Ask about use of enemas, antacids. Newborns with reduced GFR and children with chronic renal failure are susceptible.

Symptoms develop when magnesium >1.8mmol/l.
- CVS: hypotension, peripheral vasodilatation;
- GI: nausea, vomiting;
- CNS: Lethargy, weakness, hypotonia, areflexia.

Investigations ECG: prolonged PR, QRS, and QT; heart block (📖 p.193).

Treatment

- If normal renal function, IV fluids ± loop diuretics.
- If impaired renal function, dialysis.

Hypomagnesaemia

Magnesium <0.6mmol/l. Clinically concerning when under 0.3mmol/l as impairs the release of PTH, resulting in hypocalcaemia. Secondary hypokalaemia can also arise, especially with renal disease. Symptoms of isolated hypomagnesaemia resemble those of hypocalcaemia, but arrhythmias are unlikely if there are no cardiac anomalies. Causes include:
- GI loss: vomiting, diarrhoea, protracted inanition, malabsorption conditions, e.g. coeliac, CF, IBD.
- renal loss: tubular disease, e.g. nephritis, Barrter's, Gitelmann's; osmotically active agents, e.g. glucose, mannitol; medications, e.g. diuretics (loop and thiazides); nephrotoxic, e.g. amphotericin, cyclosporin.

Investigations ECG: stunted T waves; prolongation of ST (📖 p.193).

Treatment

- Urgent: IV magnesium sulphate 0.1–0.2mmol/kg/dose (2.5–5mg/kg of elemental magnesium) via slow infusion. N.B. Caution with use if renal disease. Reduce infusion rate if flushing, vomiting, or sensation of warmth (excessive vasodilatation).
- Long term: oral supplementation in divided doses to reduce likelihood of diarrhoea. Age-dependent doses—confer with pharmacy on preparations available.

Urea and uric acid

Urea is created to remove ammonia, a toxic by-product of protein catabolism that is not readily excreted. Uric acid is generated by purine metabolism, e.g. the breakdown of DNA. Uric acid is measured as urate, its salt form.

Both urea and uric acid are toxic if they accumulate.

Elevated urea >6mmol/l.
Urea is soluble in water so is easily excreted by the kidney. Thus high levels of urea seldom arise in isolation, and usually reflect impaired renal function, secondary to reduced glomerular filtration rate (GFR). Persistently high levels will cause itching and GI irritation, such as vomiting and bleeding.
Causes include:

- **increased production**. GI: upper GI bleed, high protein diet; medications: steroids, diuretics;
- **impaired excretion**. Renal: pre-renal (dehydration); renal (renal failure); post-renal (obstruction, e.g. urethral valve, stone).

Treatment

- Renal failure (see 🕮 p.261).
- Assess hydration (🕮 p.239). Rehydrate if necessary.
- Review medication.

High uric acid Urate >0.35mmol/l. Uric acid ceases to be soluble in water at high concentration. Crystals are deposited in the kidney causing renal stones; in the joints causing gout; and, ultimately, in the nerves with resultant neuropathies. Precipitation is exacerbated by dehydration or acidosis.
Causes include:

- **increased cell turnover:** malignancy, cyanotic heart disease, hereditary anaemia, psoriasis;
- **associated syndromes:** Lesch–Nyhan (X-linked, progressive developmental delay and spasticity, self-mutilation especially biting) Down syndrome; glycogen storage disorders I, III, IV, V.

Treatment

- Increasing fluid intake ± IV rehydration.
- Allopurinol 5mg/kg/dose bd to qds PO (maximum 600mg/day) to reduce production; probenecid 10mg/kg/dose qds PO to increase excretion.
- Consider alkalinization of urine.

Ammonia

Ammonia is a toxic by-product of protein catabolism. It is lipid-soluble so readily affects cerebral metabolism. In order to be excreted, ammonia must be converted to urea by the liver.

> Ammonia samples may require a specific tube; must be placed on ice and necessitate lab notification

Hyperammonaemia >100μmol/l neonates; >60μmol/l after 1 month.

Hyperammonaemia can arise from urea cycle defects or secondary to other pathologies, e.g. liver failure, organic acidaemias. These may be distinguished by the degree of hyperammonaemia, e.g. ammonia:

- 50μmol/l = transient hyperammonaemia of newborn (arises day 1 of life and resolves spontaneously);
- <500μmol/l = liver failure;
- >1000μmol/l = urea cycle defects.

However, these levels are not absolute and it is advisable to also check:

- UEC, LFT, glucose;
- venous blood gas;
- urine for metabolic screen.

These should distinguish the causes and direct further management.

- Liver failure; hypoglycaemia.
- Metabolic acidosis = organic acidaemia.
- Normal/ mild respiratory alkalosis = urea cycle defect (See below)

All cases should be discussed with metabolic/endocrine team. Dialysis may be necessary.

Urea cycle defects

These arise from one of six possible enzyme mutations—the commonest being ornithine transcarbamylase (OTC) deficiency.[1] The severity of clinical manifestations is variable, depending on the duration of exposure to ammonia, rather than the level of hyperammonaemia. Thus, chronic exposure may cause developmental delay and/or failure to thrive with possible hepatomegaly which presents at any age!

But all can develop the life-threatening acute hyperammonaemic crises, rapidly progressing from vomiting and irritability to acute confusional states and ultimately coma. Affected neonates will feed poorly (thereby minimizing the protein load) and develop seizures, which can lead to them being erroneously investigated for asphyxia or sepsis.

1 X-linked partially dominant, so predominantly affects boys but female carriers can also present.

The distinguishing features of hyperammonaemia include:
- tachypnoea;
- normal pH or mild respiratory alkalosis;
- ± hepatomegaly, failure to thrive, developmental delay.

REMEMBER
Acutely unwell child with tachypnoea ***without*** acidosis
Think Ammonia!

Management

The aim of management is to prevent further protein catabolism and to provide the substrates for the urea cycle so that the block can be overcome.
- ABC. Intubate if GCS <8.
- IV access. Consider long line if child stable.
- IV 10% glucose.
- Obtain plasma citrulline; urinary orotic acid.
- Confer with metabolic/endocrine team.
- Further treatment may involve:
  - IV benzoate; IV phenyl acetate; IV arginine;
  - IV lipids ± IV essential amino acids;

Phototherapy if neonates jaundiced.

Acid–base metabolism

When dealing with acid–base anomalies, remember the carbonic acid equation.

$$H^+ + HCO_3^- = H_2CO_3 = H_2O + CO_2$$

If one constituent of the equation increases, the equation should flow in the other direction to equilibrate.

Acidosis

Acidosis is defined as arterial pH < 7.35; venous pH < 7.3. It is detrimental to cellular function, e.g. denaturing proteins such as the Bohr effect on haemoglobin, impairing metabolic reactions.

Acid is generated by metabolism, e.g. anaerobic respiration, protein degradation, and is buffered by serum proteins and bicarbonate. Acid excretion is via the kidneys and exhaled as carbon dioxide.

Metabolic pCO_2 < 40mmHg, HCO_3 < 21mmol/l as compensatory hyperventilation with consumption of buffers, e.g. Kussmaul's breathing in DKA.

To determine the source of the acidosis, calculate the anion gap.

$$\text{Anion gap} = (Na^+ + K^+) - (Cl^- + HCO_3^-) = 8-16$$

An increased anion gap indicates increased endogenous acid production or increased consumption. A useful mnemonic is MULEPACK:

- **M**etabolic defects, e.g. organic acidaemia, fatty acid oxidation defects.
- **U**remia (📖 p.261).
- **L**actic acidosis, e.g. tissue ischaemia in shock.
- **E**thanol, methanol (📖 p.168).
- **P**araldehyde.
- **A**spirin (📖 p.161).
- **C**arbon monoxide.
- **K**etones, e.g. DKA (📖 p.404).

Treatment

- Calculate anion gap. If >16, think **MULEPACK** for causes. Treat accordingly. IV sodium bicarbonate is only given as a last resort (child must be able to excrete the CO_2 generated).
- If metabolic acidosis with a normal anion gap, this indicates:
  - bicarbonate loss: diarrhoea, proximal renal tubular acidosis (RTA);
  - impaired acid excretion: distal RTA.

Diarrhoea is the commonest cause. Otherwise consult with a nephrologist to determine RTA investigations.

Respiratory pCO_2 > 40mmHg as respiratory failure; HCO_3 increases slightly.

Treatment CPAP or intubate if child is for resuscitation.

Alkalosis

Alkalosis is defined as arterial pH > 7.45; venous pH > 7.5. It is not commonly seen in emergencies.

Metabolic HCO3 > 40mmol/l; pCO2 may rise >50mmHg with hypoventilation, particularly if there is renal compromise. Typically, potassium and chloride levels fall.

Metabolic alkalosis arises from acid loss or, rarely, alkali gain from increased consumption. The latter is usually accommodated by normal renal function. Acid loss is either from the gut or kidney.

- GI:
  - excessive vomiting, e.g. pyloric stenosis;
  - diarrhoea, e.g. carbohydrate intolerance, laxative abuse.
- Renal—extreme sodium retention by increased aldosterone.
  - Chronic reduction of circulating volume.
  - Adrenal disorders—CAH, Cushing's, renal artery stenosis.
  - Thiazide and loop diuretics.
  - Liquorice consumption.
  - Rare renal tubular disorders such as Barrter's, Gitelmann's syndrome.

Treatment

- Assess hydration (📖 p.239). IV rehydration should correct anomalies; potassium can be added once renal compromise excluded.
- Check BP—hypertension secondary to elevated renin.
  - If hypertensive, assess for adrenal disorders and perform UEC, glucose, random cortisol. If confirmed, start potassium supplementation and discuss further investigations with endocrinology.
- If not improving, discuss with renal team—renal tubular disease requires specific investigations.

Respiratory pCO_2 < 25mmHg; HCO_3 decreases minimally because of buffering. Usual cause is hyperventilation, secondary to anxiety. Often accompanied by tingling around the mouth and of the fingers and a sensation of feeling light-headed.

Other causes to consider:

- fever, pain, hypoxia, hyperthyroidism;
- poisoning: hepatic coma; urea cycle defects (📖 p.452); aspirin (📖 p.161) CNS disorders: infection, CVA.

Treatment

- Check oxygen saturations to exclude hypoxia.
- Rebreathing using a paper bag. N.B. Seldom available. Using an oxygen mask not attached to oxygen supply will suffice.
- Try to find source of anxiety.

Chapter 27

Procedures

General principles

For the purposes of this chapter, it is assumed that you know the indications of when to do these procedures. With all procedures, have senior supervision until you feel competent—you may suddenly need a pair of helping hands! Table 27.1 gives a kit list for each of the procedures. It is good practice to keep a log of every procedure you perform, as well as being impressive information to provide for interviews.

Cleanliness

Procedures can be done either as:

- clean—wash hands, use gloves, alcohol skin swabs;
- sterile—sterile gloves, no touch, chlorhexidine and/or betadine solution;
- full sterile—gown, gloves, green drapes, strict sterile precautions.

Equipment

The most important 'piece' of equipment you can have is your assistants. The number given is a minimum: you may well need more to act as entertainers.

A 'dressing pack' contains a sterile field, swabs, a tub for cleaning fluid, and tongs to hold your cleaning swabs. Some procedures commonly have a dedicated pack available, e.g. umbilical line kit, chest drain tray, central line kit.

Analgesia and sedation

There is a large array of options available: always use an appropriate method for the age of the patient. A good play specialist is a very effective tool!

- Neonates settle well with 1ml of 20% dextrose orally.
- Topical local anaesthetics, e.g. EMLA® or Ametop® cream, work well in most children. But some children seem to be resistant to them, or develop vein-hiding skin swelling.
- Ethyl chloride spray is good in children who can differentiate between extreme cold and pain.
- Lignocaine is the drug of choice for local anaesthesia (maximum dose 0.3ml/kg of 1%). Lignocaine may sting, so administer slowly and consider buffering with sodium bicarbonate—9ml 1% xylocaine with 1ml 8.4% sodium bicarbonate.
- Adrenaline/cocaine gel can be used for wounds that are not on distal extremities.
- Inhaled nitrous oxide is an excellent anxiolytic. Requires oximetry and use within 30 minutes to limit nausea.

Other versions of deep conscious sedation include:
- midazolam (intranasal, buccal, or IV); ± morphine or fentanyl IV;
- ketamine IV; give midazolam to minimize hallucinations.

(See 🕮 p.488). However, these drugs may cause respiratory compromise and should be only given under supervision of a doctor confident in airway management. N.B. Midazolam can cause altered behaviour (including agitation) in low doses.

Table 27.1 What do I need?

	Vene-puncture	**Cannula**	**Central line**	**Umbilical line**	**Arterial line**	**IO line**	**LP**	**SPA**	**Intubation**	**Crico-thyroid-otomy**	**Chest drain**	**Femoral nerve block**
Assistants	1	1	1	1	1	1	2	1	2	2	1	1
Special equipment	Needle 22G Bandaid	Cannula T-Piece Splint	Central line. Dressing	2.5–5 Fr Cord tie scalpel	22/24G cannula	IO Needle	Needle Bandaid	Needle 22G Bandaid	Endotracheal tube, Magill's forceps, laryngoscope, suction, tapes	Big cannula or dedicated kit	Largest possible chest drain	Needles (infuser, 22G), scalpel, steristrip
Analgesia	Topical	Topical	Sedate	Nil	Top	Nil	Top	Nil	Sedate	Nil	Local/ sedate	Local/ sedate
Sterility	Clean	Clean	Gown	Gown	Sterile	Sterile	Sterile	Clean	Clean	Sterile	Gown	Sterile
Gloves	Yes	Yes	Sterile	Sterile	Sterile	Sterile	Sterile	Yes	Yes	Sterile	Sterile	Sterile
Suture			4/0	4/0						4/0	4/0	
Needle	1							1			1	2

Table 27.1 (*Contd.*)

	Vene-puncture	Cannula	Central line	Umbilical line	Arterial line	IO line	LP	SPA	Intubation	Crico-thyroid-otomy	Chest drain	Femoral nerve block
Alcohol wipe	1	1						1				
Cardboard tray	1	1						1				
Dressings pack		1	1	1			1					1
Dedicated pack			Yes	Yes						1	Yes	
Extra gauze			2	2	1		1			1	2	
Sample bottles	Yes	Yes					Yes	Yes				
Saline flush		Yes	Yes	Yes	Yes	Yes						
5ml syringe		1	3	2	1	1		1		1	1	2

Venepuncture and cannulation

Contraindications Unstable airway, e.g. severe croup, epiglottitis, asthma.

Complications Pain for the patient, even with EMLA®. Small risk of local infection.

Principles This is a clean procedure. You should explain what will happen to the parents and child. Do not persist after three failed attempts—get help! When sampling blood, excessive suction will collapse a vein. Ensure the cannula tube itself (not just the tip of the needle) is in the vein before advancing the cannula tube over the needle.

Procedure: points to remember

- Wear gloves. It will feel natural with practice.
- Ensure the tops are off your sample bottles prior to starting.
- Options for venepuncture include:
  - a needle;
  - a butterfly—either the tube cut off or with a syringe attached;
  - an 'in/out' cannula.
- Ensure the skin is taut.
- Insert the point of the needle just under the skin. Pause and then advance the needle into the vein. This minimizes the risk of the vein 'bouncing' off the needle, and children often move as skin pierced.
- For cannulation, after seeing flashback, advance the needle a few millimetres further before advancing the cannula tube. Anchor with one piece of tape.

It is best to drip the blood into the bottles to minimize haemolysis. To collect blood cultures, aspirate from the hub with a drawing up (blunt) needle attached to a syringe. Do not attach a syringe to the hub of the cannula as you may lose the cannula if the child moves.

- Dispose of the needle safely.
- Tape down securely and splint to minimize flexion. Ensure assistant understands how you want this done.

Troubleshooting venepuncture and cannulation.

- '**My patient has mobile veins.**' Try approaching a vein from one side, or at a Y-junction of 2 veins, to minimize movement.
- '**I'm sure I'm in the vein, but nothing's coming out.**' Try moving the cannula out a little as the tip may be at a valve. Or you have missed.
- '**I'm trying to aspirate blood and nothing happens.**' Don't apply excessive negative pressure: the vein will collapse. Try letting the blood flow freely.
- '**I can't find a vein.**' Long saphenous is usually a finger's breadth proximal to medial malleolus. Only attempt scalp veins after telling parents.
- '**I have looked again and found a vein on the scalp. What do I do now?**' Shave a small amount of hair over the vein. Use the fingers of your left hand to dam the blood flow, and your thumb to tauten the skin. Insert cannula always pointing towards the heart. Tape and bandage securely.

Central venous access

In paediatrics, the femoral vessels are most frequently accessed as the neck is usually too short. N.B. The umbilical vessels can be used up until 14 days of age (📖 p.464).

Contraindications Pelvic fracture.

Complications Damage to femoral vein ± artery.

Principles

Ideal for:
- secure access;
- large lumen access for multiple or rapid infusions;
- giving drugs that are damaging to peripheral veins, e.g. inotropes.

This is a fully sterile procedure. Your line is likely to remain *in situ* for up to 2 weeks.

Procedure: points to remember

- The femoral artery is always lateral to the vein. Remember **NAVY**—**N**erve, **A**rtery, **V**ein, **Y** = Y-fronts! as you move medially over the groin.
- In babies and toddlers use a 4 Fr. gauge double lumen line; in older children a 5 or larger gauge is used. For both of these, a 20G cannula should suffice—if in doubt, check the wire goes through the cannula before starting.
- Use lignocaine to numb the skin if your patient is conscious.
- Insert using Seldinger technique.
  - Fill femoral line with 0.9% saline.
  - Insert needle of cannula into femoral vein—medial to artery, aim for patient's head, at 45° angle to skin.
  - Once flashback is obtained, thread cannula all the way in as if cannulating vein—this makes it less likely that the cannula will be dislodged as wire threaded in. Alternatively, remove needle without threading and occlude hub.
  - Insert Seldinger wire into vein via cannula.
  - Remove cannula taking care not to lose hold of end of wire.
  - Nick skin with scalpel blade—this facilitates dilator insertion. Thread dilator, which often needs firm pressure. Remove dilator; then thread catheter over wire into the vein. Hold wire securely throughout!
  - Remove wire, occluding end of catheter.
- If blood flows, check not pulsatile! Flush each line and attach 3-way taps to all lumens.
- Suture line in place, cover with clear sterile dressing, and attach infusion tubing.

Umbilical access

Contraindications Gastroschisis.

Complications

- Increased risk of necrotizing enterocolitis.
- Thromboembolism.
- Accidental haemorrhage.

Principles

- This is a fully sterile procedure.
- If possible, explain to parents why procedure is necessary.
- The cord is like a smiley face: two small round eyes (arteries) and one large floppy mouth (vein).
- The venous line should end up past the liver (not in the heart); the arterial line above T10 (ideal T8), and below the arch of the aorta.
- ***Securing the line is critical (Fig. 27.1).***

Procedure: points to remember

- Ask an assistant to hold the cord clamp up in the air. Clean the stump thoroughly with cleaning fluid; then hold the clean end and wash the end your assistant has just held.
- A long stump enables more attempts but makes it more difficult to thread your line.

UAC insertion

- The artery will need to be dilated to a depth of around 1cm. Do this very gently, or the artery will tear.
- Fill the umbilical line with 0.9% saline.
- Insert gently to distance of (weight (kg) x 3) + 9cm. There should not be much resistance.
- Carefully suture line in. A good method is using an elastoplast flag at the base of the line, and suture this to the stump.

UVC insertion

- Locate the vein, and measure distance from tip of umbilical stump to diaphragm.
- Carefully slide in line. You will rarely need to dilate the vein.
- Suture this in, taking extreme care not to damage the arterial line.
- Ask the nurses to tape 'goalposts' and label the lines (Fig. 27.1).

Check position of lines with an AXR—the venous line goes straight up, and the arterial line goes inferiorly towards the iliac vessels and then turns up.

Troubleshooting umbilical catheterization

- **'My arterial line has stopped threading at 4cm'**. You have blown it.
- **'My arterial line has ended up at T12. Do I really have to move it?'** Yes. The renal arteries are at L1, and the tip of the line could obstruct them.
- **'My venous line has ended up in the liver. What do I do now?'** Withdraw so that approximately 5cm is in the baby (the 'low' position).

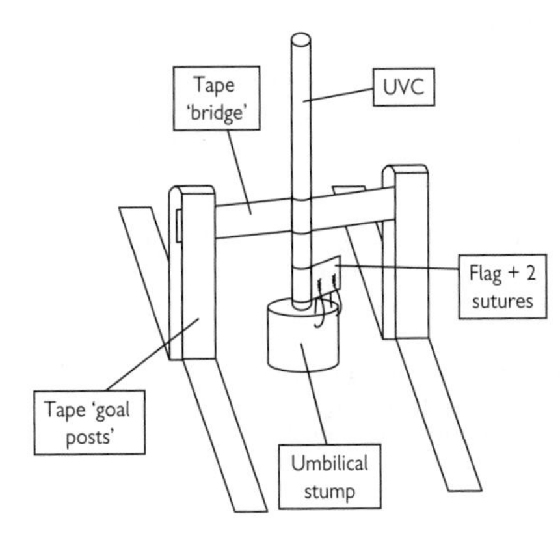

Fig. 27.1 UVC taping.

Exchange transfusion

Exchange transfusion will rapidly remove toxins such as unconjugated bilirubin, or haemolytic antibodies. It is a labour-intensive procedure, requiring the undivided attention of a doctor and nurses and usually takes over two hours to perform.

Ensure everything is prepared prior to getting blood from lab—if the blood passes its expiry time, it will require a new cross-match and delay a tedious procedure even further.

The commonest indication is neonatal jaundice which does not respond to phototherapy and fluid. Exchange transfusion is necessary to prevent kernicterus, and will also allow correction of the concomitant haemolytic anaemia.

Contraindications

Caution if haemodynamically unstable.

Complications

- Catheter-related:
  - emboli; clot or air;
  - thrombosis; venous or arterial;
  - local haemorrhage or infection;
  - associated with increased risk of NEC.
- Haemodynamic: if haemostasis not maintained.
- Metabolic:
  - hypoglycaemia;
  - hypocalcaemia; secondary to use of citrated blood. ECG monitoring mandatory and check frequently and correct as necessary;
  - hyperkalaemia; secondary to cell haemolysis in stored blood;
  - metabolic acidosis; secondary to acidic stored blood.

Principles

- Insertion of lines is a sterile procedure.
- Blood is removed and replaced at approximately the same rate.

Procedure

- Usually a double exchange, to swap >90% of baby's blood volume (of 85ml/kg)
- Insert UVC (📖 p.464) or peripheral IV.
- Insert UAC (📖 p.464) or peripheral arterial line (📖 p.468).
- Calculate the volume to be exchanged; 85 × 2 × weight (kg) ml of blood.
- Calculate the time to remove that volume in 10 ml aliquots every 2 minutes e.g. to double exchange a 4kg baby will require 680ml to be removed. This will take sixty eight 10ml aliquots every 2 minutes, or 136 minutes.
- Check baseline FBC, UEC, bilirubin, glucose and gas.

- Set infusion of (fresh) bank blood to run in through vein over 140 minutes.
- Remove 10ml blood from arterial line and discard. Then flush line with 0.5ml heparinized saline. The flushes will amount to a considerable volume over the course of the transfusion. This 'flush' volume is usually ignored in calculations, but should be incorporated into the fluid balance of haemodynamically unstable babies.
- Record every aliquot removed.
- Every 30 minutes, check the following and correct as necessary:
  - FBC; increase or reduce volume of blood infused to attain required target haemoglobin;
  - gas; rarely need to use bicarbonate to correct metabolic acidosis. Ensure adequate ventilation to remove CO_2;
  - UEC; potassium (📖 p.446);
  - Bilirubin;
  - Glucose (📖 p.442);
  - Ionized calcium; (📖 p.448).
- Repeat FBC, gas, UEC, bilirubin, glucose at end of procedure, before discarding remaining blood.
  - Top up transfusion may be required;
- Remove lines once no longer needed.

Arterial access

- Needed to enable:
  - frequent blood sampling, e.g. in DKA;
  - real time blood pressure monitoring.
- This is a sterile procedure.
- Common sites are the radial, posterior tibial, or dorsalis pedis arteries. ***Never*** attempt both arteries supplying an extremity, e.g. radial and ulnar arteries: hypoperfusion may result.
- Avoid end arteries if possible, e.g. the brachial artery.

Technique

- Palpate artery. Then occlude artery with direct pressure and check distal perfusion is still adequate. If perfusion OK, artery can be used.
- Go through skin. N.B. Radial artery is more superficial than it feels.
- Enter artery or even go right through. Remove needle.
- Attach saline flush and withdraw cannula slowly until flashback.
- Thread cannula.
- Flush gently. Skin may blanch transiently.
- Tape securely but do not obscure.
- Remember to attach a hard-walled extension tube to aid blood sampling.
- Arteries have more 'bounce' than veins. Transfixing the vessel often helps.
- If you have blown it, apply strong pressure for 5 minutes.

Intraosseous access

Contraindications

Fracture of the target bone; osteogenesis imperfecta.

Complications

- Risk of osteomyelitis.
- Extravasation may cause compartment syndrome and/or necrosis.
- Growth arrest if the growth plate is damaged.

Principles

- This is a sterile procedure.
- Consent is not needed, as this is an emergency procedure to obtain access in a critically ill child, when cannulation has failed.

This is the first access to be attempted in a baby or child who has collapsed

Procedure

- Analgesia is seldom used as any delay in obtaining access may compromise the child further. Use your discretion.
- With a scalpel, make a 0.5cm cut in the skin 1cm below and 1cm medial to the tibial tuberosity.
- Place the tip of the intraosseous needle though the cut and angle at 90° to the plane of the tibia. Applying firm downward pressure, turn the handle clockwise and anticlockwise.
- You will feel a give. Stop pushing and unscrew the stylet.
- You can aspirate blood for sampling, including blood cultures. Warn haematology that the blood is an intraosseous sample—blasts will be seen on the film.

Do not put this blood into a blood gas machine as it will clog it up

- Tape securely and/or assign someone to hold on to the line and do nothing else. It must ***not*** fall out before alternative IV access is obtained.
- Access can be used as a normal IV port; however, fluids must be syringed in manually.
- Medications can be given IO, except bretylium. Extreme care is required with sodium bicarbonate and calcium, which must be diluted to avoid necrosis with extravasation.
- Once perfusion has improved, try again for peripheral IV access or consider central access.
- When adequate venous access is obtained, remove intraosseous cannula.

Lumbar puncture

Contraindications

- Suspicion of raised intracranial pressure (risk of coning).
- Any acute neurological abnormality—GCS < 13.
- Known coagulopathy, e.g. platelets <50.
- Meningococcal illness with a non-blanching rash—LP at the initial presentation will not change management.

Complications

- Risk of neurological damage (quoted at 1:20 000).
- Risk of infection (very low).
- Risk of headache (common).
- Risk of apnoea in small babies due to holding position: must be monitored.

Principles

- This is a sterile procedure.
- You should obtain verbal consent prior to starting.
- Positioning is crucial—experienced nurses invaluable.

Procedure: points to remember

- If you have time, consider using topical anaesthetic cream. Holding causes most distress.
- Under 8 years, use 22G short needle. For adolescents, use adult needle.
  - Distance to dura: under 10kg 1.5mm/kg; 10–40kg 1.0mm/kg.
- Position child either lying on side, with hips and neck flexed; or sitting and bent forwards.
- Feel for L3/4, in line with the iliac crests. Feel the gap, and if you wish, mark ***around*** this with a pen. Never put a needle through ink or you will tattoo the patient.
- The needle should be:
  - midline ***and*** horizontal;
  - in the L3/4 space;
  - pointing towards the umbilicus.
- Advance needle until you feel 'a give' as you go through the ligamentum flavum.
- Never advance the needle without the stylet.
- If you meet firm obstruction, withdraw to skin, re-align, and try again.
- To measure CSF pressure, use a manometer. N.B. Inaccurate if child cries or moves.
- Remember to seal your needle hole with Opsite spray or equivalent.
- Samples can be sent for microbiology assessment, glucose and protein, lactate, neurotransmitters, virology, and PCR if indicated.

Troubleshooting LPs

- '**My patient is too mobile**.' Try to get your most expert nurse to hold. LPs in mobile patients are like playing darts on a boat.
- '**I only got blood out**.' Is your needle perpendicular to the back? Try advancing your needle whilst looking at it from the head of the patient, ensuring that your angle is correct.
- '**The CSF is coming out at one drip per hour**.' CSF flow can be very slow in babies. Otherwise, rotate the needle to align the bevel with the best flow.
- '**I can't hit the space**.' L4/5 can be attempted. Do not go above L3/4 as there is a risk of hitting the spinal cord.
- '**I got zero red cells!!!**' Remember to claim a bottle of wine from the supervising doctor!

Suprapubic aspiration

Contraindications

Peritonitis.

Complications

- Pain and distress.
- Theoretical risk of abdominal bleeding: very rare.

Principles

- This is a clean procedure.
- You should obtain verbal consent prior to starting.

Procedure: points to remember

- Ask the parents when the baby last passed urine. If you have an ultrasound scanner, you can check that the bladder is full.
- Have open sterile container to hand—cleaning skin often precipitates micturition. It is frustrating to miss a clean catch specimen!
- Insert a 22G needle attached to a syringe 2cm above the pubic symphysis. Angle at 30 degrees from the perpendicular, pointing towards the umbilicus.
- Aspirate whilst advancing.
- Ensure the sample stays sterile whilst transferring into a sample pot.

Troubleshooting SPAs

- '**I can't get a sample**.' Stop trying. The bladder may be empty, or you are missing. Try a clean catch or an in/out catheter. Urine bags or cotton wool have a higher chance of being contaminated.

Endotracheal intubation

Contraindications Nil.

Complications

- Loss of airway; oesophageal intubation.
- Circulatory collapse with induction drugs.
- Tracheal stenosis in medium–long term with large tubes.

Principles

- Inform parents if possible.
- Monitor patient with cardiac tracing and oximetry. Assign someone to tell you when saturations are <90% or the heart rate is falling
- Make sure a colleague can supervise and intervene if necessary.
- Unless experienced, secure airway with oral ET tube. A nasal ET tube can replace an oral ET tube later.

Procedure: points to remember

- Have your endotracheal tubes (ETT) ready: estimated size (age/4) + 4. Have one size larger and one size smaller available.
- Have suction, oxygen, bag, Magill's forceps, introducer, bougie, and laryngoscope to hand. Prepare tapes for securing tube.
- Pre-oxygenate so oxygen saturations 100%.
- If possibility of aspiration, ask assistant to apply cricoid pressure.
- Give IV drugs for rapid sequence induction (see box):
  - avoid thiopentone if blood pressure is likely to be a problem. Use ketamine;
  - avoid suxamethonium if burns, myopathies, hyperkalaemia. Use vecuronium or rocuronium.
- When you have your scope in position, pull it upwards along the line of the handle.
  - **Do not lever backwards: you will damage teeth or gums**.
- Do not force the tube through the cords. Try a smaller size.
- Insert **oral** ETT to (age ÷ 2) + 12cm; **nasal** ETT to (age ÷ 2) + 15cm.
- Release any cricoid pressure.
- Ask assistant to attach Laerdal bag with oxygen to tube.
- Check chest movements and auscultate axillae to ensure bilateral and equal air entry. If in doubt, auscultate over abdomen.
- Check length again and ensure that tube does not move!
- Secure tube at correct length. Nursing staff will have preferred technique.
- Always check tube position with CXR.
- When oxygen saturations are below 80%, stop intubation attempt, insert Guedel airway, and start bag/mask ventilation. When child stable, try again. N.B. Expect rapid desaturation in babies.

Rapid sequence induction

- Thiopentone 2–4mg/kg/dose
- Atropine 0.02mg/kg/dose (minimum 100mcg, maximum 600mcg)
- Suxamethonium 1–2mg/kg/dose

Troubleshooting intubation

- '**I can't see the cords**.' Ask assistant to increase, then lessen cricoid pressure. If necessary, hold their hand and manoeuvre it until the cords are in view; then ask them to maintain that position. It may help to have a towel under the patient's shoulders.
- '**I can't get through the cords**.'
  - Try smaller ETT.
  - Get suitably sized bougie and pass through the cords. Then railroad the ETT over the bougie, being careful not to withdraw bougie until ETT through the cords.

Cricothyroidotomy

Principles

Only indicated if all other attempts at gaining an airway have failed, and there is no other way to ventilate the patient. It is a difficult procedure as the patient will be attempting to breathe despite airway obstruction, so the target area will be moving. However, the patient will die if no attempt is made.

There are two methods: the needle cricothyroidotomy (either with a cannula or a special kit) and a surgical airway. The latter is a fully sterile procedure, involving cut down and inserting a tracheostomy tube. It should only be performed on children over the age of 12 years, ideally by ENT surgeons.

Procedure: points to remember

- Locate the cricothyroid membrane—the soft bit below the thyroid cartilage and above the cricoid cartilage. Clean the overlying skin.

Needle cricothyroidotomy

- Place your finger on the cricoid cartilage.
- Aim cannula towards chest at 45° angle.
- Advance the needle whilst aspirating back.
- Once you have a flashback of air, advance cannula tube, and discard needle.
- Attach cannula to oxygen via oxygen tubing and Y connector.
- Oxygen flow rate is child's age in years as litres per minute.
- Ventilate by occluding one end of Y connector for 1 second then release for 4 seconds.
- If no chest movement:
  - check for surgical emphysema;
  - increase oxygen flow rate.
- Secure cannula and prepare for inserting tracheostomy.

The cricothyroidotomy kit uses the Seldinger technique to insert a tracheostomy tube.

Chest drains

There are two types of chest drain available: the conventional rigid drain and the pigtail catheter. The latter are easier to insert, less painful, and can drain anything other than blood.

If there are signs of a tension pneumothorax, insert a cannula or butterfly vertically in the mid-clavicular line above the second rib. There should be a rush of air, and immediate clinical improvement. Then proceed to formal chest drain insertion

Contraindications Diaphragmatic hernia.

Principles

- A chest drain will not fix the cause of the pneumothorax.
- If clinically possible, it is always better to confirm on a CXR.

Procedure: points to remember

- For a rigid chest drain, this is a fully sterile procedure. Ensure adequate sedation and analgesia.
- Always incise parallel and above a rib: it heals better and misses the neurovascular bundle.
- The usual insertion place is the anterior axillary line of the 5th space.
- Be very careful where you site your drain: this child may grow up to be a teenager with body image issues.

N.B. If chest full of fluid, e.g. pleural effusion, [illegible] do n[illegible]
fluid off too quickly. [illegible]
may also [illegible]
fl[illegible]

Pig-tail drain

- Insert cannula with negative suction on attached syringe through chosen intercostal space.
- Once fluid or air aspirated, advance cannula over needle.
- Insert wire through needle and remove cannula.
- Nick skin and thread dilator over wire—***never*** lose sight of wire, or the surgeons will have to open child up to find it.
- Remove dilator and thread pigtail over and in required distance.
- Pigtail will have its own hollow rigid introducer inside—the whole thing goes over the wire.
- Remove the wire and the introducer.
- Some have locking mechanisms to allow pigtail to curl up once inserted.
- Stick or suture securely.
- Attach chest tube to a water seal, with suction if indicated.
- Perform a CXR to check position of drain.

Femoral nerve block

These are most effective if the femoral fracture is in the proximal two-thirds. The block is performed prior to application of a Thomas splint and provides excellent analgesia without repeated doses of IV opiates.

Contraindications Malignant hyperthermia.

Complications

- Damaging femoral artery or nerve.
- Injecting local anaesthetic into femoral vessels.
- Osteomyelitis.

Principles

- Only performed when the patient is clinically stable.
- Two local anaesthetics are used: lignocaine with its swift onset of action for superficial anaesthesia; bupivacaine for the block as it provides analgesia for hours.
- This is a sterile procedure.

Procedure: points to remember

- IV access must be available as inadvertent IV administration of local anaesthetic can result in cardiovascular collapse.
- IV analgesia ± sedation before starting may be helpful.
- Position injured limb so that femur abducted as much as possible.
- As the femoral nerve is lateral to the artery, it may be easier to work from the opposite side of the bed.
- Draw up 0.5% bupivacaine 0.3–0.4ml/kg (maximum 15ml) and attach blunt infuser needle. Draw up 1% lignocaine for superficial infiltration and attach 22G needle.
- Palpate the artery and, lateral to this point, raise a bleb of lignocaine under the skin. Once the skin is numb, position needle at 90° to skin and infiltrate sequentially downwards, aspirating prior to every administration.
- Resistance will be encountered at the inguinal ligament. Stop infiltration and withdraw syringe.
- Where needle entered skin, make a small incision with scalpel.
- Insert bupivacaine syringe with infuser needle through incision and advance carefully until inguinal ligament is reached. Apply gentle pressure to traverse ligament—be wary of underlying vessels.
- On entering the femoral triangle, there will be a slight give. The needle may move with femoral artery pulsations.
- Aspirate before infusing bupivacaine. If blood is aspirated, apply pressure and abandon procedure. Start continuous cardiac monitoring and monitor distal perfusion for the next 4 hours.
- If resistance is met during infusion, the needle may have entered the femoral nerve. Withdraw the needle slightly, aspirate, and try again.
- On completion of infusion, withdraw needle and seal skin with Steristrips.

Bier's block prior to reduction of distal fractures of the forearm is not described here. Children are seldom able to tolerate the procedure, compromising its safety. Reduction under general anaesthesia is recommended.

Chapter 28
Formulary

Introduction

This chapter is not intended to supplant the excellent paediatric formularies already available. The doses quoted are for general use and are adapted from *British national formulary for children* (ISBN 0 85369 626 8 Royal Pharmaceutical Press), with permission.

Quoted doses are age-specific and may not be appropriate for those children:

- under 3 months of age;
- with renal compromise;
- with hepatic dysfunction;
- with immunocompromise.

In such cases, consultation of more detailed paediatric or neonatal formulary, or your hospital pharmacy, is mandatory.

Be sure you know the common side-effects of the drug you are about to prescribe and remember drug interactions.

Analgesia

Topical and wounds

- EMLA®, Ametop®.
- Lignocaine 1%—maximum dose 0.3ml/kg. Lignocaine may sting so administer slowly and consider buffering with sodium bicarbonate—9ml 1% xylocaine with 1ml 8.4% sodium bicarbonate.
- Lignocaine gel for sore mouth/throat.

Femoral nerve block

- Bupivacaine 0.5% 0.3–0.4ml/kg, maximum 15ml, with xylocaine for topical analgesia.

> Bier's block for reduction of distal fractures of the forearm is not described in this book. Children are seldom able to tolerate the procedure, compromising its safety. Reduction under general anaesthesia is recommended

Oral preparations

- Paracetamol.
    - Neonate: 20mg/kg once, then 10–15mg/kg 8–12 hourly. Maximum 30mg/kg/day—halve if jaundiced or baby under 28 weeks' gestation.
    - Over 1 month: 20mg/kg once, then 15–20mg/kg 6 hourly. Maximum 90mg/kg/day and 1g/dose. Maximum 60mg/kg/d in 1–3 month olds.
- Ibuprofen 5–10mg/kg/dose 4 hourly. Maximum 400mg/dose or 2.4g/day.
- Naproxen 5–7.5mg/kg 12 hourly. Maximum dose 500mg.
- Codeine phosphate 1mg/kg 4 hourly. Maximum <1 year 3mg/kg/day >1 year 6mg/kg/day, (maximum 240mg/day).

Rectal preparations

- Paracetamol.
    - Neonate–3 months 30mg/kg then 20mg/kg 8 hourly (maximum 60mg/kg/day; halve if jaundiced).
    - Over 3 month: 40mg/kg loading dose (maximum 1g), then 15mg/kg 6 hourly. Maximum 90mg/kg/day or 4g/day.
- Diclofenac 1mg/kg/dose 8 hourly. Maximum 3mg/kg/day or 150mg/day.

IV preparations

Single dose

- Morphine. Neonate: 40–100mcg/kg; >1 month 100–200mcg/kg, maximum 10mg. Then follow with infusion of 20mcg/kg/h, titrating to response and monitoring for respiratory depression.
- Fentanyl 1mcg/kg, maximum 50mcg.
- Paracetamol—infuse over 15 minutes. 10–50 kg: 15mg/kg 4–6 hourly, maximum 60mg/kg/d; >50kg: 1g 4–6 hourly, maximum 4g/d.

Infusions

Excellent for severe pain, e.g. burns over 10% BSA, but only to be used if nursing staff confident about monitoring patient.

N.B. Give IV bolus before starting infusion.

Morphine

- Ventilated patient: infusion 20–40mcg/kg/h.
- Non-ventilated: neonate: 5–10mcg/kg/h; >1 month: 10–20mcg/kg/h.

Infusion: 1mg/kg morphine made up to 50ml with 0.9% saline; 1ml/h is = 20mcg/kg/h.

Sedation

See Chapter 25, for emergency treatment of:
- delirium (📖 p.425);
- aggression and assaultative patient (📖 p.431).

Conscious sedation is an excellent tool in ED, but should only be used if staff are confident in its use and able to monitor for adverse effects. Many departments will have their own policies.

Inhaled

Best for procedures that can be performed in under 30 minutes—nitrous causes nausea. Requires scavenger system to dissipate exhaled gases; otherwise staff will be affected too!

N.B. Will diffuse into gas-filled cavities so not recommended if pneumothorax, recent sinus, or middle ear surgery.

- 'Entonox': nitrous oxide with oxygen.

Oral

Useful for light sedation where analgesia not required, e.g. for CT scans.

- Chloral hydrate 30–100mg/kg 45 minutes before procedure; maximum 2000mg.
- Triclofos 30–100mg/kg ; maximum 2000mg.
- Alimemazine (trimeprazine–vallergan) 2mg/kg, maximum 60mg.
- Midazolam sublingual 1mg/kg (maximum 15mg).

Intravenous

Child must be fasted for at least 2 hours. Advisable to use with continuous cardiac and oximetry monitoring, with easy access to airway support equipment, e.g. bag–valve–mask. Only use if nursing staff are available to assist.

- Midazolam (over 2–3 minutes).
  - 1 month–6 years 100mcg/kg, increase in steps to maximum total 6mg.
  - 6–12 years 50mcg/kg, increase in steps to maximum total 10mg.
  - >12 years 2–2.5mg, increase in steps to maximum total 7.5mg (i.e. less than for younger children).

Deep sedation is required for relocation of fractures. Give drug as a slow push over 1 to 2 minutes, then wait for 3 to 5 minutes to observe effect before giving other drug.

- Morphine 0.1mg/kg ***plus*** midazolam 0.05mg/kg.
- Fentanyl 1mcg/kg (maximum 50mcg) ***plus*** midazolam 0.05mg/kg (maximum 2.5mg).
- Ketamine 1mg/kg ***plus*** midazolam 0.05mg/kg (maximum 2.5mg).

Antidotes

- Flumazenil 5–10mcg/kg IV (maximum dose 250mcg) to maximum of 1mg.
- Naloxone. Neonate, 10mcg/kg, repeat every 2–3 minutes.
  1 month–12 years, 10mcg/kg, then subsequent dose 100mcg/kg.
  12–18 years, 1.5–3mg/kg, then increase in increments of 100mcg/kg every 2 minutes.

Common antibiotic regimens

For specific doses, see 📖 pp.496–502.

Respiratory system

Epiglottitis Cefotaxime or ceftriaxone.

Community acquired pneumonia

- <6 months benzylpenicillin + gentamicin.
- 6 months–5 years—oral amoxil or macrolide.
- 5–18 years oral macrolide.

IV flucloxacillin, if *Staphylococcus* suspected (e.g. after recent 'flu' or measles).

If severe:

- neonate benzylpenicillin + gentamicin;
- 1 month–18 years: cephalosporin or co-amoxiclav ± flucloxacillin.

Benzylpenicillin if lobar, or streptococcal.
Macrolide if penicillin allergic, or suspect atypical cause.

Hospital acquired pneumonia Cefotaxime or ceftazidime.

Cardiovascular system

Endocarditis

- Blind therapy: IV benzylpenicillin + gentamicin ± vancomycin if prosthetic valve. If penicillin allergic, use vancomycin + rifampicin.
- Known staphylococcal: IV flucloxacillin, or vancomycin + rifampicin.
- Known streptococcal or enterococcal: IV benzylpenicillin or vancomycin, plus gentamicin

Gastrointestinal

Gastroenteritis

- Anti-bacterials rarely indicated, as self-limiting and often viral.
- Campylobacter enteritis—macrolide or ciprofloxacin.
- Salmonella—only in invasive or severe disease, or susceptible child (immunocompromised, <3 months, or haemoglobinopathy): ciprofloxacin or trimethoprim.

Antibiotic-associated (pseudo-membranous) colitis Oral metronidazole or vancomycin.

NEC in neonate IV benzylpenicillin or IV 3rd generation cephalosporin + gentamicin + metronidazole.

Peritonitis Cephalosporin + metronidazole.

Urinary tract

Mildly unwell >3 months Oral trimethoprim, cephalosporin, or coamoxiclav for 5–7 days (3 in adolescent females).

Seriously unwell or <3 months IV amoxicillin + gentamicin , or cephalosporin alone.

Central nervous system

Meningitis blind therapy

- GP may give IM penicillin, or IM cefotaxime, or IM ceftriaxone.
- Consider dexamethasone prior to, or with first dose (except in septic shock, meningococcal disease, immunocompromised, or post-surgery).
- <3 months: IV cefotaxime or ceftriaxone plus amoxicillin.
- >3 months: IV cefotaxime or ceftriaxone.

Once cause of meningitis identified:

Group B Streptococcus meningitis IV benzylpenicillin + gentamicin, or cefotaxime or ceftriaxone alone, for 14 days.

Listeria meningitis IV amoxicillin + gentamicin for 14 days.

Meningococcus meningitis—IV benzylpenicillin or cefotaxime or ceftriaxone, for 5 days.

Pneumococcus or Haemophilus meningitis

- IV cefotaxime or ceftriaxone for 14 days.
- IV benzylpenicillin if sensitive; vancomycin ± rifampicin if very resistant).
- Consider steroids early.
- For *Haemophilus*, give oral rifampicin for 4 days before discharge.

Septicaemia

Neonate <48 hours IV cefotaxime/ceftriaxone + gentamicin, ± acyclovir.

Neonate >48 hours IV cefotaxime/ceftriaxone/ampicillin ± gentamicin.

1 month–18 years, community-acquired

- IV amoxicillin + gentamicin, or cefotaxime/ceftriaxone alone.
- Add IV metronidazole if anaerobes suspected.
- Add IV flucloxacillin or vancomycin if Gram-positive suspected.

1 month–18 years, hospital-acquired

- Broad spectrum anti-pseudomonal, e.g. IV ceftazidime, Tazocin®, meropenem.
- Add IV aminoglycoside if Gram-negative suspected.
- Add IV metronidazole if anaerobes suspected.
- Add IV flucloxacillin or vancomycin if Gram-positive suspected.

If vascular device IV vancomycin.

If meningococcaemia IV cefotaxime/ceftriaxone or benzylpenicillin.

- GP should give IM before transfer to hospital.
- Rifampicin (see below) before hospital discharge.

Meningococcal prophylaxis

- Rifampicin
  - *Neonate*–1 year: 5mg/kg bd for 2 days.
  - *1–12 years*: 10mg/kg (maximum 600mg) bd for 2 days PO.
  - *12–18 years*: 600mg bd for 2 days PO.
- ***Or*** ciprofloxacin (unlicensed indication).
  - *5–12 years*: 250mg once PO.
  - *12–18 years*: 500mg once PO.

- ***Or*** ceftriaxone.
  - <12 years 125mg once IM.
  - >12 years: 250mg once IM (unlicensed indication but preferred in pregnancy).

If pregnant, use

- ceftriaxone (unlicensed indication).
  - 12–18 years: 250mg once IM.

ENT

Throat infections

Antibiotics not always necessary. Avoid if glandular fever likely. Give phenoxymethylpenicillin, or amoxicillin if:

- valvular heart disease;
- systemically unwell;
- peritonsillar cellulitis;
- immunocompromised.

Sinusitis

Antibiotics not always necessary. If discharge purulent and persistent, give

- 7 days oral amoxicillin or erythromycin. Change to co-amoxiclav if no improvement after 48 hours.
- If severely unwell or complications, give IV cefuroxime and metronidazole.

Otitis externa

- Sofradex ear drops.
- Oral flucloxacillin or erythromycin, if severe.
- Ciprofloxacin eye drops if *Pseudomonas* suspected.
- Locorten vioform drops if fungal suspected.

Otitis media

Antibiotics not always necessary. If no improvement after 48 hours:

- <1 year.
- Severe pain.
- History of complications.

Give oral co-amoxiclav or erythromycin for 5 days. If systemically unwell; IV cefuroxime or co-amoxiclav, initially.

Musculo-skeletal

Osteomyelitis

- IV flucloxacillin and benzyl penicillin.
- IV clindamycin, if penicillin-allergic.
- Add IV cefotaxime if not immunized against *Haemophilus influenzae*.
- Add IV vancomycin with either oral fusidic acid or oral rifampicin if prostheses or critically ill.

Septic arthritis

- IV benzylpenicillin + flucloxacillin ± fusidic acid.
- Clindamycin alone, if allergic.

Eye

Purulent conjunctivitis

- Antibiotics not always necessary.
- Neonate: neomycin eye drops after culture to exclude STD (📖 p.347).
- 1 month–18 years: chloramphenicol or gentamicin eye drops.

Skin

Impetigo

- Topical fusidic acid (mupirocin if MRSA), for 7 days.
- Oral flucloxacillin or erythromycin if widespread, or ill.
- Add penicillin if streptococcal.

Erysipelas

- Phenoxymethylpenicillin, or erythromycin.
- Add flucloxacillin if staphylococcal.

Cellulitis

- Oral flucloxacillin if well.
- Benzylpenicillin + flucloxacillin, or erythromycin if unwell.

Bites

- If in area likely to become infected, e.g. hand, ciprofloxacin and clindamycin. Otherwise wait and watch.
- Consider tetanus status (and rabies where prevalent).

Septic spots or paronychia

- Oral or IV flucloxacillin.
- Add gentamicin if septic.

Surgical wound infection IV flucloxacillin.

Steroid potencies

Table 28.1 Topical steroids

Topical steroid	Cream	Ointment	Lotion	Apply per day	Site
Mid-potency					
Hydrocortisone 0.5% 'Derm-aid'	✓			1 to 3	Face Closed flexures
Hydrocortisone 1.0% 'Egocort'	✓			1 to 3	Nappy area
Hydrocortisone 1.0% 'Sigmacort'	✓	✓		2 to 4	
Moderate					
Betamethasone valereate 0.02%, 0.05%, 'Betnovate'	✓	✓		2 to 3	Trunk Limbs Open flexures
Triamcinolone acetonide 0.02%, 0.05%, 'Aritocort'	✓	✓		2 to 3	
Potent					
Betamethasone valerate 0.1% 'Celestone V'	✓	✓	✓	1 to 2	Lichenified dermatitis Nummular dermatitis
Betamethasone dipropionate 0.05%, 'Diprosone'	✓	✓	✓	2	Palmoplantar dermatitis
Methylprednisolone aceponate 0.1%, 'Advantan'	✓	✓		1	Allergic contact dermatitis
Mometasone furoate 0.1% 'Elocon'	✓	✓	✓	1	
Very potent					
Betamethasone dipropionate 0.05%, 'Diprosone OV'	✓	✓		1 to 2	Palmoplantar

Equivalent anti-inflammatory doses of different steroids

Prednisolone 1mg is equivalent to:

- Betamethasone 150mcg
- Cortisone acetate 5mg
- Deflazacort 1.2mg
- Dexamethasone 150mcg
- Hydrocortisone 4mg
- Methylprednisolone 800mcg
- Triamcinolone 800mcg

Don't forget to give a steroid treatment card to anyone on more than a week of steroids—there is a small risk of adrenal suppression and susceptibility to overwhelming infection (e.g. chicken pox).

Antibiotics

Doses quoted are for children aged 1–18 years, unless cited otherwise. They may not be appropriate for children:
- under 1 month of age
- with renal compromise
- with hepatic dysfunction
- with immunocompromise.

In such cases, consultation of more detailed paediatric formularies or your hospital pharmacy is mandatory.

Acyclovir

Topical
- HSV on skin splodge 5 times a day for 5 days.
- HSV in eye small splodge 5 times a day until 3 days after lesion healed.

Oral
- Chicken pox, herpes zoster:
  - 1 month–12 years: 20mg/kg qds for 5 days. Maximum 800mg/day.
  - 12–18 years: 800mg 5 times a day for 7 days.
- HSV infection:
  - 1 month–2 years: 100mg 5 times a day until all lesions healed.
  - 2–18 years: 200mg 5 times day until all lesions healed.

Intravenous
- Chicken pox and herpes zoster:
  - 3 months–12 years: 250mg/m^2 tds for 5 days (📖 p.517).
  - 12–18years: 5mg/kg tds for 5 days.
- Disseminated HSV:
  - 3 months–12 years: 250mg/m^2 tds for 5 days (📖 p.517).
  - 12–18 years: 5mg/kg tds for 5 days.
- Meningitis:
  - Double dose for disseminated HSV and treat for 21 days.

Amoxycillin

Oral
- 40mg/kg tds. Double if severe infection.
- Endocarditis prophylaxis (📖 p.189).

Intravenous
- 50mg/kg 6–8hrly. Give 4hrly if severe infection.

Ampicillin

- 25mg/kg IV qds. Double dose if severe infection and give 4–6hrly
- Endocarditis prophylaxis (📖 p.189).

Augmentin (co-amoxiclav)

Dose expressed as mg amoxillin/mg clavulanic acid.

Oral

- 1 month–6 years: 0.25ml/kg of 125/31 suspension tds.
- 6–12 years: 0.15ml/kg of 250/62 suspension tds.
- 12–18 years: one 250/125 tablet tds.

Intravenous

- 1 month–12 years: 30mg/kg tds.
- 12–18 years: 1.2g tds.

All doses can be doubled for severe infection—beware liver toxicity. Infusions can be given 6-hourly if severe infection.

Azithromycin

Oral

- 10mg/kg daily for 3 days.
- STD 20mg/kg; maximum 1g single dose.

Benzathine penicillin see penicillin (intramuscular)

Benzyl penicillin see penicillin (intravenous)

Cefalexin

- 1 month–12 years: 12.5mg/kg bd; maximum 1g qds.
- 12–18 years: 500mg bd/tds; maximum 1.5g qds.

Dose can be doubled for severe infection.

- Endocarditis prophylaxis (📖 p.189).

Cefotaxime

Intramuscular

- Gonorrhoea 500mg once.
- Pre-transfer of suspected meningococcus 50mg/kg.

Intravenous

- 50mg/kg tds 5–7 days. Can give 50mg/kg qds if severe infection.

Ceftazidime

Intravenous

- 25mg/kg tds; double dose if severe infection.

Ceftriaxone

Intramuscular

- Meningococcus prophylaxis for pregnant women (unlicensed indication), 250mg once.
- Pre-transfer of suspected meningococcus:
    - If <50kg 50mg/kg.
    - If >50kg 1000mg.
- STD 125mg single dose

Intravenous

- Child < 50kg: 50mg/kg daily for 5 to 7 days; up to 80mg/kg if severe infection. Infuse over 5 minutes.
- Child > 50kg: 1g daily for 5 to 7 days; up to 2–4g if severe.

Cefuroxime

- IV 20mg/kg tds; maximum dose 1.5g qds if severe infection.

Ciprofloxacin

Oral

- 1 month–12 years: 7.5mg/kg bd.
- 12–18 years: 250–750mg bd.
- Gonorrhoea 500mg single dose.
- Meningococcal prophylaxis (unlicensed indication).
  - 5 –12 years: 250mg once.
  - 12–18 years: 500mg once.

Intravenous

- 4mg/kg bd for 7 days; maximum dose 400mg. Infuse over 60 minutes

Clarithromycin

Oral

- 1 month–12 years: 7.5mg/kg bd for 7 days.
- 12–18 years: 250–500mg bd for 7 days.

Intravenous

- 1 month–12 years: 7.5mg/kg bd for 7 days; maximum dose 250mg bd for 14 days.
- 12–18 years: 500mg bd for 7 days.

All infusions are given over 60 minutes through a large vein.

Clindamycin

Oral

- 1 month–12 years: 3–6mg/kg qds.
- 12–18 years: 150–300mg qds; maximum dose 450mg qds if severe.
- Endocarditis prophylaxis (📖 p.189).

Intravenous

- 1 month–12 years: total daily dose 15–25mg/kg, given in 3 to 4 divided doses.
- 12–18 years: 0.6–2.7g/d given in 2 to 4 divided doses.
- Endocarditis prophylaxis (📖 p.189).

Co-amoxiclav see augmentin

Erythromycin

Oral

- 1 month–2 years: 125mg qds.
- 2–8 years: 250mg qds.
- 8–18 years: 500mg qds.

Doses can be doubled in severe infection.

coplanin

hree loading doses of 10mg/kg bd; maximum 400mg. Then 6mg/kg
aily; maximum 200mg.

methoprim

mg/kg bd; maximum 200mg.
ng/kg nocte as prophylaxis for UTI.

ncomycin

l

ntibiotic-associated colitis:
- 1 month–5 years: 5mg/kg qds for 7 to 10 days.
- 5–12 years: 62.5mg qds for 7 to 10 days.
- 12–18 years: 125mg qds for 7 to 10 days.

avenous

ng/kg tds; maximum 2g/day.
ndocarditis prophylaxis (📖 p.189).
lonitor levels and adjust dose accordingly.

Intravenous
- 12.5mg/kg qds; maximum 4g a day.

Ethambutol

- Unsupervised treatment: 15mg/kg daily for 2 months.
- Supervised: 30mg/kg 3 times a week for 2 months.

Fansidar®

Fansidar is initiated only after treatment with quinine. It is not used in children who are G6PD deficient.
- <4 years: ½ tablet daily.
- 5–6 years: 1 tablet daily.
- 7–9 years: 1 ½ tablet daily.
- 10–14 years: 2 tablets daily.
- 15–18 years: 3 tablets daily.

Flucloxacillin

NB flucloxacillin is contraindicated if liver disease.

Oral
- 1 month–2 years: 62.5–125mg qds.
- 2 –10 years: 125–250mg qds.
- 10–18 years: 250–500mg qds.

Intravenous
- 12.5–25mg/kg qds; maximum 2g qds.

All doses can be doubled in severe infection.

Fluconazole

Oral
- Oral candidiasis:
  - 1 month–12 years: 3mg/kg daily for 7 to 14 days; load with double dose on day 1.
  - 12–18 years: 50mg daily for 7 to 14 days; double dose if severe infection.
- Tinea pedis/corpora/cruris or dermal candidiasis:
  - 3mg/kg daily for 14 to 28 days; Tinea pedis may require 6 weeks.

Intravenous
- Invasive candidiasis.
  - 6–12mg/kg daily. Maximum 400mg/day.

Fusidic acid (sodium fusidate)

Oral
- 1 month–1 year: 15mg/kg tds.
- 1–5 years: 250mg.
- 5–12 years: 500mg.
- 12–18 years: 750mg.

Intravenous
- 6–7mg/kg tds. Maximum 500mg.

Gentamicin

IM

- Single dose regimen:
  - <10 years: 7.5mg/kg.
  - >10 years: 6mg/kg.

Intravenous

NB Peak and trough levels must be checked.

- Either 7mg/kg daily.
- Or 1–12 years: 2.5mg/kg day tds; 12–18 years: 2mg/kg tds.
- Endocarditis prophylaxis (📖 p.189).

Griseofulvin

When topical treatment has failed.

- 1 month–12 years: 10mg daily; double dose if severe.
- 12–18 years: 500mg daily; divide dose if unpalatable.

Isoniazid

- Unsupervised: 5–10mg/kg daily for 6 months; maximum dose 300mg.
- Supervised: 15mg/kg 3 times a week for 6 months; maximum dose 300mg.

NB Pyridoxine prophylaxis against neuropathy only required if child malnourished.

Meropenem

- <50kg: 10mg/kg tds.
- >50kg: 500mg tds.
- Meningitis 2g tds.

Dose can be doubled if severe infection; infuse over 5 minutes.

Metronidazole

Oral

- 1–12 years: 7.5mg tds; maximum 400mg/day.
- 12–18 years: 400mg tds.
- PID 400mg bd for 14 days.

Intravenous

- Loading dose 15mg/kg; 7.5mg/kg tds.

Penicillin

Oral 'Phenoxymethylpenicillin'

- 1 month–12 years: 12.5mg/kg qds.
- 12–18 years: 500mg qds; maximum 1g qds.
- Strep throat 250mg bd.

Intramuscular 'Benzathine penicillin'

- Pre-transfer of suspected meningococcus:
  - <1 year: 300mg.
  - 1–9 years: 600mg.
  - 10–18 years: 1.2g.
- Syphilis 1.8g.

Intravenous 'Benzyl penicillin'

- 30–50mg/kg qds; maximum dose 2.4g.

Pyrazinamide

- Unsupervised treatment: 35mg/kg daily for 2 months; 1.5g if under 50Kg; 2g if over 50kg.
- Supervised: 50mg/kg daily 3 times a week for 2 months; 2g if under 50kg; 2.5g if over 50kg.

Pyridoxine

- Drug-induced neuropathy prophylaxis in malnourished cl daily.

Quinine

Oral

- 10mg/kg tds for 5 days then treat with Fansidar®
  - G6PD deficient, treat with Quinine for 14 days. Do n Fansidar®

Intravenous

- 10mg/kg; maximum 600mg; double dose if consciousness Dilute to 2mg/ml in 5% dextrose and infuse over 4 hours later start 10mg/kg tds (diluted to 2mg/ml, infused over 4 tablets can be tolerated.

Rifampicin

Oral

- 1 month–1 year: 5–10mg bd
- 1–18 years: 10mg/kg bd; Maximum 600mg bd
- Meningococcal prophylaxis:
  - Under 1 year: 5mg/kg bd for 2 days.
  - 1–12 years: 10mg/kg bd; maximum 600mg bd for 2 day
  - 12–18 years: 600mg bd for 2 days.

Intravenous

- 1–12 years 20mg/kg.
- 12–18 years 600mg.
- Dilute in 0.9% saline to concentration of 600mg/500ml anc 2–3 hours.

Roxithromycin

- 2.5–4mg/kg bd for 7 days.

Sulphadoxine/pyrimethamine–see Fansidar®.

Tazocin®

- 90mg/kg qds; maximum 4.5g qds.

Appendices

Appendix 1

Fluids and electrolytes

Children need glucose as well as electrolytes in their fluid requirements. The composition of fluids varies between countries, e.g. 0.45% saline is with 5% dextrose in US, and 0.18% saline is not used in Australia. If the fluid in the text differs from the one available to you, use the version with the nearest proportion of saline.

- 0.9% saline = normal saline.
- 0.45% saline = N/2 + 2.5% dextrose.
- 0.18% saline = N/5 + 4% dextrose.
- 5% dextrose—often used as base solution for infusions.
- Hartmann's—good for surgical conditions.

Other preparations include:

- 10% dextrose—used for neonates, arrest treatment of hypoglycaemia. N.B. Hypertonic;
- Colloid: 4% albumin, Gelofusin®. No longer favoured for use in resuscitation. However, albumin infusions still used for treatment of nephrotic syndrome, liver failure.

Glucose

Maintenance saline + dextrose should meet a child's metabolic need for glucose and sodium. However, in resuscitation, normal saline is used which is why the need to check glucose is emphasized.

Neonates and children with certain metabolic conditions where gluconeogenesis is impaired, e.g. fatty acid oxidation disorders, require 10% dextrose. If this does not exist in your department, supplementation of the lower concentration dextrose is necessary.

Calculation

To convert 500ml 2.5% dextrose to 10% dextrose:

- have 2.5% dextrose containing 2.5g glucose per 100ml, i.e. 12.5g per 500ml bag;
- want 10% dextrose containing 10g glucose per 100ml, i.e. 50g per 500ml bag;
- therefore, need to add 37.5g glucose (50–12.5);
- 50% glucose contains 50g dextrose per 100ml, so 75ml of 50% dextrose contains 37.5g;
- ***therefore, need to add 75ml of 50% glucose to 500ml bag 2.5% dextrose to convert to 500ml of 10% dextrose.***

Potassium

Potassium supplementation should only be started if you are certain that renal function is not impaired and child is passing urine; check serum potassium every 4–6 hours to assess response

Routine supplementation of maintenance fluids is seldom necessary. However, if the child is on medications known to lower potassium, e.g. salbutamol, insulin, frusemide, amphotericin, or is losing potassium, e.g. gastroenteritis, then supplementation/correction is indicated.

- Maintenance is 2mmol/kg/day.
- 10–20mmol KCl can be added to a 500ml bag of saline. It is not advisable to exceed 4mmol KCl per 100ml, nor 0.2mmol/kg/hour.

- **Emergency treatment.** If hypokalaemia symptomatic or with ECG changes, give KCl IV 0.2mmol/kg (maximum 40mmol). Dilute in at least 50ml saline and give through a large vein, preferably central. Cardiac monitoring mandatory, ideally on HDU/PICU.
- Check potassium levels daily and adjust supplementation accordingly.
- If long-term therapy, consider continuous potassium infusion but confer with PICU for composition and measure regularly.
- If hypokalaemia secondary to frusemide, add spironolactone 1mg/kg bd.

Fluid prescription

Maintenance fluids

There are several regimens for maintenance fluid calculation. The easiest to remember is given in Table A1.1.
Thus a 14kg child requires (10 x 100) + (4 x 500) = 1200ml/24h, i.e. 50ml/h maintenance fluid.

Fluids when dehydrated

Child will need maintenance fluids + replacement of deficit.
- Assess degree of dehydration—usually 5% if IV fluids necessary.
- Replacement = weight (kg) x % dehydration x 10.

Thus 14kg child with 5% dehydration requires:
14 x 5 x 10 = 700ml replacement
plus 1200ml maintenance = 1900ml/24h, i.e 79.2ml/h.

N.B. Certain conditions, e.g. hypo/hypernatraemia, or severe DKA (when often 10% dry) necessitate rehydration ***over 48 hours*** to lessen the risk of cerebral oedema developing. Thus 14kg child with 5% dehydration in such circumstances requires: maintenance of 1200ml each 24 hours, plus 700ml deficit 1200 + 1200 + 700 = 3100ml over 48h, i.e. 64.6ml/hr

Points to remember

- ***Never*** abbreviate when prescribing IV fluids: 'N/S' can be interpreted as 'N/**5**'.
- ***Remember*** two bags of 5% dextrose do not make 10% dextrose!

- Hypotonic fluids may produce fatal hyponatraemia
- SIADH causes hyponatraemia and is not rare
- Hypo/hyperkalaemia may be life-threatening

Children require electrolyes to be checked daily if on IV fluids and nil by mouth.

Table A1.1 Fluid requirement for a given weight

Weight	Fluid requirement
0–10kg	100ml/kg
10–20kg	1000ml ***plus*** 50ml/kg for every kg over 10kg
Over 20kg	1500ml ***plus*** 20ml/kg for every kg over 20kg

Normal values: haematology, coagulation, biochemistry, urine, CSF

Most pathology laboratories will issue results along with their own accepted normal ranges. However, these are not always paediatric or neonatal ranges and may differ from other laboratories. Different labs may quote in different units. It is imperative therefore, to interpret laboratory values in light of the local normal ranges, but also look at the child in front of you. Beware (and repeat) results that do not fit the clinical picture. When ordering investigations, ask yourself if the result will really change what you do and beware ordering tests simply to put your mind at rest.

Table A2.1 Normal haematology values

Age	Hb (g/dl)	Haematocrit	MCV (fl)	WCC ($\times 10^9$/l)	Neutrophils	Lymphocytes	Eosinophils	Basophils	Platelets	Reticulocytes
Birth	15–23	0.45–0.75	100–125	10–26	2.5–14	2–7	0–0.9	0–0.1	150–450	110–450
2 weeks	13–20	0.4–0.65	88–110	6–21	1.5–5.5	3–9	0–0.9	0–0.1	170–500	10–80
6 months	10–13	0.3–0.4	73–84	6–17	1–6	3–11	0.5–0.9	< 0.2	210–560	15–110
12 months	10–13	0.3–0.4	70–80	6–16	1–8	3–10	<0.9	< 0.13	200–550	20–150
2–5 years	11–13	0.3–0.4	72–87	6–17	1.5–9	2–8	<1.1	<0.12	210–490	50–130
5–12 years	11–15	0.3–0.4	76–90	4–14	1.5–8	1.5–5	<1	<0.12	170–450	50–130
>12 years										
Female	12–15	0.35–0.45	77–95	4–13	1.5–6	1.5–4.5	<0.8	>0.12	180–430	50–130
Male	12–16	0.35–0.5	77–92	4–13	1.5–6	1.5–4.5	<0.8	>0.12	180–430	50–130

Table A2.2 Clotting indices

Coagulation tests (mean values)	1–5 years	6–10 years	11–18 years
PT	11	11.1	11.2
INR	1	1	1
APTT (seconds)	30	31	32
Fibrinogen (g/l)	2.75	2.8	3
Bleeding time (mins)	6	7	5

Table A2.3 Normal biochemical values

Albumin		
<1 month	25–45g/l	
1–12 months	30–50g/l	
>1 year	32–50g/l	
Alanine aminotransaminase (ALT)		
Infant	10–80u/l	
Child	10–40u/l	
Alkaline phosphatase (ALP)		**Increases at times of rapid growth**
Newborn/infant	140–1100u/l	
Child	250–800u/l	
Ammonia		
Newborn	50–90μmol/l	
Child	20–50μmol/l	
Amylase		
Infant	<50u/l	
Child	100–400u/l	
Aspartate aminotransferase (AST)		
Newborn	10–75u/l	
Child	10–45u/l	
Base excess	+/– 2.5mEq/l	
Bicarbonate		
Newborn	18–23mmol/l	
Child	20–26 mmol/l	

Table A2.3 (*Contd.*)

Bilirubin		**<10% conjugated in newborn period**
Cord blood	<60μmol/l	
First 3 days	See charts on neonatal unit	
3–10 days	<250μmol/l	**Raised in breast fed babies. Should settle by 2 weeks**
>2 months	<25μmol/l	
Blood volume	Approx. 80ml/Kg	
Calcium (serum)		
1st week	2–3mmol/l	**Lower in bottle-fed**
Child	2.2–2.7mmol/l	
Calcium (ionized)	1–1.3mmol/l	**Measured if concerned about hypocalcaemia**
CO_2: partial pressure (pCO_2)	4.7–6kPa 35–45mmHg	**To convert from kPA to mmHg, multiply by 7.6**
Chloride	95–106mmol/l	
Creatine kinase (CK)		
Newborn	<300u/l	
Child	<200u/l	
Creatinine		
Newborn	20–100μmol/l	
Child	20–80μmol/l	
Glucose		
Fasting	3.5–5.5mmol/l	
Newborn	2.2–4.4mmol/l	
Child	4–7mmol/l	
Lactate		
Newborn	<3mmol/l	
Child	1–2mmol/l	
Lactate dehydrogenase (LDH)	60–240u/l	
Magnesium		
Newborn	0.6–1mmol/l	
Child	0.6–0.9mmol/l	
pH (arterial)	7.35–7.42	**0.03 lower if venous**

Table A2.3 (*Contd.*)

Oxygen (PaO_2)		**To convert from kPA to mmHg, multiply by 7.6**
Newborn	9–13kPa 68–99mmHg	
Child	11–14kPa 84–106mmHg	
Phosphate		
Newborn	1.2–3mmol/l	**Lower if breast fed**
<1 year	1.3–2mmol/l	
>1 year	1.2–1.9mmol/l	
Potassium		**If sample haemolysed, will get spurious higher level**
Newborn	4–7mmol/l	
Child	3.5–5.5mmol/l	
Sodium		
Newborn	132–145mmol/l	
Child	135–145mmol/l	
Thyroid stimulating hormone (TSH)		
<3 days	<40mu/l	
3–7 days	<25mu/l	
7–14 days	<10mu/l	
>14 days	<5mu/l	
Thyroxine: T4		
Newborn	140–440nmol/l	
Infants	90–195nmol/l	
Child	70–180nmol/l	
Free T4	9–23picomol/l	
Triiodothyronine: T3		
Newborn	0.8–6nmol/l	
Child	1.5–3.8nmol/l	
Urate (uric acid)	0.12–0.42mmol/l	
Urea	2.5–6.6mmol/l	

Table A2.4 Drug therapeutic ranges

Drug	µmol/l (unless stated)	
Carbamazepine	12–50	
Digoxin		
Infants	<5.1nmol/l	
Child	1–2.6nmol/l	
Gentamicin		
Peak	8–18	15 minutes post IV dose (tds regime)
Trough	<2	Pre–dose
Phenytoin	30–70	
Theophylline		
Asthma	55–110	
Preterm apnoea	30–70	
Tobramycin	11–21	
Sodium valproate	300–600	
Vancomycin		
Trough	<10mg/l	
Peak	25–40mg/l	

Table A2.5 Normal urinary composition

Cells		
Erythrocytes	0–10 x 10^6/l	
Leucocytes	0–4 x 10^6/l	Up to 20 x 10^6/l in females
Creatinine clearance		
Newborn	90–180µmol/l/24h	
Child	45–350µmol/l/24h	
Osmolarity		
Newborn	80–120mOsmol/kg	Maximum 600mOsmol/kg
Child	Up to 1200mOsmol/kg	(mOsmol/kg = mmol/kg)
pH		
Newborn	>5	
Child	5.3–7.2	
Sodium		
Newborn	<0.4 mmol/kg/24	
Child	<3.7 mmol/kg/24	40–225mmol/24h
Volume: minimum	**0.5–1ml/kg/h**	

Table A2.6 CSF values

	Normal		Bacterial meningitis			
	Child	**Newborn**	**Untreated**	**Partially treated**	**Viral meningitis**	**Tuberculous meningitis**
Appearance	'Gin' clear	'Gin' clear	Turbid	Clear or turbid	Often clear	Cloudy
Polymorphs (cells/ml)*	0	0–10[†]	>10–10 000	10–1000	5–500 in early stages	>10–10 000
Lymphocytes (cells/ml)*	0–6	0–30	0–20	10–1000	10–1000	10–1000
Gram stain	Absent	Absent	Often see organism	Rarely see organism	No organisms	May see AAFB on ZN stain
Glucose (mmol/l)	2.5–4	>1[‡]	<2/3 blood level	Low or normal	>2/3 of blood level	Very low
Protein (g/l)	0.15–0.5	0.61–2.0[§]	0.5–4	0.15–0.5	<1.0	1–6

* May be up to 100/ml if intracranial haemorrhage. Will be associated with CSF glucose <1mmol/l.

† If traumatic tap, calculate from peripheral blood ratio of red to white cells. Approximately 1:500 white to red cells. If in doubt, treat as significant. Xanthochromia suggests old intracranial haemorrhage.

‡ Must compare to blood sugar.

§ Up to 3 in pre-term infant.

Body surface area estimation and BMI

Body surface area (BSA) estimation

BSA is only required in ED for management of nephrotic syndrome and newly diagnosed leukaemics. If possible, obtain the child's weight and height and use the formal nomogram.

If the child cannot stand, Table A3.1 provides useful approximations.

Table A3.1 Estimation of body surface area based on age and weight

Age (years)	Weight (kg)	Surface area (m^2)
0	3	0.2
1	10	0.4
3	15	0.6
6	20	0.8
10	30	1.0
14	50	1.5
Adult	70	1.7

Body mass index

$$\text{BMI} = \frac{\text{weight in kg}}{\text{height (m)} \times \text{height (m)}}.$$

Ideal BMI = 20 to 25kg/m^2.

Appendix 4

Neurology

Children's modified GCS and AVPU

Table A4.1 Children's modified Glasgow coma scale(GCS)

Eyes open			**Score**
Spontaneously			4
To speech			3
To pain			2
No response			1
Best verbal response			
Under 2 years	**2–5 years**	**>5 years**	**Score**
Smiles, coos, cries appropriately	Appropriate words and phrases	Orientated; Converses	5
Cries but consolable	Inappropriate words	Confused	4
Persistent cries	Cries ± screams	Inappropriate words	3
Grunts	Grunts	Incomprehensible sounds	2
No response	No response	No response	1
Best motor response to pain			
<1 year	**>1 year**		**Score**
Spontaneously moves	Obeys command		6
Localizes pain	Localizes pain		5
Flexion—withdrawal	Flexion—withdrawal		4
Flexion—abnormal	Flexion—abnormal, 'decorticate'		3
Extension	Extension, 'decerebrate'		2
No response	No response		1

AVPU

- **A**lert.
- **V**oice (responds to).
- **P**ain (responds to).
- **U**nresponsive.

GCS of 8 = responsive only to **P**ain = intubation necessary

Developmental milestones

Table A4.2 Developmental milestones—the easy ones to elicit!

Age	Gross motor	Fine motor	Social	Hearing
Newborn		Fixates; follows briefly		May respond to sound
6 weeks	Lifts head briefly	Hands open at times	Smiles	Quiets to sound nearby
3 months	Takes weight on forearms	Holds items; hand regard	Laughing	Turns head to sound
6 months	May sit unsupported	Transfers objects; mouthing	Fear of strangers	Looks for origin of sound
9 months	Crawls; stands holding on	Pincer grip	Plays peek-a-boo. Looks for fallen toy	Tries to babble responsively
12 months	Walks ± one hand held	Casts objects on floor	Knows own name	2 to 3 word vocabulary
18 months	Walks backwards	Scribbles	Points to 2–3 parts of the body	5 to 20 words
2 years	Runs; kicks ball	Copies vertical and circular lines	Knows first name	2 to 3 word phrases
3 years	Stands on one foot	Copies circle	Knows own sex	Uses plurals
4 years	Can hop	Draws person with 3 parts	Knows name and address	Can count to 4
5 years	Can skip	Draws person with 6 parts	Knows difference between morning and afternoon	Grammatical speech

Appendix 5

Normal values: vital signs

Table A5.1 Normal values of respiratory rate

Age (years)	Respiratory rate (breaths/min)
<1	30–40
1–2	25–35
2–5	25–30
5–12	20–25
>12	15–20

Table A5.2 Normal values of heart rate

Age (years)	Heart rate (beats/min)
<1	110–160
1–2	100–150
2–5	95–140
5–12	80–120
>12	60–100

Table A5.3 Normal values of systolic blood pressure and blood pressure threshold for hypertension

Age (years)	Systolic pressure (mmHg)	Hypertension
<1	70–90	115/75
1–2	80–95	115/75
2–5	80–100	115/75
5–12	90–110	125/80
>12	100–120	135/85

Appendix 6

Cardiorespiratory arrest

Rapid sequence induction (RSI)

- Thiopentone, 2–4mg/kg/dose.
- ***Plus*** atropine, 0.02mg/kg/dose (maximum 1mg).
- ***Plus*** suxamethonium, 1–2 mg/kg/dose.

Ketamine (IV 1–2mg/kg/dose) can be used instead of thiopentone if child shocked or in status asthmaticus.

If possibility of hyperkalaemia or myopathies, use rocuronium (IV 0.6–1.2mg/kg/dose).

Infusions for transfer of intubated child

- Vecuronium, 100–200mcg/kg/h.
    - 5mg/kg vecuronium made up to 50ml with 5% dextrose.
    - 1ml/hr = 100mcg/kg/h.
- Morphine, 20–40mcg/kg/h.
    - 1mg/kg morphine made up to 50ml with 5% dextrose.
    - 1ml/hr = 20mcg/kg/h.
- Midazolam, 100–200mcg/kg/h.
    - 5mg/kg midazolam made up to 50ml with 5% dextrose.
    - 1ml/hr = 100mcg/kg/h.

Infusions for a shocked child

- Adrenaline, noradrenaline.
    - 0.3mg/kg of drug made up to 50ml with 5% dextrose.
    - 1ml/hr = 0.1mcg/kg/min.
    - Start at 0.05–1.0mcg/kg/min.
- Dobutamine, dopamine.
    - 15mg/kg of drug made up to 50ml with 5% dextrose.
    - 1ml/hr = 5mcg/kg/min.
    - Start at 5mcg/kg/min and increase up to 20mcg/kg/min.

Equipment and drug doses

- Estimation of weight.
  - Newborn: 3.5kg.
  - 6 months: 6.0kg.
  - Over 1 year: (age in years + 4) × 2kg.
- Endotracheal tube.
  - Size: 4 + (age in years ÷ 4).
  - Length for oral tube: 12 + (age in years ÷ 2) cm.
  - Length if nasal tube: 15 + (age in years ÷ 2) cm.
- DC shock: 4J/kg.

Table A6.1 Drug doses

Drug	Dose
Bolus of fluids	20ml/kg, 0.9% saline
Adrenaline (enpinephrine)	0.1ml/kg, 1 in 10 000 (10mcg/kg)
10% Dextrose	5ml/kg
Amiodarone	5mg/kg over 20 minutes
Atropine	20mcg/kg (minimum 100mcg, maximum 600mcg)
10% Calcium chloride	0.2ml/kg
Lignocaine	1mg/kg
Sodium bicarbonate 8.4% (1mmol/ml)	1mmol/kg

Index

P

Q

R

S

T

U